Clinical Nutrition

for pain, inflammation and tissue healing

David R. Seaman, DC, MS, DABCN

NutrAnalysis, Inc.
Hendersonville, NC

NutrAnalysis, Inc
P.O. Box 306
Lake Lure, NC 28746
(800) 377-7978, Fax (828) 625-8081

ISBN 0-9667211-0-1

Library of Congress Card Catalog Number: 98-88132

Contents

.

PREFACE

Members of the chiropractic profession have always urged their patients to exercise regularly and eat properly. When I went through chiropractic college, the need for exercise and good nutrition was acknowledged and promoted; however, effective methods of implementation were not taught. Fortunately, in recent years this has begun to change and is particularly evident in the field of rehabilitation. Numerous chiropractic colleges now offer course work in rehabilitation and there are many postgraduate certification programs available to field practitioners.

Compared to rehabilitation, students and doctors do not embrace nutrition with nearly the same level of interest or excitement. Perhaps this is because our college curriculums have historically offered classes that are introductory and not very practical. Subsequently, many students graduate from chiropractic college without much interest in making nutrition an integral part of their practices. This lack of interest is demonstrated by the fact that postgraduate programs in nutrition are not nearly as popular or successful as other disciplines such as rehabilitation, sports injuries, orthopedics or neurology.

My interest in nutrition began when I was in junior high school. In part, this was probably because I was somewhat of a sickly child with allergies who had a hard time gaining weight. I received regular allergy shots for several years during my early youth, without any concurrent nutritional recommendations. I eventually grew out of my allergies, but was still somewhat sickly, prone to injury, and unable to gain weight. As I went through junior and senior high school, my mission was to gain weight so I could be more competitive on the basketball court and baseball diamond. This lead me to a local health food store

in search of some answers. Unfortunately, none were to be found.

I entered undergraduate college with the hope of pursuing a career in the field of nutrition. Despite majoring in biology/nutrition, I was unable to find one course that offered any practical information. An exercise physiology elective provided my first encounter with applied science. I thought this practical application of science would continue in chiropractic college; however, I soon discovered that the developing science of chiropractic was still in its infancy during the early 1980s when I went to school.

Upon graduating from chiropractic college in 1986, I began a masters program in nutrition. Surely this would provide me with practical nutrition knowledge I could apply in the clinical setting. Once again, I was mistaken.

In 1988, at about the time I needed to decide on a final research project, I happened to attend a weekend lecture taught by Dr. Barry Wyke, who for years was a leading researcher at the Neurological Unit, Royal Academy of Surgeons of England. He directed the Unit's research focus into the field of articular neurology, a very chiropractic-related topic. During that lecture, Wyke outlined what was understood about nociceptor and mechanoreceptor innervation of the musculoskeletal system. He explained that nociceptors were depolarized by mechanical trauma and the chemical mediators that were released by injured tissues, including lactic acid, potassium ions, histamine, prostaglandins, 5-hydroxytryptamine and kinins.

At that point in time, I was aware that nonsteroidal anti-inflammatory drugs (NSAIDs) and certain nutrients could inhibit prostaglandin production, which is why they offered an analgesic and anti-inflammatory effect. However, not until that lecture by Dr. Wyke, did I make the connection that NSAIDs and certain nutrients could reduce back pain by altering the excitability of spinal nociceptors.

After that lecture, I began to collect articles that discussed each of the chemical irritants and their relationship to inflammation and nociception. Additionally, I sought out articles that explained how dietary and nutritional factors could influence the production of each chemical irritant. I also called researchers at various universities around the country and ask questions about each of these topics. To my surprise, experts in the area of nociception were unaware that nutritional factors could influence nociception and inflammation. Similarly, while nutrition researchers understood that certain nutrients could inhibit pain and inflammation, they were unfamiliar with nociceptors and the nature of nociceptor sensitization and thus, had little appreciation for how nutrition could influence the activity of central nociceptive pathways.

In the past ten years I have collected thousands of articles devoted to subjects of nociception, inflammation and nutrition. About six years ago, I began presenting this information to chiropractors and students at various meetings around the country. Most had either forgotten or never learned the details about nociception and inflammation, and most were also unaware of the nutritional factors that could influence these two important processes. Without this information, it is very difficult to appreciate how nutrition can support chiropractic care, tissue healing and the functional restoration of musculoskeletal structures.

The purpose of this text is to address these topics. The first four chapters provide foundational information and focus on nociception, inflammation, pharmacology, and important conceptual issues related to chiropractic and nutrition. The remaining chapters are devoted to clinical nutrition topics that relate directly to nociception, inflammation, and several conditions encountered in chiropractic practice.

David R. Seaman

Chapter 1

NOCICEPTIVE PROCESSES AND SPINAL DYSFUNCTION

A text devoted to clinical nutrition will naturally require a clinical focus. If this were a text for cardiologists, the focus would be heart disease. If the intended audience were to be gastroenterologists, the clinical focus would obviously be devoted to nutrition factors related to the digestive system. However, this clinical nutrition text is designed primarily for chiropractors and our clinical focus is the neuromusculoskeletal system. In particular, chiropractors endeavor to restore function to the neuromusculoskeletal system, usually through various methods of manual care. Accordingly, our nutritional approach should be designed with the same goal in mind and therefore, nutritional interventions should complement our manual care.

Since the inception of the chiropractic profession, the nervous system has been a chief center of interest. For many years, chiropractors tried to understand and explain how a subluxation could impinge upon nerves and promote body dysfunction. Subluxation was not viewed as a type of spinal injury; instead, it was believed that subluxations were injurious to the nervous system. This focus took precedence for years, to the exclusion of other important areas. For example, there was never any real effort to understand how spinal structures are *innervated* by the nervous system, which would lead us to investigate how injury to spinal tissues might alter the function of neurological receptors within those tissues and subsequently affect body function. It is somewhat surprising that this topic was ignored for so many years, especially when we consider that Sherrington first spoke of nociceptors before 1906.

It is now well-known that nociceptors and mechanoreceptors represent the neurological link between musculoskeletal structures and the central nervous system. In particular, nociceptors are specifically designed to respond to injurious stimuli. Considering that patients primarily present themselves to our offices with injured spines, our focus should be directed at nociceptor function. Figure 1-1 lists the various chemicals that stimulate nociceptors, which also happen to be the same chemicals which drive the inflammatory process.

Research has clearly demonstrated that our dietary habits can directly influence the production of the various chemical irritants, which means that our diet can influence nociception and inflammation. Additionally, a great deal of evidence suggests that nociception and inflammation can promote spinal dysfunction. For this reason, individual chapters have been devoted to both nociception (Chapter 1) and inflammation (Chapter 3). Subsequent chapters discuss the nutritional modulation of nociception and inflammation.

NOCICEPTION AND THE SUBLUXATION COMPLEX

For years, the five component model of the subluxation complex was described by Dr. L. John Faye[135, 136]. The five pathological components included: neuropathophysiology, kinesiopathology, myopathology, histopathology and inflammatory biochemical changes. Lantz[256] revised Faye's description of the subluxation complex to include the following eight pathological components: kinesiopathology, neuropathology, myopath-ology, connective tissue pathology, vascular abnormalities, an inflammatory response, histopathology and biochemical abnormalities. More recently, Lantz slightly modified his model of the subluxation complex[256a].

Although the various pathological components of the subluxation complex have been elucidated to a considerable degree, a cause and effect relationship has yet to be clearly defined. It should be mentioned that one of the major problems encountered in trying to define the cause-effect relationship in a dynamic process, is that a beginning point must almost be arbitrarily chosen, and such a task is difficult.

As illustrated in *Figure 1-1*, nociceptive activity can result in sympathetic hyperactivity, reflex muscle spasm, autonomic symptoms or concomitants, and pain. Autonomic concomitants refer to symptoms which are induced by nociceptive bombardment of the brain stem and hypothalamus, such as digestive, cardiovascular, and respiratory symptoms.

It is likely that sympathetic hyperactivity and muscle spasm are the segmental responses that promote segmental hypomobility and the various pathological components of the subluxation complex. It should be understood that nociceptive-induced sympathetic hyperactivity and muscle spasm may be present without symptoms, such as

autonomic concomitants and pain. In this case, a patient could be asymptomatic yet the subluxation complex and other diseases might be present. Thus, it should be remembered that *nociception does not equate with pain.* Kandel, Schwartz & Jessel provide a clear definition of nociception[228-p.385]:

> "Nociception refers to the reception of signals in the central nervous system evoked by activation of specialized sensory receptors (nociceptors) that provide information about tissue damage. Not all noxious stimuli that activate nociceptors are necessarily experienced as pain."

As described in this definition, noxious stimuli (i.e., tissue damage/injury) activate nociceptors. The prefix noci comes from the Latin word *nocere* which means "to injure"[118]. Thus, nociceptors are actually injury receptors. Dorland's Medical Dictionary defines injury as, "...damage inflicted to the body by an external force." This definition is extremely general and covers the gamut of potential injuries from asymptomatic repetitive microtrauma, such as sitting all day in front of a computer, to symptomatic trauma such as whiplash. Ultimately, each type of injury stimulates local nociceptors which transmit such information to the CNS through nociceptive afferent pathways

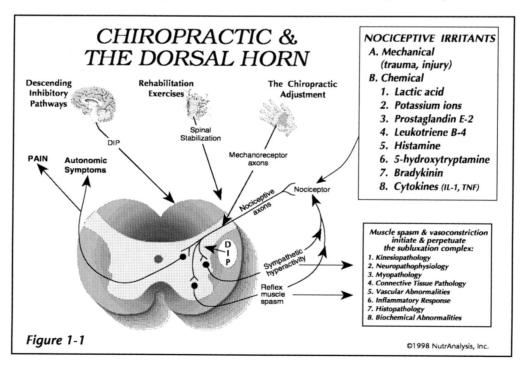

Figure 1-1

(A-delta and C fibers). Type A-delta fibers range in diameter from 1-5 microns and conduct impulses at velocities ranging from 5-30 meters per second. Type C fibers range in diameter from .5-1.5 microns and conduct impulses at velocities ranging from .5-2.0 meters per second[228-p.351].

Nociceptors are located in nearly every tissue in the body. Most researchers agree that virtually all structures in the spine are innervated by nociceptors. These structures include skin; subcutaneous and adipose tissue; fibrous capsules of zygapophyseal and sacroiliac joints; synovial folds; longitudinal, spinal, interspinous, flaval and sacroiliac joints; periosteum covering vertebral bodies and arches and attached fasciae, tendons and aponeurosis; dura mater and epidural fibro-adipose tissue; walls of blood vessels supplying spinal and sacroiliac joints, and the vertebral cancellous bone; walls of epidural and paravertebral veins; and walls of intramuscular arteries[42, 43, 44, 175-p.51-52, 180, 490, 491, 493]. Whereas Wyke and earlier researchers maintained that the adult disc was not innervated by nociceptors[493], more recent work by Bogduk describes nociceptive innervation of the disc[41, 42, 43, 44]. Slosberg provided an easy way to remember the spinal structures with nociceptive innervation; only the articular cartilage, the nucleus pulposus and the inner two-thirds of the annulus are not innervated by nociceptors[423].

In summary, nociceptors specifically receive injurious tissue damaging stimuli which is transmitted into the central nervous system via nociceptive axons. The result of such nociceptive activity may include sympathetic hyperactivity, reflex muscle spasm, autonomic concomitants and pain[47, 48, 137, 206, 356, 491]. The remainder of this section will describe how the various pathological components of the subluxation complex may develop from sympathetic hyperactivity and reflex muscle spasm.

Sympathetic hyperactivity

Nociceptive input will excite sympathetic preganglionic fibers which enter into the sympathetic chain and synapse with postganglionic fibers. The postganglionic fibers enter the peripheral tissue where they innervate blood vessels, sweat glands and piloerector muscles.

The precise mechanism by which the sympathetic nervous system promotes pain, inflammation and reflex sympathetic dystrophy is not known[665]. Therefore it would be impossible to definitively state how the sympathetic nervous system influences the pathogenesis of the subluxation complex.

Originally, I thought that vasoconstriction was the main outcome of segmental sympathetic hyperactivity and resulted in tissue hypoxia. Although this may be the case, there are many potential mechanisms and interactions which need to be considered regarding vasomotor control. Additionally, it is likely that sympathetic hyperactivity promotes tissue injury by mechanisms other than vasoconstriction.

Any discussion about the sympathetic nervous system demands that we have a basic understanding of the receptor subtypes for norepinephrine and epinephrine. So, for the purpose of better understanding how segmental sympathetic hyperactivity may influence joint dysfunction, we will go on a temporary detour and examine some of the basics related to the sympathetic nervous system and its regulation of blood flow.

Postganglionic sympathetic nerve terminals, i.e., gray rami C fibers, are known to release norepinephrine[749], while the adrenal medulla releases 80% epinephrine and 20% norepinephrine[176-p.279]. So, when we try and figure out how the sympathetic activity might influence joint dysfunction, we need to consider the local release of norepinephrine and the systemic release of epinephrine. Before examining this topic it is important to develop an understanding about the adrenergic receptors.

There are 4 main types of adrenergic receptors: $\alpha 1$, $\alpha 2$, $\beta 1$, and $\beta 2$[570-p.102]. Norepinephrine excites mainly α-receptors, and can also excite β-receptors to a slight extent. Epinephrine excites both receptors approximately equally. The relative effects of norepinephrine and epinephrine on different effector organs is determined by the types of receptors in the organs. Obviously, if they are all betareceptors, epinephrine will be the more effective excitant[176-p.277].

Confusing the issue of adrenergic receptor function is the fact that certain α functions are excitatory while others are inhibitory. Likewise, certain β functions are excitatory and others are inhibitory. Therefore, α and β receptors are not necessarily associated with excitation or inhibition but simply with the affinity of the hormone for the receptors in the given effector organ[176-p.277]. Adding to this confusion is the fact that different metabolic states can alter adrenergic receptor distribution. The relationship between circulating levels of thyroid hormone and the expression of β-receptors is a good example that has both physiological and clinical relevance[749].

Patients with pathological elevations of circulating thyroid hormones show manifestations typical of adrenergic activation: tachycardia, increased thermogenesis, and sweating. The symptoms can be successfully treated with b-receptor antagonists. Experimental studies point to increased numbers of β-receptors in some, though not all tissues during thyrotoxicosis. Interestingly, α-receptors appear to be reduced. In contrast, hypothyroid patients show some symptoms that could be attributed to impaired adrenergic function. In hypothyroidism, there appear to be fewer β-receptors[749].

Irrespective of the above mentioned factors which are involved in adrenergic receptor function, there are some general relationships which are described in standard neurology and physiology texts. For example, it is often stated that skeletal muscle blood vessels contain β2-receptors, while the skin contains α-receptors[570-p.378]. Consequently, during the "fight or flight" response, sympathetic stimulation leads to *vasodilation* of vessels in the somatic muscles [contains β-receptors], but it leads to *vasoconstriction* of cutaneous vessels (α-receptors) and the vessels of the digestive system (α-receptors) and lungs[570-p.379]. This same scenario is often applied to the blood flow changes that occur during exercise. However, we cannot apply this scenario to sedentary states and during tissue injury, inflammation, pain, and joint dysfunction. This is because there are additional adrenergic receptors within blood vessels that need to be considered.

The smooth muscle cells within blood vessels contain α1- receptors, α2- receptors, and β2-receptors[749]. Recall that α-receptors promote vasoconstriction while β-receptors promote vasodilation[749]. Under normal resting situations, i.e., during conditions where we have resting heart rates, epinephrine will not be released from the adrenal gland to any significant degree. Therefore, the main catecholamine interacting with vascular receptors will be norepinephrine from postganglionic sympathetic terminals. As norepinephrine mainly excites α-receptors, rather than β-receptors, there would be a tendency towards vasoconstriction during segmental sympathetic stimulation, i.e., during injury states in which inflammation and nociceptive input is enhanced. As an example, research related to reflex sympathetic dystrophy (RSD) suggests that sympathetic hyperactivity will cause vasoconstriction and hypoxia. Accordingly, a treatment option for RSD is a sympathectomy, which is known to result in a restoration of blood flow into the affected limb[650].

There is additional information that needs to be considered regarding peripheral blood regulation. Many people in chiropractic believe that it is entirely controlled by the nervous system. This notion is patently incorrect. Guyton discusses blood flow regulation in some detail. He begins by discussing the nature of smooth muscles.

Multi-unit smooth muscle is similar to skeletal muscle in that each fiber operates entirely independently of the others and is often innervated by a single nerve ending; also, a basement membrane-like substance separates individual fibers. This type of smooth muscle is found in the iris and ciliary muscle of the eye, as well as piloerector muscles[167-p.312].

Single-unit smooth muscle, or syncytial smooth muscle, refers to a whole mass of hundreds to millions of muscle fibers that contract together as a single unit. It is often called visceral smooth muscle because it is found in the gut, bile ducts, ureters, uterus, and many blood vessels[167-p.312].

The major share of the control over visceral smooth muscle is by *non-nervous stimuli*. Indeed, probably half or more of all smooth muscle contraction is initiated, *not by action potentials* but by stimulatory factors acting directly on the smooth muscle contractile machinery, including (a) local tissue factors and (b) circulating hormones.

Arteries, arterioles, veins and venules are all innervated. However, meta-arterioles, precapillary sphincters and capillaries have little or no nerve supply, yet they are highly contractile[167-p.331]. These vessels respond rapidly to local conditions in the surrounding interstitial fluid. Low oxygen levels, CO_2, hydrogen ions, adenosine, lactic acid, reduced Ca^{++} concentration, and *increased potassium ion concentration* function to cause vasodilation[167-p.317]. As it turns out, potassium is one of the most important local regulators of blood flow. For example, Thomas et al. recently concluded that, muscle contraction activates potassium channels, i.e., ATP-sensitive potassium (KATP) channels, which results in the release/extrusion of intracellular potassium. The subsequent increase in extracellular potassium is thought to be "a major mechanism underlying metabolic inhibition of sympathetic vasoconstriction in exercising skeletal muscle"[828]. Nitric oxide may also play a role in the regulation of blood flow in exercising skeletal muscles by opposing sympathetic vasoconstriction via the activation of KATP channels[829]. An entire section is devoted to potassium in Chapter 5.

Most of the circulating hormones in the body will also affect smooth muscle contraction at least to some degree, and some have profound effects. Some of the more important blood-borne hormones that affect contraction are *norepinephrine, epinephrine,* acetylcholine, angiotensin, vasopressin, oxytocin, serotonin, and histamine[167-p.317]. On a side note, one reason why sympathectomies often fail to reduce sympathetic hyperactivity and pain is because catecholamines from the adrenal medulla stimulate the local neural and tissue α-receptors and re-ignite the painful syndrome.

So far, we have discussed only the segmental control of vasomotor tone. It is important to realize that local sympathetic outflow is greatly influenced by the descending control exerted by structures found in brain stem. Guyton offers a succinct explanation of suprasegmental vasomotor control. He describes a *vasomotor center* in the reticular formation of the upper medulla and lower pons that controls the vasoconstrictor system[176-p.331-37].

A *vasoconstrictor area* (sometimes called area C1)

is located in the anterolateral portion of the upper medulla. The neurons in this area project throughout the cord and release norepinephrine which excites the so-called vasoconstrictor neurons in the intermediolateral cell column (IML). There is also a *vasodilator area* (sometimes called area A1) in the anterolateral portion of the lower medulla. Fibers project from A1 to the vasoconstrictor area where they cause inhibition, thus causing vasodilation (which probably means that there is less vasoconstrictor excitation of the IML). Moment to moment activity in both vaso-constrictor and vasodilator areas are determined by vagal and baroreceptor input via the nucleus tractus solitarius.

Under normal conditions the vasoconstrictor area is tonically active, causing the IML to fire at a rate of 1/2 to 2 impulses per second. These impulses maintain a partial state of contraction in blood vessels, i.e., a state of vasomotor tone. Guyton describes an experiment that illustrates vasomotor tone. Complete spinal anesthesia was caused in a laboratory animal, which inhibited CNS neuron activity, i.e., both segmental and suprasegmental. Arterial pressure fell from 100 to 50 mm Hg. Norepinephrine was then injected intravenously and the arterial pressure rose to a level greater than normal, and then subsequently fell as the catecholamine was catabolized. This experiment suggests that norepinephrine release from local sympathetic terminals probably promotes vasoconstriction. For a far more detailed description of brain stem control of sympathetic outflow see Guyenet[644].

After considering all of the information discussed in the above paragraphs, it should be clear that we cannot make definitive statements about the sympathetic nervous system and subluxation/joint complex dysfunction. However, enough information is available to suggest that local tissue hypoxia can be promoted by sympathetic hyperactivity. Now lets get back to our discussion about tissue hypoxia and how it may promote joint dysfunction.

Tissue hypoxia is probably the most common result of vasoconstriction, and it [hypoxia] is regarded as a very common cause of cell injury[92-p.2]. Cotran[92-p.4-5] provides a detailed description of the events that occur as a consequence of tissue hypoxia, a summary of which follows. A decrease in blood flow equates with a reduction in oxygen delivery and reduced ATP synthesis. Thus, the aerobic pathways of the cell, including the Krebs Cycle and the Electron Transport Chain, will no longer function properly. As a result of decreased oxygen availability, the cell shifts toward anaerobic metabolism (i.e., glycolysis) which provides significantly less ATP than the aforementioned aerobic pathways. Reduced ATP production is associated with an influx of Ca^{++}, an efflux of K^+, decreased intracellular pH, mitochondrial swelling, ER (endoplasmic reticulum) swelling, clumping of nuclear chromatin, decreased protein synthesis and lipid deposition. It should be understood that all of these signs of injury are reversible if oxygenation is restored. However, at some point irreversible injury will occur if hypoxia continues. An important point to appreciate is that, "the duration of hypoxia necessary to induce irreversible injury varies considerably according to the cell type and the nutritional and hormonal status of the animal[92-p.8]." Based on this fact, *hypoxic cell damage is an individual experience and no two cases are the same.* All patients will have different degrees of tissue damage.

Irreversible cell injury is characterized by two events which occur in addition to those associated with reversible injury[92-p.8]. The first being an intracellular release of lysosomal enzymes, which is associated with a falling pH (acidic) that occurs as a consequence of a shift to anaerobic metabolism. The second is the development of profound disturbances in cell membrane function, which is thought to be due to continued ATP depletion. As ATP disappears, so does the cell's ability to keep calcium concentrated in the extracellular fluid. It is important to understand that the ATP-driven calcium pump creates a calcium ion gradient of about 10,000-fold, leaving an internal concentration of calcium ions of about 10^{-7} M in contrast to an external concentration 10^{-3} M[176-p.73]. Reduced ATP synthesis allows for an influx of calcium which results in the activation of phospholipase enzymes which initiate cell membrane-phospholipid degradation and prostaglandin production. Increased cytosolic calcium is also associated with cytoskeletal damages which promote cell membrane damage.

The continuum of vasoconstriction-induced hypoxic injury does not end with lysosomal enzyme release and ATP depletion. At no precisely specified time, vasoconstriction is ultimately associated with a restoration of blood flow which brings in a host of partially reduced oxygen free radicals[92-p.9]. This event is known as reperfusion injury[92-p.9, 301] and has been associated with arthritis[309], as well as ischemic diseases of the heart, bowel, liver, kidney, and brain[301]. Below is a quote from Cotran[92-p.9] that provides an excellent description of free radicals and illustrates the degree to which free radical pathology is linked to disease:

"Free radicals are chemical species that have a single unpaired electron in an outer orbital. In such a state, the radical is extremely reactive and unstable and enters into reaction with inorganic or organic chemicals — proteins, lipids, carbohydrates — particularly with key molecules in membranes and nucleic acids. Moreover, free radicals initiate autocatalytic reactions, whereby molecules with which they react are themselves converted into free radicals to thus propagate the chain of damage...It is emerging as a final common pathway of cell injury in such varied processes as chemical and radiation injury, oxygen and other gaseous toxicity, cellular aging, microbial killing by phagocytic cells, inflammatory damage, tumor destruction by macrophages, and others."

Understand that the information cited from Cotran[92] concerning hypoxia is general information and can be applied to all cells. We as chiropractors are of course most intimately involved with the musculoskeletal system. In this regard, consider the following data concerning fibromyalgia and myofascial pain. Research suggests that the muscles of patients with primary fibromyalgia (PF) exist in a state of hypoxia due to sympathetic vasoconstriction[1, 197]. A histological evaluation of muscles compromised by PF revealed moth-eaten fibers, ragged-red fibers, mitochondrial abnormalities, Z-streaming and cytoplasmic bodies[197]. A biochemical analysis revealed decreased levels of both ATP and phosphocreatine[197]. It is thought that long periods of partial hypoxia occur in painful muscles, and that free radicals could possibly damage the mitochondrial membranes[197]. Travell & Simmons[449] provide similar histological and biochemical data regarding trigger points. A similar biochemical review of triggers points is also provided by Schneider and Cohen from a chiropractic perspective[399]. We should recall that trigger points are generally described as focal areas of muscle which manifest increased metabolic rate and decreased circulation (i.e., local hypoxia)[449].

So far, hypoxia has been described from a microscopic viewpoint. On a more macroscopic and practical level, Lantz states that "experimental arterial occlusion is known to lead to joint stiffness[256]." In other words, in some manner, decreased ischemia/hypoxia can lead to joint hypomobility (kinesiopathology). Cotran offers the beginning of a physiological explanation:

"Depending on the severity of the hypoxic state, cells may adapt, undergo injury, or die. For example, if the femoral artery is narrowed, the skeletal muscle cells of the leg may shrink in size (atrophy). This reduction in cell mass achieves a balance between metabolic needs and the available oxygen supply. More severe hypoxia will induce injury and cell death."[92-p.2]

This quote has interesting practical implications for chiropractors. How often do you as a chiropractor find atrophic changes in the postural muscles of the spine? I am sure that you will agree that it is quite common, and reflex vasoconstriction is mostly likely a contributing factor. Kirkaldy-Willis[234] describes how vasoconstriction in the multifidus muscle results in a cascade of events that begins with decreased circulation and ends with sustained multifidus contraction (i.e., hypomobility of the associated zygapophyseal joints). We are told that as this pathological cycle continues, muscle atrophy will occur, and ultimately the result will be fibrosis and chronic pain.

Thus far we have described vasoconstriction-induced hypoxia as it relates to microscopic and macroscopic alterations in muscular tissue. We should all appreciate that sympathetic hyperactivity

has effects other than vasoconstriction. Sympathetic efferent fibers, in addition to vasomotor innervation, are thought to innervate intrafusal fibers of striated muscle[144, 210], such that sympathetic hyperactivity can lead to muscle spasm[210, 243, 244].

There is an additional way in which sympathetic hyperactivity may influence subluxation/joint complex dysfunction. In 1986, Levine et al. demonstrated that chemical sympathectomy significantly reduced the severity of joint injury in experimentally induced arthritis and also prevented the development of arthritis[701]. Several articles have reviewed this topic [655, 665, 701]. These articles go into great detail and are important to study. I will highlight some of the points that are applicable to our current topic of discussion.

Chemical sympathectomy is known to reduce signs of inflammation including plasma extravasation and vascular permeability. Spontaneously hypertensive rats (SHR), i.e., rats with increased SNS activity are known to develop much more severe arthritis than normotensive rats. The reason why sympathetic hyperactivity can promote inflammation, and subsequently enhance nociception, is because of the mediators released by sympathetic terminals. While classic descriptions of sympathetic terminals may lead us to believe that norepinephrine is the only mediator, research has demonstrated that postganglionic fibers release many additional mediators including prostaglandins, purines, neuropeptide Y and perhaps other substances[655]. Not only does the sympathetic terminal release a variety of mediators, it also contains numerous membranous receptors for substances such as prostaglandins, bradykinin, serotonin, hydrogen ions, and opiate peptides [655]. Additionally, sympathetic terminals have α2- and β2-adrenergic receptors[655]. The β2-receptors are thought to be activated by epinephrine release from the adrenal medulla. Via this interaction it is thought that β2-receptors may play a role in promoting neurogenic inflammation [655].

At this point in time, all of the interactions between the chemicals released by sympathetic terminals and those that stimulate sympathetic terminals are not known. What is known, however, is that somatic tissue injury, inflammatory mediators, epinephrine, and nociceptive input serve to stimulate sympathetic efferent fibers which then, in turn, promote/enhance inflammatory and nociceptive processes at the site of injury.

It should be mentioned that all of these articles which discussed sympathetic fibers, also reviewed how the nociceptor participates in the inflammatory process. In short, it appears that both nociceptors and sympathetic terminals must be present for an appropriate inflammatory response to occur after tissue injury. Nociceptor involvement will be discussed in the next section entitled, "Physiology and biochemistry of nociceptors."

Based on the information presented thus far, it appears clear that nociceptive-induced sympathetic hyperactivity may promote histopathological changes within spinal joints in at least three ways. First, sympathetic hyperactivity can cause vasoconstriction within muscles and lead to hypoxia-induced myopathology. Second, sympathetic hyperactivity can promote muscle spasm, which may result in myopathology and joint hypomobility. Third, sympathetic hyperactivity can promote inflammation and enhance tissue injury.

Before ending this discussion about sympathetic hyperactivity, the term "somatovisceral reflex" will be discussed. This term is "thrown around" a lot by chiropractors during attempts to describe how subluxation causes viscera disease. The typical explanation proposes that subluxation of a particular spinal segment will interfere with the spinal nerve at the segmental level and result in dysfunction of the related organs. A common suggestion is that subluxation of the first and/or second thoracic vertebrae will lead to heart dysfunction. The work of Dr. Irvin Korr is typically cited to support such a suggestion. Indeed, Korr suggests that sympathetic hyperactivity has been associated with the development of a variety of diseases including neurogenic pulmonary edema, peptic ulcer and pancreatitis, arteriopathy, and cardiovascular-renal syndromes[245]. Unfortunately, very little work has been done to verify the possibility that segmental vertebral lesions can cause related visceral disease. Whether these diseases develop because of vasoconstriction in the respective tissues or because of trophic changes is not clear. In actual fact, it is very difficult to tell

if subluxation/joint dysfunction at a given segment will specifically influence organs innervated by nerves from that level. Lewit states that the evidence which proposes that disturbances of a vertebral segment will cause visceral disease is *conjectural* [271a]. In addition, a recent review of the literature, by Nansel and Szlazak, presents compelling evidence which suggests that such a segmental relationship between subluxation and visceral disease is very unlikely[329a]. However, Lewit and Nansel & Szlazak state that dysfunction of the vertebral column may cause symptoms that are mistaken for visceral disease, which most likely involves a suprasegmental relationship.

Although Bonica suggests that segmental sympathetic hyperactivity can reduce tone of the GI tract which may progress to ileus[47], he spends a great deal more time discussing the relationship between segmental nociceptive input and the subsequent stimulation of suprasegmental centers[48]. Segmental nociceptive input enters the cord and travels up the anterolateral pathway and terminates in the brain stem, hypothalamus, thalamus and cerebral cortex. Bonica states that,

"suprasegmental reflex responses result from nociceptive-induced stimulation of medullary centers of ventilation and circulation, hypothalamic (predominantly sympathetic) centers of neuroendocrine function, and some limbic structures. These responses consist of hyperventilation, increased hypothalamic neural sympathetic tone, and increased secretion of catecholamines and other catabolic hormones."[48]

Bonica goes on to mention that cortisol is one of the catabolic hormones that is released. Cortisol will be a focus of discussion in Chapter 6.

Research by Sato et al. provides a vivid explanation for why our focus should be directed on the suprasegmental effects of nociceptive input from dysfunctional joints. Sato et al. induce inflammation in the knee joint of anesthetized cats. The knees were then moved through their normal ranges of motion. The nociceptive input from such movement was sufficient to stimulate activity in the inferior cardiac nerve and increase blood pressure[387a]. Quite conceivably, nociceptive input from the sacroiliac joints and lumbar spine, or any other dysfunctional joint, could also have such an effect. For a long list of symptoms induced by nociceptive input from spinal structures see Feinstein[136a] and Nansel & Szlazak[329a]. After reading these papers, it will become obvious why we should abandon the segmental theories of yesteryear.

Reflex muscle spasm

Dvorak and Dvorak[607-p.44-45] review the work of Schmidt et al. who studied the response of alpha-motor neurons to painful stimuli. They found that nociceptive afferents have direct entry to the alpha- and gamma-motor neurons. Dvorak and Dvorak theorize that this relationship may explain the muscle tension/spasm that we see in association with spinal dysfunction. Bonica states that nociceptive-induced stimulation and sensitization of somatomotor neurons results in muscle spasm[48]. *Figure 1-1* illustrates the connections between nociceptive afferents and somatomotor neurons.

It should be understood that muscle spasm is not really a precise clinical term. There is actually an ongoing debate about the existence of muscle spasm in spinal dysfunction. This is probably because spasm is typically associated with the spastic changes that occur after an upper motor neuron lesion. Perhaps muscle tension or muscle guarding would be better terms. In the mean time, many respected researchers still use the term muscle spasm in context with spinal pain. I have elected to use the term muscle spasm as well.

There are two fundamental consequences of muscle spasm which include vascular compression and joint hypomobility. With respect to vascular compression, consider the following quote from Guyton[176-p.128]:

"Muscle spasm is a very common cause of pain, and is the basis of many clinical pain syndromes. This pain probably results partially from the direct effect of muscle spasm in stimulating mechanosensitive pain receptors. However, it possibly results also from the indirect effect of muscle spasm to compress the blood vessels and cause ischemia. Also, the spasm increases the rate

of metabolism in the muscle tissue at the same time, thus making the relative ischemia even greater, creating ideal conditions for release of chemical, pain-inducing substances."

McCardle provides us with information to help us better understand the relationship between muscle spasm and vascular compression. He states[298-p.350]:

"When a muscle contracts to about 60% of its force generating capacity, blood flow to the muscle is occluded due to elevated intramuscular pressure. With a sustained static or isometric contraction, the compressive force of the contraction can actually stop the flow of blood."

Based on this information, it is reasonable to suggest that nociceptive-induced muscle spasm exists in patients to varying degrees and contributes

Joints
  Shrinks joint capsules
  Increased compressive loading
  Leads to joint contracture
  Increased synthesis rate of glycosaminoglycans
  Increase in periarticular fibrosis
  Irreversible changes post-8-wk immobilization
Ligament
  Lowers failure or yield point
  Decreased thickness of collagen fibers
Disc biochemistry
  Decreased oxygen
  Decreased glucose
  Decreased sulfate
  Increased lactate concentration
  Decreased proteoglycan content
Bone
  Decreased bone density
  Eburnation
Muscle
  Decreased thickening of collagen fibers
  Decreased oxidative potential
  Decreased muscle mass
  Decreased saromeres
  Decreased cross-sectional area
  Decreased mitochondrial content
  Type 1 muscular atrophy
  Type 2 muscular atrophy
  20% loss of muscle strength per week
Cardiopulmonary
  Increased maximal heart rate
  Decreased VO2 maximum
  Decreased plasma volume

Table 1-1. Negative effects of immobilization (reprinted with permission from Liebenson C. Pathogenesis of chronic back pain. J Manipulative Physiol Ther 1992; 15:299-308).

to pain and hypoxic tissue damage. It appears that muscle spasm also promotes degenerative changes in the zygapophyseal joint and disc. Kirkaldy-Willis[234] illustrates how muscle spasm is the determining factor that leads to facet strain and annular tearing. Lantz, in his treatise on The Vertebral Subluxation Complex indicates that joint degeneration, as a consequence of joint hypomobility, begins with muscle spasm. He states[256]:

> "In studies of immobilization of the knee it was shown that in the early stages of joint degeneration, restricted joint mobility was due almost exclusively to the muscle/tendon component. Cutting the muscle away restored movement to normal ranges. This was not true of later stages in joint degeneration where joint mobility appears to be restricted due to capsular and ligamentous stricture."

Lantz has written another excellent paper which describes the connective tissue degeneration that occurs as a consequence of joint immobilization[255]. He discusses the changes that occur in articular cartilage, synovium, articular capsule, periarticular ligaments, subchondral bone, the intervertebral disc and the meninges. More recently, Liebenson reviewed the literature and listed the pathological

changes that develop when musculoskeletal tissues are immobilized (see *Table 1-1* on the previous page). It is important to understand that this information is appreciated by members of many professions including chiropractic, medicine, osteopathy, and physical therapy. In the case of chiropractic, we commonly refer to these changes as the pathological components of subluxation.

Figure 1-2 represents Lantz's effort to portray how these pathological components interact. Understand that it is difficult to portray complex pathophysiological interactions on paper.

Figure 1-3 on the following page illustrates a proposed dynamic relationship between the pathological components. The problem with the dynamic diagram is that it breaks down a pathological process into a step by step sequence of events. In reality, the various pathological changes may occur simultaneously and/or at different rates. One could also argue that there is a greater relationship between the various pathological changes, and thus, the dynamic diagram needs more arrows. This argument is probably true, however, more arrows could make the diagram more confusing for the practitioner who rarely reads texts devoted to pathology, physiology and biochemistry. The purpose of the dynamic diagram

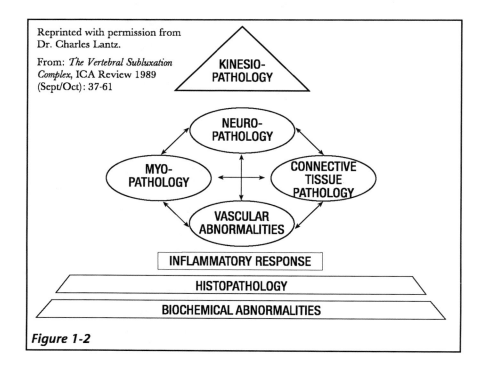

Reprinted with permission from Dr. Charles Lantz.

From: *The Vertebral Subluxation Complex*, ICA Review 1989 (Sept/Oct): 37-61

KINESIO-PATHOLOGY

NEURO-PATHOLOGY

MYO-PATHOLOGY

CONNECTIVE TISSUE PATHOLOGY

VASCULAR ABNORMALITIES

INFLAMMATORY RESPONSE

HISTOPATHOLOGY

BIOCHEMICAL ABNORMALITIES

Figure 1-2

is not to demonstrate every possible connection; rather, its purpose is to demonstrate that a continuum does indeed exist.

As the dynamic illustration demonstrates, tissue damage results in mechanical and chemical irritation of nociceptors. Nociceptive afferents stimulate sympathetic efferents and alpha-motoneurons, which constitutes part of the NEURO-PATHOPHYSIOLOGY component of the

subluxation complex. The result of such stimulation is Sympathetic Hyperactivity and Muscle Spasm. As the arrows indicate, Sympathetic Hyperactivity and Muscle Spasm lead to the development of VASCULAR ABNORMALITIES and MYOPATHOLOGY, both of which promote KINESIOPATHOLOGY and CONNECTIVE TISSUE PATHOLOGY.

At this point, look at the arrows that go from

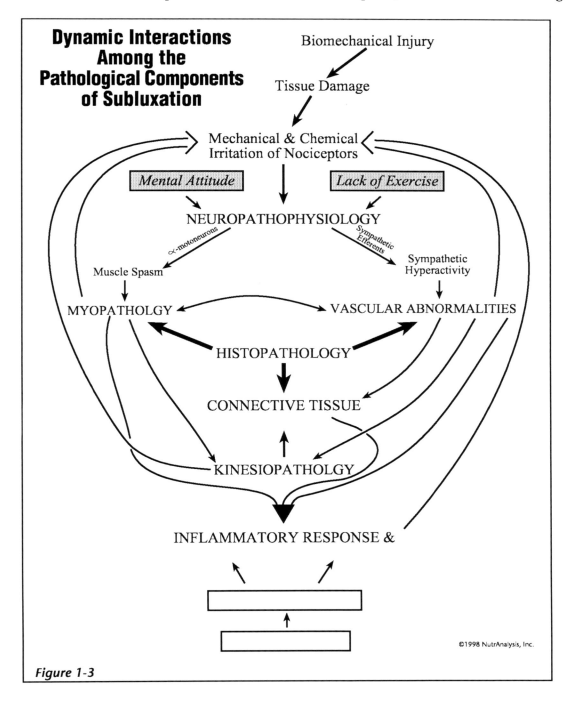

Dynamic Interactions Among the Pathological Components of Subluxation

Biomechanical Injury

Tissue Damage

Mechanical & Chemical Irritation of Nociceptors

Mental Attitude   Lack of Exercise

NEUROPATHOPHYSIOLOGY

∝-motoneurons   Sympathetic Efferents

Muscle Spasm   Sympathetic Hyperactivity

MYOPATHOLGY   VASCULAR ABNORMALITIES

HISTOPATHOLOGY

CONNECTIVE TISSUE

KINESIOPATHOLGY

INFLAMMATORY RESPONSE &

©1998 NutrAnalysis, Inc.

Figure 1-3

MYOPATHOLOGY and KINESIOPATHOLOGY to the word mechanical, which means to indicate that both pathologies act as mechanical irritants that stimulate nociceptors to perpetuate the subluxation complex continuum. The diagram further illustrates how VASCULAR ABNORMALITIES, MYOPATHOLOGY and CONNECTIVE TISSUE PATHOLOGY promote the development of an INFLAMMATORY RESPONSE and BIOCHEMICAL ABNORMALITIES, both of which produce chemical irritants that go on to stimulate nociceptors to perpetuate the subluxation complex continuum.

As illustrated in the center of the diagram, HISTOPATHOLOGICAL changes occur in blood vessels, muscles and connective tissues which are compromised in the dysfunctional joint. Such changes in these structures most likely contribute to the development of the already described mechanical and chemical irritation of nociceptors.

Treatment considerations

The adjustment appears to intervene in the subluxation complex continuum in two ways. First, the adjustment helps to restore normal biomechanical integrity to vertebral joints and thus, reduces mechanical irritation and mechanically-induced chemical irritation of articular nociceptors. Second, the adjustment causes a reflex inhibition of vasoconstriction and myospasm and therefore, reduces mechanical and chemical irritation of extra-articular nociceptors.

An extremely important point to understand is that, although the INFLAMMATORY RESPONSE and BIOCHEMICAL ABNORMALITIES are generated as part of the subluxation complex continuum, both components can also be influenced by the nutritional status of the tissues. In the bottom box below the dynamic diagram, write in the words Nutritional Status. In the box above Nutritional Status, write in the words Inflammatory Potential. Now the diagram suggests that our Nutritional Status determines how the Inflammatory Potential of our tissues can influence the production of chemical irritants. It should be understood that the Inflammatory Potential of our

tissues develops as an independent component and is not influenced by the chiropractic adjustment. It should also be understood that if the Inflammatory Potential is "pro-inflammatory" in nature, then the pathogenesis of the subluxation complex may continue despite good chiropractic care. A "pro-inflammatory" Inflammatory Potential denotes a state in which our tissues are predisposed to produce excessive amounts of chemical irritants. Such is thought to be the case with arthritis[35, 237], Alzheimer's disease[237] and probably most other degenerative diseases such as heart disease, cancer and autoimmune diseases[614].

In summary, this section discussed how nociceptive reflex responses can play a role in the pathogenesis of subluxation/joint complex dysfunction. It should now be obvious why a good understanding of nociceptor function is important. The next section provides a detailed description of the physiology and biochemistry of nociceptors, which will help to deepen your understanding of this clinically important topic.

PHYSIOLOGY AND BIOCHEMISTRY OF NOCICEPTORS

Having a general understanding of receptor physiology is important before one can truly appreciate the individual aspects of nociceptor physiology. It should be understood that, to a large extent, sensory receptor activity dictates central nervous system activity. According to Guyton[176-p.85], "most activities of the nervous system are initiated by sensory experience emanating from sensory receptors, whether they be visual receptors, auditory receptors, tactile receptors on the surface of the body, or other kinds of receptors."

Guyton classifies receptors into five main categories which include mechanoreceptors, thermoreceptors, nociceptors, electromagnetic receptors and chemoreceptors[176-p.103]. As you can see, the term proprioceptor was not used. Proprioceptor is a catch-all term that really describes tissue mechanoreceptors that are involved in proprioception. Proprioception has recently been described in the following manner:

> "Proprioception as defined by Sherrington (in 1906), refers to perception of joint and body movement as well as position of the body, or body segments, in space. More specifically, proprioception enables us to check on the spatial orientation of our bodies or body parts in space, the rate and timing of our movements, how much force our muscles are exerting, and how much and how fast a muscle is being stretched. Although Sherrington identified the muscle afferents, joint receptors, and vestibular labyrinth as proprioceptors, we have considered the vestibular receptors as a special class of proprioceptors and will confine our discussion in this section to the non-vestibular proprioceptors[142-p.84]."

This quote provides an excellent definition of proprioception, but fails to help clarify proprioceptive terminology. This author places vestibular receptors into a special class of proprioceptors, which is not helpful because other texts, such as Guyton[176-p.103], do not consider proprioceptors to be a class of sensory receptors. This is only one example of the confusion that exists in this area of physiology. So that you do not get confused, simply remember that there are a variety of tissue mechanoreceptors (joint receptors, muscle receptors and vestibular receptors) which provide sensory information to proprioceptive centers within the central nervous system.

Our discussion about receptors will center around mechanoreceptors and nociceptors. It should be understood that all sensory receptors are associated with an afferent nerve fiber. Action potentials travel along the afferent fiber carrying sensory information (i.e., information from the environment) into the central nervous system. The process by which sensory information is converted into an action potential is called transduction[176-p.103]. In this respect, sensory receptors act as biological transducers.

Below, the terms receptor potential, receptor adaptation, receptor threshold, peripheral nociceptive sensitization, and central nociceptive sensitization are defined. These are five very important aspects of receptor physiology that should be understood.

Receptor potential: A change in the membrane potential of a receptor is referred to as the receptor potential. When the receptor potential exceeds the excitation threshold of its associated afferent nerve fiber, then action potentials appear in the afferent fibers[176-p.103-104]. Let's say, for example, the resting membrane potential of the afferent fiber is -90mV, and -60mV is the threshold that must be reached before an action potential fires. When the receptor is stimulated, positive ions (Na^+) will rush into the nerve fiber and make the membrane potential less negative. If the receptor continues to be stimulated, then more positive ions will rush in. When enough positive ions enter the afferent fiber, the membrane potential will reach -60mV and an action potential will fire. From this explanation you can see that receptors respond to stimuli in a graded fashion. In other words the receptor potential will increase with increasing stimulation. In contrast, action potentials are not graded; rather, they are an all-or-none phenomena.

Receptor Adaptation: Adaptation is the process by which a receptor stops responding to a stimulus. For example, when a stimulus is applied to a receptor it will usually respond at a very high impulse rate at first, and then at a progressively lower rate until finally it may not respond at all, despite the continued presence of the stimulus[176-p.105]. In other words, over time, a receptor potential will diminish despite the continued presence of a stimulus. To differentiate the adaptive nature of receptors, they are classified as rapidly adapting (phasic receptors), slowly adapting (tonic receptors), or non-adapting.

Receptor threshold: Receptors are characterized as having either low or high thresholds of activation. Receptors that respond to very subtle forms of stimuli, such as light touch, are classified as low threshold receptors. On the contrary, certain receptors that respond only to intense forms of stimuli or noxious stimuli are characterized as high threshold receptors.

The relationship between receptors and afferent fibers: The following section discusses the nerve fibers which are associated with various joint receptors. As you will soon see, each receptor is associated with a different size afferent fiber. In fact, it is easy to get confused by the different classification systems for joint receptors and nerve fibers. For example, some are mislead to believe that Type I joint receptors are associated with Group I afferent fibers, and so on. In fact, the authors of a recent article claimed that Type III joint receptors, i.e., Golgi tendon-like mechanoreceptors, were associated with Group III afferent fibers, i.e., A-delta nociceptive afferents. This lead the authors to incorrectly conclude that Golgi tendon organs have a nociceptive function[775, 793]. To help avoid such a mistake, carefully read the following paragraphs which describe the differences between joint receptors and nerve fiber types.

Characteristics of joint receptors: The zygapophyseal joints of the vertebral column [as well as other synovial joints] are thought to have four different types of joint receptors, which are loosely classified as Type I, Type II, Type III, and Type IV joint receptors[56-p.46-59, 304, 482]. Types I, II, and III are all mechanoreceptors which respond to tension generated within connective tissue structures. Type IV receptors are nociceptors which respond to tissue damaging stimuli.

Type I joint receptors are found in the superficial layers of joint capsules and in periarticular ligaments and tendons. They often vary in appearance and may resemble Ruffini's endings, Golgi-Mazooni endings, Meissner's corpuscles, and basket or flower spray endings[304, 492]. Type I receptors are slow to adapt and also have very low thresholds, such that they are stimulated by the normal tension sustained in non-moving joints. Their activity increases as greater tension develops in the respective tissue. Because Type I receptors are active when joints are at rest and during movement, they can function as static and dynamic receptors[492]. The nerve fiber that is thought to be associated with Type I joint receptors is the A-beta fiber type of the Erlanger/Gasser classification system and Group II fiber type of the Loyd/Hunt classification system[492].

Type II joint receptors are found within the dense connective tissue in the deeper layers of joint capsules and ligaments. Type II receptors also vary in appearance and may look like Pacinian corpuscles, Vater-Pacinian corpuscles, modified Pacinian corpuscles, Paciniform corpuscle, Meissner's corpuscle, Golgi-Mazzoni bodies, bulbous corpuscles, and club-like endings[304]. They are rapidly adapting mechanoreceptors which fire brief bursts of impulses when joint tissue tension is augmented at the onset of movement. They have low thresholds and are thought to act exclusively as dynamic receptors[492]. The nerve fiber that is thought to be associated with Type II joint receptors is the A-beta fiber type of the Erlanger/ Gasser classification system and Group II fiber type of the Loyd/Hunt classification system[492].

Type III joint receptors were originally thought to be located exclusively in joints of the appendicular skeleton[492]. A recent study revealed that Type III joint receptors are present in the zygapophyseal joints of the cervical spine. Type III receptors were found in ligaments, tendons, and in dense fibrous connective tissue of the joint capsule[304]. Type III receptors are often described as Golgi tendon-like receptors. They are similar in appearance to Golgi's ending and Golgi-Mazzoni corpuscles[304]. Type III receptors are slow adapting and have very high thresholds of activation, such that they respond only when high tensions are generated in joint capsules and ligaments[492]. The nerve fiber that is thought to be associated with Type III joint receptors is the A-alpha fiber type of the Erlanger/Gasser classification system and Group I fiber type of the Loyd/Hunt classification system[492].

Type IV joint receptors, like all other tissue nociceptors, respond to tissue damaging stimuli. As mentioned earlier, they are located in all spinal tissues except for the articular cartilage, nucleus pulposus and the inner two-thirds of the annulus fibrosis. Unlike slowly adapting and rapidly adapting receptors, nociceptors do not adapt[176, 304, 492]. In fact, excitation of the nociceptive afferent fiber may actually increase as stimulation of the nociceptor continues over time[176]. The nerve fibers that are thought to be associated with Type IV joint receptors are the A-delta and C fiber types of the Erlanger/Gasser classification system and Group III and Group IV fiber types of the Loyd/

Hunt classification system[492].

In normal situations, nociceptors have very high thresholds of activation. Light touch and normal joint movements do not stimulate nociceptors. Nociceptors become activated when tissues are exposed to sufficiently severe mechanical distortion (high-threshold stimulation) or sufficiently marked alterations in the chemical composition of the tissue fluid that bathes them[491], which is characteristic of the inflammatory process. At this point it should be understood that nociceptors are thought to be the most sensitive to chemical irritants[337-p.25, 505].

Peripheral nociceptive sensitization: Unlike other receptors, nociceptor thresholds can be lowered. This occurs when nociceptors undergo a sensitization process. Sensitization refers to an abnormally low nociceptor threshold that develops due to the presence of an acidic pH and irritant chemicals such as prostaglandin E-2, leukotriene B-4, histamine, 5-hydroxytryptamine, bradykinin and perhaps norepinephrine[73, 137, 187]. Lactic acid and potassium ions also stimulate nociceptors; however, they are not thought to be sensitizing agents. Some papers and texts state that substance P is a sensitizing agent. A close examination of such writings will reveal that most authors actually state that substance P is an indirect sensitizer of nociceptors. This is because substance P, after it is released by stimulated nociceptors, will cause local tissues to release some of the sensitizing agents mentioned above. Substance P is discussed in more detail in an upcoming paragraph.

In a sensitized state, nociceptors will be activated by normal, low-threshold innocuous movements[392], such as normal head turning. This results in nociceptive bombardment into the spinal cord dorsal horn. Not only are sensitized nociceptive receptors more sensitive to stimulation, due to a lowered threshold of activation, they also display prolonged and enhanced responses to such stimulation[47-p.95]. Thus, it appears that a sensitized nociceptor will initiate the firing of excessive action potentials in nociceptive afferents. The term peripheral nociceptive sensitization can be used to refer to sensitized nociceptors. The term central sensitization is used to describe the sensitization of synaptic connections within the CNS. Central

sensitization will be discussed shortly.

In recent years, it has been demonstrated that the nociceptor itself may play a role in the sensitization process. Research has demonstrated that upon stimulation, nociceptive receptors release various neuropeptides including neuropeptide Y, galanin, met-enkephalin, leu-enkephalin, calcitonin gene related peptide (CGRP) and substance P[392]. The most well studied of these are CGRP and substance P, both of which are thought to work synergistically to produce plasma extravasation (i.e., the escape of fluids into the surrounding tissue, as in inflammation)[392]. Other research suggests that the release of substance P by activated nociceptors will cause vasodilation, increased vascular permeability, pavementing of leukocytes in venules, PMN phagocytosis, local prostaglandin synthesis, and mast cell release of histamine, serotonin and leukotrienes[268], all of which can promote local inflammation and further nociceptor stimulation.

As discussed earlier in the section devoted to sympathetic hyperactivity, it is known that sympathetic efferent discharge back into the area of injury can promote inflammation by enhancing the release of various chemical mediators. Neurogenic inflammation is the term used to describe the inflammation that is driven by nervous system processes, including substance P release from nociceptors and sympathetic efferent activity. By promoting neurogenic inflammation, the nervous system can enhance the production of chemical mediators involved in peripheral sensitization.

Central nociceptive sensitization: Woolf[487] was the first to demonstrate experimentally that central neurons are sensitized, or facilitated, as a consequence of noxious input. Current research maintains that nociceptive input results in central changes:

"Brief stimulation of afferent C fibres caused changes of excitability in motor reflexes and expansions of receptive fields of dorsal horn neurones which outlasted the actual stimulus. The presence of 'central changes' implies that there are not only alterations in the afferent drive of central neurones, but that the sensitivity to afferent inputs in the central neurones themselves is enhanced."[392]

In the laboratory, this enhanced activity of central neurons can be studied by inducing inflammation in animals by injecting various substances such as Freund's complete adjuvant (FCA), kaolin and carrageenan. Changes in the discharge properties of spinal neurons during inflammation were first documented in 1983 in rats with FCA-induced chronic polyarthritis[487]. Various terms can be applied to the enhanced activity of central neurons due to nociceptive input, such as hyperexcitability, amplification, facilitation, and sensitization. Recently, the term "wind up" has been used to characterize a state of C-fiber input dependent central sensitization[364].

Many processes are thought to be involved in the development of central sensitization of the nociceptive system. According to Schaible[392], the processes involved may include: (1) changes in the ionic environment of central neurons, (2) the effects of fast-acting transmitters and slow acting modulators, (3) the activation of intracellular second and third messenger systems, and (4) additional mechanisms such as gene expression. Dubner and Ruda[124] recently published a paper on spinal cord plasticity that describes some of these changes in detail. It appears that spinal cord plasticity is responsible for the development of central nociceptive sensitization.

Based on the information described in this section, it should be clear that the released chemical irritants are directly responsible for the peripheral sensitization of nociceptors and indirectly responsible for the central nociceptive sensitization that occurs in the central nervous system. The result of such sensitization is increased reflex/synaptic activity[392]. Based on this data, examine the illustration of *Chiropractic and the Dorsal Horn* (*Figure 1-1*) and consider how peripheral nociceptor sensitization and central sensitization of the spinal cord can promote the pathogenesis of the subluxation complex. It should be remembered that *chemical irritants* are responsible for the sensitization process.

Nociception in clinical practice: An important point to understand is that sensitized nociceptors can be evaluated clinically during the physical examination and chiropractic analysis. Many times a clinician will find that patients are abnormally sensitive to innocuous mechanical pressure during an evaluation. Such a condition, in which pain is produced by normally painless stimuli, is known as allodynia[73]. Often times, clinicians will also find that patients experience almost unbearable pain and sensitivity to mechanical pressure that would normally be characterized as just painful and uncomfortable. Such a condition, in which abnormally intense pain is produced by normally painful stimuli, is known as hyperalgesia[73]. When either condition is present in a patient, the clinician can be relatively sure that the patient's tissues are exposed to excessive chemical irritants which results in sensitized nociceptors. Additionally, these patients often say they take NSAIDs to help reduce pain and inflammation. These patients, in particular, need the nutritional interventions described in this book.

Chapter 2

TERMINOLOGY AND CONCEPTUAL ISSUES

At times, journal editors will invite researchers to provide commentary on a given article and debate issues with the author. This commentary/debate usually follows the article of focus. In the same fashion, the present chapter will discuss some of the chiropractic terminology and conceptual issues that were highlighted in Chapter 1. Additionally, Chapter 1 provided the neurological foundation for a chiropractic approach to nutrition. The present chapter will introduce this approach and also discuss conceptual issues related to nutrition with a focus on food allergies, candida, body detoxification, and food combining.

TERMINOLOGY AND CONCEPTUAL ISSUES RELATED TO SUBLUXATION/JOINT COMPLEX DYSFUNCTION

Chapter 1 focussed on how nociception could promote the subluxation complex. The purpose of the next chapter, i.e., Chapter 3, is to distill the clinically important aspects of inflammation and apply them to the pathogenesis of joint complex dysfunction, which in reality, is a chiropractic term to describe a *soft tissue injury of the vertebral column.*

The information in Chapters 1 and 3 essentially represent a departure from the way subluxation is typically described. The subluxation complex is mostly viewed as a static condition, rather than a dynamic pathophysiological continuum involving nociception and inflammation. As an example, neither the so-called Mercy guidelines[308] or the so-called Windham guidelines[486] provide dynamic functional definitions for the subluxation complex.

Mercy defines the vertebral subluxation complex as "an aberration of normal spinal biomechanics, usually involving a restriction or loss of normal movement of a motion segment, and associated aberrations in the tissues which support articular motion (e.g., nerve, muscle, connective and vascular)"[308]. Very little, if any, additional discussion is devoted to the subluxation complex.

Mercy states that the subluxation syndrome, "is defined here to mean the clinical signs and symptoms that relate to pathophysiology or dysfunction of spinal and pelvic motion segments or to peripheral joints that may be amenable to manipulative/adjustive procedures"[308]. We are not provided with a name for the lesion which causes the syndrome, nor are we provided with insight regarding the manner in which the lesion can produce symptoms or what the symptoms may be.

Windham[486] states that a vertebral subluxation is "a misalignment of one or more articulations of the spinal column or its immediate weight-bearing articulations, to a degree less than a luxation, which by inference causes alteration of nerve function and interference to the transmission of mental impulses, resulting in a lessening of the body's innate ability to express its maximum health potential." Windham[486] also tells us that the term vertebral subluxation "has referred to the event in which a moveable vertebra was caused to fixate outside its normal juxtaposition with the vertebra above or below," and that "...as a result of the numerous structural and functional studies, these general effects of the vertebral subluxation have been focused into five categories." Windham goes on to list five different aspects of subluxation including kinesiopathology, neuropatho-

---

The Subluxation Complex

- A pathomechanical joint lesion (usually hypomobility) that develops as a consequence of (1) micro and/or macrotraumatic tissue injury and associated inflammatory response, (2) inflammatory damage that may be perpetuated by a nutritional status that is pro-inflammatory in nature, (3) degenerative changes in muscular and connective tissues due to sedentary living, (4) decreased descending inhibitory pathway activity due to aberrant psychological states, and (5) dysafferentation (i.e., increased nociception and decreased mechanoreception which are caused by 1-4).

- Evaluation of hypomobile joints consistently reveals histopathological changes within the associated neuromusculoskeletal tissues, which demonstrates that a hypomobile joint manifests as a structural disease that chiropractors call the subluxation complex.

- This disease called the subluxation complex, may produce a variety of patient-specific symptoms depending upon (1) specific end organ changes initiated by nociceptive reflex activity, and (2) which central autonomic, endocrine, limbic, motor and/or sensory nuclei are most affected by increased nociception and/or decreased mechanoreception.

Table 2-1   © 1998 NutrAnalysis, Inc.

---

physiology, myopathology, histopathology and pathophysiology. According to Windham, the subluxation complex is defined as an "event" that has "certain effects" and thus, subluxation is not characterized as an entity in and of itself.

Clearly, the Mercy and Windham guidelines fail to define subluxation in a functional fashion. The same holds true for the model put forth by Lantz, which was described as a static model in the last chapter. This is probably because the nociceptive processes are absent from all three descriptions of subluxation. Indeed, it seems impossible to define subluxation in a dynamic fashion unless nociception and inflammation are included in the model.

Table 2-1 provides a definition of subluxation that is based on the dynamic nature of nociception and inflammation. This definition suggests that the subluxation complex is a disease because it is characterized by pathological tissue changes, and can result in many different symptomatic presentations. The view that subluxation is a disease, rather than the cause of disease, may contradict what many DCs believe about the nature of subluxation. It should be understood that the belief that subluxation is the cause of disease is inconsistent with how chiropractors define subluxation, i.e., a condition associated with pathological changes.

We should all remember that back in 1910, D.D. Palmer stated that "the determining causes of disease are traumatism, poison and autosuggestion"[342-p.359]. *Figure 2-1* illustrates how subluxation is caused by trauma (mechanical irritants), poison (chemical irritants), and autosuggestion (reduced descending inhibition).

Modern pathology texts basically agree with D.D. Palmer's view about disease causation. The latest edition of *Robbin's Pathologic Basis of Disease* states that cell injury and death, i.e., diseases, are caused by hypoxia, physical agents such as trauma, chemical agents and drugs, infectious agents, immunologic reactions, genetic derangements and nutritional imbalances[93-p.3]. It appears that all diseases, including the subluxation complex, are caused by the same agents. This fact of pathophysiology should alert us to the fact that our view of subluxation should be updated.

Based on the above information, and much of the information in this book, I spent a lot of time thinking about terminology issues in chiropractic. This lead me to write four papers devoted to terminology issues[794, 795, 796, 797]. Three of these papers can be found in Appendix B at the back of this book. One of these papers proposed that we adopt the term "joint complex dysfunction" to

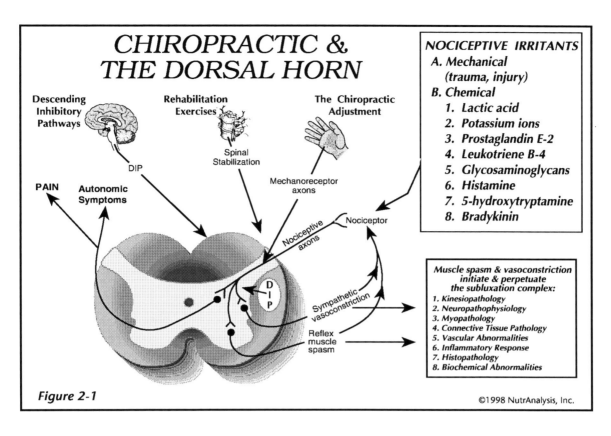

Figure 2-1

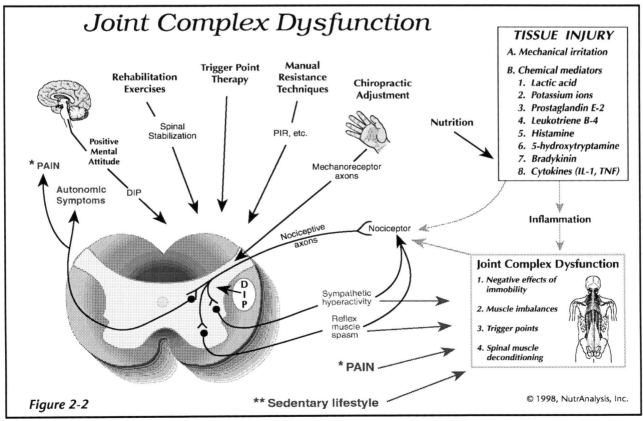

Figure 2-2

describe the spinal condition that chiropractors treat through such methods as adjustments, exercise, and nutrition[795]. *Figure 2-2* illustrates the concept of joint complex dysfunction. As you can see, the image is similar to that of Chiropractic and the Dorsal Horn, with some notable exceptions.

There are several reasons for advancing the term joint complex dysfunction. Primarily, it has to do with the way subluxation is defined and characterized. The term "subluxation" has historically been defined as a spinal misalignment that places pressure on nerves as they travel through the intervertebral foramen. This description suggests that no injury has been incurred by the musculoskeletal system; instead, we are lead to infer that nerves have been injured due to pressure from subluxation. Accordingly, when vertebral subluxation is the condition to be addressed, the primary goal is to realign the vertebrae and reduce nerve pressure. With the subluxation model of nerve pressure and nerve interference, 1) injury to the musculoskeletal system is not considered, 2) the innervation pattern in musculoskeletal tissues is not considered, 3) nociception and inflammation within musculo-skeletal tissues is not considered, 4) pain is not considered, 5) atrophic changes and weakening of the musculoskeletal system is not considered, 6) chronicity of musculoskeletal deconditioning is not considered, 7) associated cardiovascular deconditioning is not considered, 8) rehabilitation issues are not considered, 9) nutritional issues are not considered, 10) psychosocial issues are not considered, and 11) important orthopedic, neurologic, and diagnostic issues are not considered.

Clearly, the classic subluxation model does not take into consideration many issues of concern regarding pathophysiology within the musculoskeletal system. In contrast, joint complex dysfunction refers to the biochemical and neurological abnormalities that develop in response to injury of musculoskeletal tissues. Accordingly, this text is written for the purpose of defining the body's response to injury, with a focus on the nutritional biochemistry issues related to restoring integrity to injured musculoskeletal structures.

NEUROMUSCULOSKELETAL SPECIALIST

At this juncture it would be useful to discuss the term "neuromusculoskeletal specialist," which is embraced by many DCs and disliked by others. We can resolve this terminology issue by answering some simple questions.

1. What structures do we adjust?

    We adjust musculoskeletal structures that are innervated by the nervous system, i.e., a neuromusculoskeletal structures. Although adjustments excite somatic afferents which influence the CNS and visceral structures, we do not adjust CNS or visceral structures. So, to suggest that we are anything but neuromusculoskeletal specialists seems inconsistent with our current training and treatment focus.

2. Will the term neuromusculoskeletal specialist characterize us in such a way that we will only treat back pain?

    The NMS characterization will limit only those who are unfamiliar with the relationship between somatic afferents and the generation of symptoms of visceral disease. For detailed discussions see Nansel and Szlazak[329a] and Seaman and Winterstein[796].

3. Do people need neuromusculoskeletal specialists?

    Yes, neuromusculoskeletal dysfunction is the most common cause of physical disability. Arthritis, back pain, and cervicogenic vertigo are just three examples of debilitating conditions related to faulty neuromusculoskeletal function.

A common criticism levied against those who embrace the neuromusculoskeletal characterization is that such practitioners are no more than pseudomedical pain therapists. *Figure 2-2* demonstrates that this view is quite short-sighted. A chiropractor who utilizes the treatment methods outlined in this image provides patients with numerous potential long-term health benefits. For example, utilizing low-tech rehabilitation methods, i.e., spinal stabilization exercises, propriosensory training, etc., can enhance a patient's strength and coordination, and thereby help prevent future injury and disability. Additionally, improved locomotor function will give patients the chance to maintain aerobic fitness into their 40s-70s which can significantly reduce morbidity from chronic diseases such as heart disease. Utilizing nutrition can also provide patients with many long-term benefits. The nutritional protocols described in this text to reduce inflammation, pain and nociception are also known to prevent cancer, heart disease, diabetes, and many other chronic diseases.

CONCEPTUAL ISSUES RELATED TO NUTRITION

Most will agree that the main focus of chiropractic practice is to restore biomechanical integrity to spinal and extremity joints. Naturally, we do this by adjusting these joints. Many chiropractors complement their adjustments with a variety stretching techniques and low-tech rehabilitation exercises. However, when it comes to nutrition, the focus often turns away from the musculoskeletal system. As opposed to offering nutritional strategies to complement our spinal adjusting, i.e., a "nutritional adjustment", many chiropractors turn to approaches and philosophies that do not directly address the musculoskeletal system such as food allergies, Candida albicans, and detoxification. The remainder of this chapter discusses some of the pros and cons of these approaches.

Food allergies

Years ago, I thought that food allergies were a major concern for most patients. Such sentiments were based on clinical improvements I observed when patients went on partial elimination diets. I would have patients eat mostly vegetables and fruits, some grains, moderate amounts of protein and drink 1 to 2 quarts of water per day. Simultaneously, I would have them avoid things like junk food, coffee, alcohol, pizza, packaged foods, and fast food. Within a few days to a week, it was common for energy levels to significantly improve and to see pain levels drop dramatically. Today I realize that this dietary program offered anti-inflammatory benefits and thus, patient improvements were most likely derived from the anti-inflammatory nature of this diet, and not from eliminating food allergies.

In the past I would have also thought that most rheumatoid arthritis (RA) patients would have food allergies. However, research suggests that perhaps only about 1/3 of RA patients have this problem. Results from a research trial involving an extensive elimination diet suggested that only 10 of 27 RA patients had food allergies[237]. The authors stated that the results obtained by *all* 27 patients could not be explained by food allergies, and thought that the majority of patients improved due to an increased production of anti-inflammatory eicosanoids from fatty acids of vegetable origin.

It is important to realize that RA patients commonly have damaged and "leaky" guts due, in part, to prolonged NSAID therapy. This is a population that would be particularly prone to food antigen penetration and food allergies, yet only 1/3 of the RA patients had food allergies. This suggests that the average patient entering a typical private practice will not be suffering with food allergies. The main exception to this rule would be gliadin sensitivity which does appear to be somewhat common in the so-called normal population[546, 708, 724, 867]. Gliadin is found in numerous grains, such as wheat, rye and oats (see Chapter 7 for details).

Clinicians should be aware that certain populations of patients may be more inclined to have food sensitivities. For example, patients with migraine headaches, irritable bowel syndrome, Chrohn's disease, eczema, hyperactivity, and rheumatoid arthritis (as mentioned above), may be sensitive to similar foods, i.e., cereal grains, dairy products, caffeine, yeast, and citrus fruits. Avoidance of these foods often leads to symptomatic relief [661]. Hunter hypothesized that such patients may have imbalances in digestive enzymes and gut flora, and not an immunological disease. Hunter also indicates that such imbalances may be genetically passed on, such that a familial tendency towards food intolerance has long been recognized. Finally, he states that, "if food allergy is not an immunological disease, but a disorder of bacterial fermentation in the colon, it might be more appropriately named an 'enterometabolic disorder'"[661]. Assessing for digestive efficiency, gut permeability, and gut pathogens may be appropriate in these patients.

For more details about food allergy, it would be wise to acquire scientific texts devoted to the topic[567, 577]. These texts make it clear that food allergy is not a common finding in the average ambulatory patient.

Candida albicans

No discussion about conceptual issues in nutrition would be complete without at least mentioning Candida albicans. In short, Candida is misunderstood organism. Candida species are a normal component of our gut flora along with hundreds of other bacteria. Microbes are actually a normal and essential part of human existence. In fact, the number of microbial cells existing in our body at any one time, greatly exceed the number of our own cells.

The digestive tract is considered to be a reservoir for facultatively pathogenic fungi, particularly Candida albicans[689]. A recent article reviewed the incidence of Candidemia in a Canadian tertiary care hospital from 1976 to 1996, and determined that 23% of deaths could be directly attributable to Candida species[680]. Without examining the details one could be led to infer that Candida is a chronic condition that begins long before one enters the hospital, similar to cancer and heart disease. This notion has led some to believe that certain general symptoms act to signal the presence of immune-compromising Candida.

Books published for the layman, and naive doctors and nutritionists, consider numerous symptoms to be signs of Candida infestation such as fatigue or lethargy, poor memory, feeling "spacey," inability to make decisions, numbness, insomnia, muscle aches, pain, constipation, diarrhea, attacks of anxiety or crying, cold hands or feet, shaking or irritable when hungry[627]. It is thought that candidiasis can play a key role in headaches, depression, cancer, AIDS, skin rashes, low sex-drive, food allergies, sensitivity to tobacco and odors, joint and muscle pains, menstrual irregularities, digestive problems, and severe cases can even be fatal[627].

Researchers often look askance at such claims, stating that "there is no connection between the incidence of Candida in the digestive tract and multiple local symptoms like fatigue, headache, heartburn and others called 'candidiasis hypersensitivity syndrome' or 'mycophobia'"[680]. In fact, it is probably very unlikely that Candida albicans plays any role in the generation of symptoms which are present in the typical ambulatory patient. Candida commonly lurks its ugly head in patients with cancer and AIDS, for example, who undergo immunosuppressive therapy[846].

Antibiotic therapy is also known to promote the growth of opportunistic organisms; however, it is not possible to assume that antibiotic use will cause a disabling case of candidiasis. In the Canadian hospital study cited earlier, the authors explain that all patients with candidemia possessed at least 2 risk factors. The three main risk factors included antibiotic therapy, catheterization, and immunosuppression, i.e., a combination of risk factors that are not typically in clinical chiropractic practice.

It should be understood that a diagnosis of candidiasis cannot be given to a patient based upon symptoms alone, particularly the ones listed earlier. Kroker provides a list of clinical factors that might lead one to the diagnosis of candidiasis in a young to middle age female[695]. Presenting symptoms would include fatigue, mood lability, depression, inability to concentrate, headaches and loss of energy. Additionally, there would be symptoms of yeast overgrowth in the mouth, vagina, and intestine. These patients also commonly crave carbohydrates and yeast foods. A past history should reveal chronic yeast infections, chronic antibiotic use for acne or infections, oral birth control pill usage, and/or oral steroid use. Associated conditions may be present such as endocrinopathies, mitral valve prolapse, premenstrual syndrome, and inhalant, food, and chemical sensitivities. Physical examination should reveal signs of oral or vaginal yeast infection, signs of essential fatty acid deficiency and/or signs of respiratory allergy[695].

In addition to these manifestations, it is incumbent upon the practitioner to perform laboratory evaluations to determine the presence and virulence of Candida. Examples of such tests include a culture from mouth/throat, vagina and stool, a serum Candida antigen to test for potential dissemination for local reservoirs, and a candida-specific secretory IgA test of a stool sample. It should be understood that Candida cultures do not indicate that candidiasis is present. Additional specific tests, such as the ones mentioned above, are required to confirm a diagnosis.

Without going through the rigors of a thorough case history, physical examination, and laboratory evaluation, it would be impossible to confidently diagnose a case of candidiasis. Surprisingly, many will argue this point, suggesting that symptom relief, i.e., fatigue, pain, and irritability, due to dietary modifications is a sign that Candida has been eradicated. The typical "anti-Candida diet" or "Candida control diet"[695] involves the elimination of refined foods, yeast containing foods, fruit juices, sweeteners of all kinds (limited amounts of honey and maple syrup are often permitted), overripe fruits, and yeast containing grains. Sometimes a fruit-free diet is initially recommend. Otherwise, most fruits are acceptable. A liberal intake of vegetables is recommend with the exception of high-carbohydrate vegetables like corn, lima beans, potatoes, and yams. All meat, poultry and fish are usually acceptable. Most nuts and seeds are allowed, save for peanuts and cashews.

Obviously, the so-called "anti-candida diet" would be a good diet for anyone to follow who wants to feel better and prevent disease. In fact, with a few exceptions, this diet is typically recommended to patients with heart disease, cancer, diabetes, and to athletes and others who want to pursue health and fitness through nutrition. This diet is also nearly identical to the anti-inflammatory diet described in this book (see Chapters 5, 6, and 10).

Liver detoxification - Fact or fiction?

Introduction

For years, both professional and laymen involved in the so-called "natural health movement" have advocated the therapeutic concept of detoxification. For example, Bernard Jensen is probably the most well-known advocate of colon cleansing, and has been doing so for some 50 years. Jensen is also an advocate of regular exercise and eating a fruit and vegetable-diet, while avoiding refined and processed foods.

In the past 10 years, the concept of liver detoxification has been a clinical focus, attracting chiropractors, nutritionists, and medical doctors. The reason for this is obvious, the liver is the body's primary organ of detoxification. Consequently, nutritional products have been designed to detoxify the liver and laboratory tests were created to assess liver toxicity.

One laboratory[633] suggests that, "your body's natural defenses may be overwhelmed by toxins in food, water and air." They recommend that you perform a hepatic detoxification profile if more than two of the following apply to you (this is only a partial list):

* allergies, sinus problems, or joint pain

* frequently tired after a normal day

* gastrointestinal problems

* one or more alcoholic beverages per week

* used prescription drugs 2 or more times in the past year

* ever used insect sprays or herbicides

We are told that if two or more apply, we may be reacting to increased exposure and burdening the body's detoxification ability. Coincidentally, at least two or more will apply to almost all of us, which implies that we all need to run a detoxification test.

In actual fact, very little research supports the existence of designer supplements or the rational behind testing for hepatic detoxification. A review of several papers will demonstrate the fallacy of these interventions.

Review of literature

In the 1950s, it was determined that the hepatic endoplasmic reticulum, i.e., microsomes, possessed oxidative enzymes capable of metabolizing drugs and xenobiotics[555]. Initial research demonstrated that hepatic microsomes contained "a unique CO-binding pigment exhibiting an unusual visible absorption maximum at 450 nm in its CO-reduced difference spectrum"[736]. Shortly thereafter, this pigment was characterized by optical spectroscopy and given the temporary name cytochrome P450[736]. The name cytochrome P450 has stuck, even though they are not morphologically similar to mitochondrial cytochromes involved in ATP synthesis. It should be mentioned that many different organs contain P450 enzymes, such as the lung, kidney, and brain.

> "Rather than electron-funneling cytochromes in the true sense of the word, P450 hemoproteins are enzymes. Heme-thiolate protein is perhaps the most accurate term. For better or worse, the cytochrome P450 has stuck."[736]

At first, P450 was thought to represent a single enzyme. To date, well over 500 different P450s have been characterized at the level of their DNA sequences; however most species probably do not have more than 40-50 different enzymes[642]. Other authors suggest that humans may have 60 or more different P450s[736]. While cytochrome P450 is generally used to described the gene superfamily, a nomenclature system was published in 1991 to distinguish the various P450 enzymes[642]. It should also be understood that the general term "mixed function oxidase" (MFO) is commonly used when referring to the P450 enzymes

The root symbol CYP delineates cytochrome P450. Following CYP will be an Arabic numeral designating the P450 family, followed by a letter indicating the subfamily, which is then followed by another Arabic numeral to delineate the individual gene[736]. Examples include CYP1A2, CYP2C18, CYP2D6, CYP2E1, CYP3A4, and CYP4A11, which are the enzymes thought to be responsible for the metabolism of virtually all drugs[736]. Nebert provides a table which lists these enzymes, the drugs they act on, and the associated carcinogens that can be produced[736].

For reasons that should be obvious, much of the research devoted to this area of investigation centers around drug interactions. Such research helps to determine therapeutic doses, plasma drug clearance, drug-drug interactions, toxic manifestations, as well as stimulatory and inhibitory interactions. Guengerich recently wrote an article devoted to this subject, and explained that an outcome from such research is the development of drugs that avoid cancer promoting CYP1A enzymes[642]. [Regarding this CYP1A relationship, Guengerich references the work of Ioannides and Park[663], which is discussed in the next section].

Research has also led to the discovery of certain P450 polymorphisms, which have important clinical implications associated with drug therapy. For example, approximately 1/10 of the population display a fast-metabolizing phenotype for CYP1A1, which is thought to be involved in cigarette smoke-induced toxicity or malignancies[736].

Another example is the CYP2D6 gene, which is expressed in the liver and central nervous system. A polymorphism for this gene was identified in 1977, and it is now known that populations are divided into two general categories, i.e., an extensive metabolizer and a poor metabolizer. Approximately 5-10% of white individuals display the poor metabolizer phenotype, while it was observed in 16% of Nigerians, less than 2% among Asians, and only 1% in a Chinese population that was studied. This is a clinically important polymorphism because the CYP2D6 enzyme metabolizes a large number of commonly used drugs, including antiarrhythmic, beta blockers, monoamine oxidase inhibitors, morphine, antipsychotics, and tricyclic antidepressants. In fact, it is recommended that safe use of psychiatric and cardiovascular drugs depends a prudent consideration of the CYP2D6 phenotype/genotype. Research has been determined that the poor metabolizer CYP2D6 phenotype appears to be associated with idiopathic Parkinson's disease. Fortunately, 90% to 95% of the time, genotyping can accurately predict the phenotype[736].

Conditions such as multiple chemical sensitivity, food intolerance, and sick building sydrome may also be related to P450 polymorphism. It is known that certain drugs and xenobiotic agents can initiate each of these diseases, which happen to commonly occur among family members, suggesting a genetic predisposition[736].

At this point, it should be obvious that no nutritional relationships to liver function have been discussed, and there has been no mention of functional tests to assess hepatic detoxification in the average ambulatory patient. The reason for this is that standard articles and reviews of the literature do not address these issues[555, 642, 643, 663-p.93, 736]. There are some papers that discuss how diet and nutrition can influence the P450 system; however, none make general or specific recommendations to upregulate or downregulate hepatic detoxification[540, 640, 641].

Phase I and Phase II pathways

In addition to the cytochrome 450 family, often referred to as the Phase I system, there is an additional group of enzymes that are involved in detoxification, which are often referred to as the Phase II system. While Phase I enzymes typically oxidate various substrates, often into more toxic substances, the Phase II system converts these substances into non-toxic and readily-excretable substances. The specifics of the Phase II system will be discussed later in this chapter. Nebert and McKinnon provide a concise description of hepatic detoxification:

> "P450 enzymes represent the classical phase I metabolism in which a given substrate is oxygenated. Phase II enzymes often use the inserted oxygen as a site for further

metabolism (e.g., glucuronidation, or conjugation with glutathione, sulfate, or glycine). Together phase I plus phase II metabolism usually results in the detoxification of drugs and environmental pollutants. However, in the past 20 years, it has been appreciated that P450 enzymes can transform relatively innocuous agents, procarcinogens and promutagens, to hepatotoxins or the ultimate carcinogen or mutagen."[736]

Ioannides, Parke and Lewis have written some interesting papers on the differences among certain P450 enzymes[662, 663, 704, 746]. Their original work[662, 704, 746] focussed on the difference between the P450 family, now known as CYP2B and others[663], and the P448 family of enzymes, which are now known as CYP1A family[663]. The reason for this focus is because these were the first two forms of hepatic microsomal enzymes that were recognized[663]. Obviously, it is now known that many more exist[663]. In their 1986 article they stated:

> "As cytochrome P448 leads to increased toxicity it would be advisable to design drugs and other chemicals that act neither as substrates nor inducers of this form"[704].

The purpose of their study was "to determine the molecular dimensions of the active sites of cytochromes P448 and P450 from the molecular geometry of specific substrates, inhibitors and inducers of these enzymes, using computer-graphic techniques, in an attempt to define the molecular dimensions that would be associated with potential toxicity and carcinogenicity of chemicals"[704].

In 1987, Ioaniddes and Parke explained the differences between P450 and P448. The natural endogenous substrates of cytochrome P450 are thought to be steroids, sterols, and fatty acids, although it can also act on xenobiotics. Although the P450 system can create reactive intermediates and carcinogens, the cytochrome P450 oxidation of xenobiotics (drugs, pesticides, industrial chemicals, etc.) is concerned *primarily with detoxification*, as the reactive intermediates are good

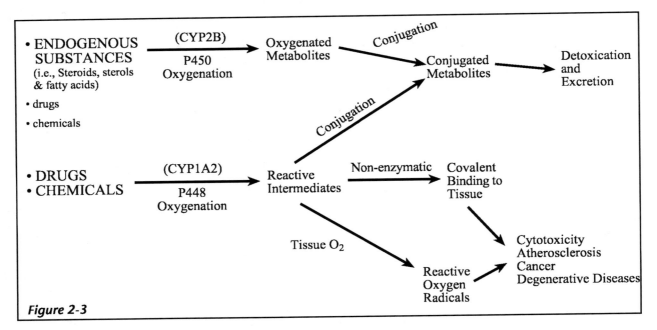

Figure 2-3

substrates for conjugation which results in the formation of more polar, biologically inactive, readily-excretable metabolites. In contrast, the reactive intermediates created by the P448 system are poor substrates for conjugation. This is because the P448 oxidation products have been rendered conformationally hindered and therefore, are unsuitable substrates for conjugation with epoxide hydroxylase or glutathione transferase. Thus, induction of the P448 system seems to be specifically involved in the activation of chemicals to reactive intermediates, and the subsequent formation of mutagens and carcinogens (see *Figure 2-3*).

Ioannides and Park provide a similar description in their 1993 article[663]. Induction of the CYP1A family results in the formation of genotoxic planar epoxides with conformationally hindered oxygens that are *much less readily conjugated* compared to non-planar epoxides with non-hindered oxygens. However, it should be understood that CYP1A induction is accompanied by the induction of Phase II conjugases, which often times leads to "the naive misconception that induction of CYP1A would increase the detoxification of carcinogens because of the induction of Phase II enzymes"[663]. For not only is the induction of Phase II enzymes far less than the induction of CYP1A, but the induced conjugases would have negligible detoxicating activity on CYP1A reactive intermediates. "Failure to detoxicate the electrophilic ultimate carcinogen allows covalent binding to nuclear DNA, with genotoxic changes to protooncogenes resulting in malignant initiation, and cytotoxic damage leading to enhance replication of the transformed cells (promotion)"[663].

Clinical issues related to Phase I pathways

It is known that caffeine is metabolized by CYP1A2[663, 736]. In fact, caffeine 3-demethylase is considered a marker for CYP1A2[663]. Brockmoller and Roots state that, "caffeine clearance is enhanced by inducers of cytochrome P448, enzymes that are now termed CYP1A1 and CYP1A2"[566]. Thus, studying caffeine clearance might provide insight into the nature of hepatic dysfunction. Indeed, studies have demonstrated that caffeine is a model compound for measuring liver function[674, 771], and that salivary caffeine clearance testing represents a highly sensitive, noninvasive, and innocuous procedure for quantifying hepatic microsomal function, and is suitable for routine use[674].

One of the first laboratories to make this test available commercially was Diagnos-Techs in 1988. The lab's application guide is consistent with the literature and explains that the test offers a high predictive accuracy in assessing cumulative damage or impairment to hepatic cells[603]. Following oral intake of caffeine, two salivary samples are collected and used to determine the half life of caffeine [T (1/2)]. Prolonged caffeine T (1/2) may reflect a suppression of P448 (i.e., CYP1A2) or a reduction in the viable number of hepatocytes such as that which occurs in cirrhosis. On the contrary, shortened T (1/2) reflects a state of P448 induction and suggests an enhanced capacity to produce reactive intermediates. P448 may be induced by xenobiotic exposure, drugs, alcohol or cigarette smoke.

Diagnos-Techs only does Phase I testing because Phase II assessment is inherently unreliable. The application guide explains why assessing liver conjugation via urinary glucaric acid measurements is imprecise and insensitive[603].

Clinical issues related to Phase II conjugation pathways

Before continuing, it is important to remember that toxicology is a complex field of study. Many readers may already be somewhat confused by the information presented thus far. This should be expected to certain degrees for toxicology "is a multidisciplinary subject, as it embraces areas of pharmacology, biochemistry, chemistry, physiology, and pathology"[831]. Without a strong background in these areas, it will be difficult to understand the intricate dynamics associated with the body's response to xenobiotic agents. Consequently, it would not take much to be mislead about diagnostic and treatment procedures related to toxicology. Concerning Phase II conjugation pathway, this problem is particularly evident. Well-meaning laboratories, instructors, nutrition companies and practitioners, with good intentions, have made Phase II pathways a major diagnostic and therapeutic focus despite the lack of sound, supporting evidence. How could something like this happen? Some of the reasons become quite obvious after examining information that is available to most of us.

At the present time, there are probably more than 100,000 foreign chemicals in the environment to which humans are exposed. These substances include therapeutic drugs, pesticides, environmental pollutants, industrial chemicals, food additives, and natural substances found in foods[831]. One only needs to watch television, read the newspaper, or listen to the radio to encounter this information. Simply stated, pollution is an issue of concern for most people.

A glaring example involves water consumption. We all know that we cannot walk down to a local river and take a drink, and now many of us refuse to drink tap water. Many people will only drink filtered or bottled water. Additionally, numerous individuals no longer eat certain foods because they contain preservatives, artificial colors, artificial flavors, chemically altered fats, and other unnecessary chemicals. These are actually reasonable concerns and practices, so it should be obvious why many people are interested in determining how pollutants and toxins may affect the body.

The caffeine clearance test represented one of the first clinical laboratory tests that could provide some insight into this issue, by directly assessing the activity of a P450 enzyme, i.e., CYP1A2, that may be involved in the transformation of various substances into carcinogens and mutagens. It is also well known that Phase II conjugation pathways play a crucial role in detoxification by converting toxic compounds into non-toxic substances that can be readily excreted. This fact of toxicology has led people to assume that we can analyze Phase II pathways as readily as CYP1A2. However, this is not the case.

What exactly are the Phase II conjugation pathways? Conjugation reactions involve the addition of an endogenous substance, i.e., carbohydrate derivatives (glucuronic acid), amino acids (glycine), glutathione and sulfate, to a foreign compound that has been acted upon by the Phase I system. The conjugated compound is rendered more polar and less lipid soluble, thus facilitating excretion and reducing the likelihood of toxicity. As you have just read, the substances donated in conjugation reactions are often involved in intermediary metabolism, which means that they should be readily available in individuals who nourish themselves satisfactorily. For details and diagrams of conjugation reactions, see Timbrel[831].

The remainder of this section is devoted to discussing some of the individual conjugation reactions and how they came to be developed by current laboratories.

Glycine conjugation

Regarding conjugation testing, at least as early as 1982, standard clinical laboratory texts explained that assessing Phase II glycine conjugation with benzoic acid is an *inaccurate* and *insensitive* procedure[551]. The oral challenge dose is 6 g of sodium benzoate which should conjugate with glycine, resulting in the production of hippuric acid. Unfortunately, when benzoate is taken orally, impaired absorption and nausea can develop, in which case an intravenous test may be used. For the oral test, at least 3-3.5 g hippuric acid should be recovered in the urine within a 4 hour period. Consider the following information carefully:

> "Amounts excreted above the limits have no significance. Excretion is normal in hemolytic jaundice and in uncomplicated gallbladder disease and obstructive jaundice. It is decreased in hepatitis, tumors, cirrhosis, and obstructive jaundice with liver impairment."[551]

Obviously, there is little utility to Phase II assessment with benzoate. The test is normal when patients have serious diseases and it is decreased by many of the conditions that cause changes in caffeine clearance. In particular, oral challenges can be flawed from the start due an impaired absorption of benzoate.

Despite the obvious shortcomings in Phase II assessment, in the early 1990s, MetaMetrix Medical Laboratory introduced a functional liver detoxification test involving caffeine clearance and the benzoate challenge test[726]. Around that time, a couple of articles were published which lauded the utility of the benzoate test as an accurate marker of Phase II detoxification efficiency[559, 762]. At the same time, this variety of liver testing was heavily promoted as an effective and accurate method to uncover hidden liver problems which may be the cause of numerous conditions including fibromyalgia, chronic fatigue syndrome, joint and muscle pain, neurodegenerative diseases, and other chronic problems. Even normal people with minor symptoms of fatigue and pain were urged to have

their Phase I and II pathways assessed to see if there was an underlying toxicity problem. Additionally, various nutrition companies began to distribute specific nutrition supplements to support hepatic detoxification (this subject will be discussed in the next section). Needless to say, this program of testing and supplementation was marketed very well and became extremely popular despite what seems to be a lack of reliability, efficacy, and rigorous scientific documentation. Moreover, this approach to hepatic testing represented a significant departure from the accepted use and clinical purpose of these tests.

Apparently, in the mid 1990s Great Smokies Diagnostic Laboratory (GSDL)[633] acquired the liver detoxification profile developed by MetaMetrix. Initially, GSDL used the caffeine clearance test and the benzoate challenge. In their application guide[633], GSDL explains that benzoate has been employed in model studies of glycination and was used by GSDL in the past as an indicator of the body's conjugation status. However, they cite research published in 1988[806] that discussed the difficulty of assessing benzoate conjugation due to an unavoidable level of analytical noise due to endogenous levels of benzoate from food and gut sources. Because they felt research suggested that patients may be exposed to additional benzoates from the environment and certain foods, such as soda, they decided to stop using sodium benzoate in favor of aspirin and acetaminophen.

In the GSDL application guide, they make a case for assessing conjugation pathways as a component of "a functional assessment" that provides "a comprehensive profile of the body's detoxification capacity and potential susceptibility to oxidative damage"[633]. Several references are offered as supportive evidence for assessing conjugation pathways. The remainder of this discussion on liver detoxification is devoted to analyzing these references to see if they support Phase II testing.

Regarding glycine conjugation, the GSDL application guide states:

> "Aspirin is readily degraded into salicylic acid and is potentially a better indicator molecule. Although salicylate is conjugated

with glycine, similar to benzoate, it also is converted to glucuronide derivatives and three oxidized derivatives. The slower glucuronidation pathway relative to glycine conjugation makes aspirin a more sensitive challenge to the glycine conjugation capability, while oxidized derivatives allow unique insights into free radical status [Patel et al[750]]."

Patel et al. explain that salicyluric acid, the glycine conjugate of salicylic acid, generally accounts for about 75% of the salicylate excreted in the urine after a therapeutic dose. However, patients with aspirin overdose typically excrete less salicyluric acid. They studied the metabolism of aspirin in 18 healthy volunteers and in 45 patients who entered the hospital because of aspirin overdose. In healthy volunteers who took aspirin, plasma glycine levels did not differ significantly from the levels detected before aspirin ingestion. In contrast, patients with aspirin overdose had plasma glycine levels that were consistently lower than normal subjects, suggesting depletion of available glycine. Treatment of aspirin overdose with glycine increases the rate of formation of salicyluric acid.

Nowhere in this article did Patel et al.[750] suggest that oxidized derivatives allow unique insights into free radical status. Nor did they discuss or imply that performing aspirin challenge tests would be useful in determining the detoxification status of the average patient with fatigue, constipation, or any other common complaint.

Sulfate conjugation

The GSDL application guide opens with what appears to be a review of the literature that supports the use of sulfate conjugation in Phase II assessment.

"Neurotransmitters, steroid hormones, certain drugs, and many xenobiotic and phenolic compounds employ sulfation as their primary route of detoxification [Levy[703]]. Acetaminophen (also known as paracetamol) is an example of a molecule detoxified primarily through the sulfation pathway. Because acetaminophen is widely available, intensely researched, and safe under most conditions, Great Smokies employs it to evaluate the sulfate conjugation pathway."

Levy[703] does not state that sulfation is the primary route of detoxification for various hormones, drugs, etc.; instead, he states that it is an important pathway of biotransformation for these substances. He also states that, "it is fortunate in many respects that the body can dispose of phenolic compounds by two major routes, sulfation and glucuronidation." Levy also explains that newborn infants primarily eliminate acetaminophen by sulfation; however, "adults convert acetaminophen mainly to the glucuronide conjugate." Additionally, Levy states that sulfation is a process of limited capacity[703], which is probably why glucuronidation plays such an important role in eliminating acetaminophen.

The GSDL application guide then states:

"Steventon identified many poor sulfoxidizers with diminished acetaminophen sulfate conjugation and reported that these individuals are most susceptible to environmental illness and problems of the nervous system, including Parkinson's disease and motoneuron disease [Steventon et al.[818, 819]]. Acetaminophen sulfate conjugation has also been shown to be reduced in patients with rheumatoid arthritis [Bradley[564]]."

In the 1989 article by Steventon et al.[818] they compared sulfoxidation in 68 patients with Parkinson's disease (PD), 121 hospital patients with nondegenerative neurologic diseases, and 200 normal volunteers who were not taking medication. Sulfoxidation is the process by which the body converts substances like cysteine into inorganic sulfate, which is the variety of sulfate utilized during Phase II conjugation. The enzyme involved in this conversion is cysteine dioxygenase and the active sulfating agent is phosphoadenosine-5'-phosphosulfate (PAPS).

Steventon et al.[818] determined that 63% of PD patients were poor sulfoxidizers, while 35.3% were non-metabolizers. Of the 121 hospital patients,

37.2% were poor metabolizers, while 4.9% were non-metabolizers. Finally, within the normal subjects, 35% were poor sulfoxidizers, while 2.5% demonstrated no sulphoxidation whatsoever. The researchers also compared sulfate conjugation between PD patients (n=27) and controls (n=35) [from the data, it appears like the controls were represented by both normal subjects and hospital patients]. Acetaminophen-sulfate values of >5% was considered to represent normal sulphate conjugation; i.e., normal inorganic sulfate levels and the presence of appropriate conjugation enzymes. A total of 16.1% of controls compared to 71.4% of PD patients failed to produce a sufficient amount of sulfate conjugates. The authors went on to explain that there can be a genetic defect that would influence P450 pathways and sulfoxidation pathways, such that PD may be the result of environmental factors superimposed on a previous genetic susceptibility to toxic metabolites. It should be understood that no mention was made in this paper that normal subjects and patient controls with depressed sulfate metabolism represented a population at risk for developing neurodegenerative diseases. Additionally, no such conclusion was made in the 1990 paper.

In their 1990 study, Steventon et al.[819] compared sulfate conjugation in patients with Parkinson's disease (PD) and motor neurone disease (MND) to that of age-matched controls. The control population consisted of volunteers who worked at the hospital or college, and a group of patients without nondegenerative neurologic diseases, who were instead suffering with lumbar disc disease, benign intracranial hypertension, and multiple sclerosis. They discovered that PD and MND patients produced less acetaminophen sulfate conjugates than controls. The only comment made about the control subjects was observational in nature:

> "The control patients with non-neurode-generative diseases showed no differences in acetaminophen metabolism from other members of the control population."

They also found out that PD and MND patients had a reduced ability to convert cysteine into inorganic sulfate. As mentioned above, the sulfoxidation of cysteine involves cysteine dioxygenase, an enzyme which appears to be underactive in patients with PD and MND. Steventon et al. also suggest that these patients may have decreased formation of phosphoadenosine-5'-phosphosulfate (PAPS), the active sulfating agent. In other words, the lack of sulfate conjugation in these patients is probably due to reduced endogenous inorganic sulfate production, and not because of dysfunctional conjugation pathways. However, reduced inorganic sulfate production would still lead to reduced sulfate conjugation. Thus, Steventon et al. concluded:

> "If, however, Parkinson's disease and motor neurone disease patients have decreased capacity to form sulfate conjugates, for whatever reason, they may be more susceptible to toxicity from either endogenous or exogenous compounds which would be detoxified via this pathway...The use of compounds (i.e., acetaminophen), currently accepted as safe, and at therapeutic doses, may therefore possibly potentiate the action of neurotoxins in certain individuals who appear to be at risk."[819]

At least according to this study, the population at risk seems to be those with neurodegenerative diseases and/or those genetically predisposed to develop neurodegenerative disease; however, normal controls and those suffering from lumbar disc disease, hypertension, or multiple sclerosis *do not appear to be at risk*. In summary, the work of Steventon et al. suggests that if you have patients with neurodegenerative diseases, make sure to assess their medications carefully and try to avoid those that will overwhelm the sulfate conjugation pathway. Also, this study suggests that research should focus on determining why these patients have problems with inorganic sulfate production. In fact, this same scenario may apply to patients with other diseases such as rheumatoid arthritis. Bradley et al. state, "the decrease in sulfate conjugate production may reflect lower phenol-sulphonotransferase levels [the conjugation enzyme] or reduced levels of availability of inorganic sulfate, but is probably due to sulfate levels; it has been shown that RA patients have less sulfated glycosaminoglycans"[564].

Clearly, none of what we have reviewed thus far suggests that assessing sulfate conjugation has utility in clinical practice as a marker of faulty detoxification in the average patient that would predispose them to develop various diseases. Later in the GSDL application guide we are told:

"Some individuals accumulate cysteine and have low sulfate levels [Heafield[654]]. In patients with neurologic disorders such as Alzheimer's disease, Parkinson's disease, and motor neuron defect, it appears that the enzyme responsible for sulfoxidation or cyteine to sulfate is often deficient, leading to an elevated plasma cysteine/sulfate ratio."

This quote applies to what was discussed above regarding deficits of inorganic sulfate production. A careful reading of Heafield et al. reveals that their research does not support routine Phase II conjugation assessment. One of the topics they focus on is the problem with an elevated cysteine/sulfate ratio. They explain that high levels of circulating cysteine may act with transition metals, such as iron, and thereby generate free radicals which may be neurotoxic.

Additionally, a by-product of depressed inorganic sulfate formation will be a reduction in Phase II conjugation of xenobiotics which may add to the toxic burden in this patient population. No mention is made of patients with non-neurodegenerative diseases and the importance of assessing Phase II pathways.

Further into the section devoted to sulfate conjugation the GSDL application guide states:

"It is worth noting that standard treatments for acetaminophen overdose are cysteine or the glutathione precursor, N-acetylcysteine (NAC) [Corcoran[588], Levy[702]]. Although usually effective if administered early in the toxification process, one might wonder if treatment failures are ever related to deficiencies in sulfoxidation [Smilkstein[813]]. These compounds, therefore, are likely candidates for nutritional supplementation."

Corcoran et al.[588] state that, "replacement of lost cellular sulfhydryl content has become the common objective in management of patients overdosed with acetaminophen." However, they go on to explain the nature of their research which involved studying the effects of NAC on hepatic necrosis in *mice*. The ability of 1000 or 1200 mg of NAC per kilogram of body weight was given to mice exposed to several different hepatotoxins. The mice weighed about 20 grams each. The authors concluded that NAC is good to treat hepatotoxicity when the toxin is known to deplete hepatic glutathione levels[588].

Levy's article[702] has absolutely nothing to do with acetaminophen overdose, cysteine, or NAC. This paper, published in 1965, is devoted solely to the pharmacokinetics of salicylate elimination[702].

Smilkstein et al.[813] mention nothing about treatment failures and their relationship to deficient sulphoxidation. In fact, their "letter to the editor" is one of many that was directed at a case history that was recently reported involving acetaminophen overdose. They suggest supplementing with 1330 mg of NAC per kilogram of body weight over a 3-day period. Several years earlier Smilkstein et al. analyzed the results from a 10-year national multi-center study to assess the efficacy of NAC therapy for acetaminophen poisoning[814]. They treated some 2500 patients with a loading dose of 140 mg oral NAC per kilogram of body weight, followed four hours later with a 70 mg/kg dose that was repeated every four hours for an additional 17 doses. Obviously, these supplemental levels represent far more than doctors in clinical practice would use. Indeed, none of the references reviewed thus far discuss the utility or protocols for cysteine or NAC supplementation in standard patient care.

Glucuronide conjugation

The GSDL application guide also begins the section on glucuronidation with what appears to be a review of the literature that supports Phase II assessment.

"Because of the ready availability of UDP-glucuronate in vivo, glucuronidation is considered an important detoxification mechanism when sulfation or glycination is diminished or saturated [Patel[751]]. For most individuals, glucuronidation is a supplemental pathway. The kinetics of glucuronidation causes it to be a secondary, slower process than sulfation or glycination."

Patel et al.[751] indicate that acetaminophen is *extensively conjugated* by glucuronic acid and sulfate, while a minor metabolic route involves P450 oxidation of acetaminophen into a hepatotoxic reactive intermediate, which subsequently undergoes conjugation with glutathione. There is no mention of glucuronidation being a slow, supplemental pathway. Quite to the contrary, Patel et al. state that sulfation is a limited pathway, which agrees with the comments of Levy[703] that were discussed in the sulfate section. Patel et al.[751] state, "saturation of elimination via sulfate conjugation is known to occur at relatively low doses of acetaminophen," which is probably why Levy stated that glucuronidation is the primary conjugation pathway for acetaminophen in the adult population[703]. The statistical data from Patel et al. indicated that for the Caucasian population, glucuronides represented 51.5% of the acetaminophen metabolites found in the urine, while 44.1% were sulfate conjugates. For the Oriental population, 51.8% of the acetaminophen metabolites were glucuronides, while 44.0% were sulfate conjugates[751].

In a more recent article, Patel et al., again explain that glucuronide conjugation is a major process[752]. Timbrell states that glucuronidation is a major conjugation pathway for a wide variety of substances[831]. Mutschler et al. explain that oral administration of acetaminophen is rapidly and completely absorbed from the digestive tract. Detoxification occurs through biotransformation with *major glucuronide* and *sulfate* metabolites[734-p.167].

The GSDL application guide goes on to state:

"Glucuronidation appears to be enhanced in obese patients, with capacity for glucuronidation related almost linearly to total body weight [Abernathy[533]]. Thus, obese people have enhanced capacity for detoxification of molecules that utilized this pathway."

As indicated, Abernathy et al.[533] do not discuss conjugation assessment in the standard population. In fact, they do not even suggest that obese patients should be tested before taking various medications. However, they do state that "intravenous lorazepam which is clinically available and exclusively glucuronidated, may provide a tool to predict capacity for drug glucuronidation in a given individual." They conclude, "in clinical terms, the findings from the present study suggest that maintenance doses of drugs biotransformed by glucuronidation should be increased approximately in proportion to total body weight in obese patients"[533].

The glucuronidation section of the GSDL application guide makes the following conclusion:

"As free radical stress can lead to damage of the mitochondrial oxidative phosphorylation mechanism, it is reasonable to suggest that people suffering from oxidative stress may have diminished capacity for Phase II glucuronide conjugation. An interesting example of decreased glucuronidation occurs in subjects with Gilbert's syndrome. It is caused by a diminished bilirubin glucuronysl transferase activity, leading to accumulation of bilirubin in vivo." [Patel[751]]

The first sentence in the above quote appears to confuse two different aspects of metabolism. Mitochondrial oxidative phosphorylation is the final component in ATP synthesis, which occurs in most cells to varying degrees. As stated earlier in this chapter, cytochrome P450 enzymes are not like the electron shuttling system involved in aerobic respiration and ATP synthesis. To suggest that oxidative damage to machinery of ATP synthesis will somehow preferentially disrupt glucuronidation seems a bit unrealistic and unreasonable. Additionally, the Patel et al.[751] article does not mention anything about oxidative stress and hepatic conjugation pathways. Furthermore, Gilbert's syndrome is not caused by oxidative stress in the fashion implied in the above statement. Gilbert's syndrome is known to be a "genetically-based impairment of bilirubin glucuronidation"[751].

Additional testing issues

Regarding elevated phase I/phase II ratios, the GSDL application guide states that elevated ratios:

"May reflect elevated (induced) Phase I processes or diminished Phase II conjugation reactions. Studies suggest the ratio of Phase I to Phase II detoxification processes is important in determining the toxicity of certain drugs and that these ratios are significant indicators of the balance of biological processes." [Dolara et al.[605]]

In fact, Dolara et al. make no such conclusion or inference anywhere in their article. They state that, "oxidation of cortisol and conjugation of paracetamol were controlled with different mechanisms, varied considerably between individuals, and were not predictive of pharmacokinetics of the inducers in treated patients."

To support certain aspects of their comprehensive detoxification profile, the GSDL application guide states:

"In addition, glutathione, glutathione peroxidase, superoxide dismutase, plasma cysteine, and plasma sulfate are assessed from fasting blood specimens taken the morning after the challenge. When glutathione, cysteine, and sulfate are measured after an acetaminophen challenge, they amount to a functional test of glutathione and sulfate reserve capacity" [James et al.[664]]. Thus, these tests are sensitive indicators of biological detoxification status."

This quote clearly implies that James et al. has done studies on humans that reveal these antioxidant markers and utility in clinical laboratory diagnosis. In fact, James et al. studied *male mice*. A marked potentiation of hepatotoxicity was produced by acetaminophen (400/mg/kg) after the mice were pretreated with the adrenergic agonist phenylpropanolamine (200 mg/kg). The authors state that, "a variety of adrenergic compounds known to deplete hepatic glutathione by a moderate 30-50% may potentiate the hepatotoxicity of acetaminophen and possibly other hepatotoxic compounds for which glutathione conjugation is an important detoxification pathway." Nothing is mentioned about "a functional test of glutathione and sulfate reserve capacity" after routine 650 mg acetaminophen challenges and subsequent testing of blood levels of glutathione, cysteine and sulfate. In fact, James et al. explain that, "the results of these experiments suggest that a 20-30% depression of hepatic glutathione, regardless of the manner in which it is produced, will potentiate acetaminophen hepatotoxicity, despite the fact that a glutathione change of this magnitude by itself is of no toxicological consequence"[664].

Summary

As described above, primary research has demonstrated that caffeine clearance testing for Phase I detoxification may be useful for routine testing. However, no such evidence seems to exit which supports the routine testing of Phase II pathways. Until more definitive information is available, Phase II testing does not appear to be a clinical intervention that should be pursued or advocated.

Nutritional modulation of hepatic detoxification

A handful of indexed review articles have been published in the last 15 years which discuss the nutritional regulation of the cytochrome P450 and conjugation enzyme systems in the liver[540, 640, 641, 858]. These articles typically state that it is difficult to determine the precise influence various nutrients will have on hepatic detoxification pathways because there are so many different enzymes which often act differently. Indeed, Yang and Yoo stated that, "a general statement that certain dietary factors increase or decrease MFO (i.e., P450 enzyme system) and drug metabolism can be misleading and cause confusion"[858]. In a 1984 review article devoted to nutritional factors related to detoxification processes, Guengerich stated[640]:

"Many of the techniques needed to carry out careful studies of the effects of nutrients are only now coming into use, and this area is still in its infancy."

Some 7 years later in 1991, Anderson authored a review article devoted to diet and cytochrome P450, which is currently cited by clinical nutritionists as *authoritative evidence* for supporting the use of powdered detoxification formulas in the treatment of liver toxicity. Anderson explains[540]:

"Deficiencies of a number of vitamins can alter hepatic mixed function oxidations in laboratory animals but have been studied little in humans...A number of other deficiencies including zinc, copper, selenium, and magnesium may influence the mixed function oxidase system in laboratory animals. Studies in humans are lacking."

In other words, the precise effect of nutritional deficiencies on MFO function in humans is unknown and therefore, specific nutritional recommendations and formulas to influence specific hepatic enzymes could only be based on speculation. By the time Anderson published this paper, detoxification products for Phase I and Phase II were already on the market for humans.

Then, in 1995, Guengerich published another review article on the influence of nutritional factors on P450 enzymes. He stated:

"Most of the available literature on vitamins and micronutrients comes from studies with experimental animals and, as mentioned above for fasting and obesity, some caution is needed in extrapolation of these results to humans. Furthermore, many of the studies with individual nutrients were done several years ago and the indexes that were measured were often not very specific for particular P450 enzymes."[641].

These comments by the experts should be considered in light of the view presented by various clinical nutritionists. For example, Pressman describes a nutritional regime involving specific macro- and micro-nutritional elements which have been demonstrated to promote upregulation of cytochrome P450 and liver conjugase activity[562].

It should be mentioned that Pressman references Anderson's 1991 paper[540] as supportive evidence for this statement. Clearly, the quote cited earlier from Anderson's paper does not support Pressman's contention. Additionally, Anderson's paper focuses on the P450 system and does not discuss the nutritional modulation of liver conjugase activity. Pressman also states that,

"this food-based program utilizes a nutritionally-balanced product consisting of an amino acid fortified rice protein concentrate, rice carbohydrate [usually rice syrup solids], medium-chain triglycerides, along with adequate vitamin and mineral enrichment to enhance hepatic cytochrome P450 activity"[562].

It should be understood that this formula is basically rice powder, amino acids, fatty acids, and a multiple vitamin/mineral. None of the articles reviewed in this chapter even remotely suggest that such a formula will alter hepatic function. Nonetheless, other similar papers describe the importance of upregulating hepatic detoxification enzymes[559, 756] which cite the 1991 Anderson article [540] as the supportive evidence.

The logic of this approach should be questioned due to the fact that purposely upregulating P450 enzymes could be lethal. Recall from earlier in this chapter that upregulation of certain P450 enzymes may promote cancer. Shimada et al. recently stated[806]:

"During the past decade [i.e., 1987-97], significant roles of several human P450 enzymes in the activation of procarcinogens and promutagens have been determined in many laboratories; CYP1A1, 1A2, 1B1, 2A6, 2E1, and 3A4 have been reported to be the major enzymes involved in the activation of most of the procarcinogens and promutagens that are metabolized by P450 enzymes in humans."

Accordingly, the cancer fighting effect of certain foods is thought to be due to their ability to *inhibit* cytochrome P450. Even the commonly cited Anderson article describes that the anticancer effect of certain food substances is due to the *inhibition* of P450 enzymes[540]. Guengerich also describes the anti-cancer effect of certain food constituents, most of which have been studied in animals. Dialyl sulfide from garlic *inhibits* certain P450 enzymes and isothiocyanates can inhibit P450 reactions and enhance conjugation reactions[641]. Certain substances like flavonoids can stimulate or *inhibit* cytochrome P450 depending on the structure of each enzyme, while indole-3-carbinol from cruciferous vegetables appears to induce P450 and conjugase enzymes[641]. More recent animal studies have shown that diallyl sulfone from garlic reduces acetaminophen hepatotoxicity by *inhibiting* P450 enzymes[705]. A human study recently showed that oxidative metabolites of acetaminophen were decreased when watercress was consumed 10 hours before taking 1 gram of acetaminophen[578]. Shimada et al. recently discovered that organoselenium compounds could *inhibit* human hepatic P450 enzymes studied in vitro[806].

Collectively, the available evidence demonstrates that it is not possible to provide definitive conclusions about the complex area of human hepatic function and its direct relationship to specific nutrients and various supplement formulations. Clearly, it is not possible to suggest that "rice protein powder, mixed with vitamins and minerals" constitutes an ideal liver detoxification product. Surprisingly, many will argue this point, suggesting that symptom relief, i.e., fatigue, pain, and irritability, due to the use of this supplement is a sign that liver toxicity has been reduced. Obviously, this argument is as weak as the one put forth by Candida advocates which was discussed earlier in this chapter.

It should also be mentioned that practitioners usually encourage extensive dietary modifications in addition to taking the rice-based detoxification formula. This diet is free of refined foods and focuses mainly on the consumption of vegetables, fruits, high quality oils (fish, flax, and olive), and high quality protein. As stated in the Candida albicans section, this diet is often recommended to patients with so-called "candidiasis", heart disease, cancer, diabetes, pain and inflammation, and to athletes and others who want to pursue health and fitness through nutrition. Even patients with rheumatoid arthritis, a supposedly "toxic condition", experienced significant relief when such a diet is followed[237]. It should be emphasized that these benefical results occured within four weeks and interventions with special detoxification formulas were not required. Clearly, the utility of these products should be questioned until objective evidence is available.

Food combining

In the mid 1980's, the topic of food combining received a great deal of press when *Fit For Life* was published. Scientists openly criticized much of what was written in *Fit For Life* because several of the explanations were not tenable. For example, just fruit until lunch is not appropriate for very many people because fruits are low in fat and protein, both of which are needed to maintain blood glucose levels for extended periods of times. The book also suggested that dairy products are unfit for human consumption. This may be the case for processed dairy products; however, unprocessed dairy products have been consumed over the ages and have proven to be quite health promoting.

From a practical clinical perspective, food combining is often very beneficial for patients. The main combination of concern seems to be the mixing of fruits with vegetables and/or proteins (meats, nuts, legumes). Such combinations often promote gastrointestinal distress, i.e., bloating, gas and pain.

The exact reason why *certain* patients develop symptoms is not known. The main theory that has been promoted over the years has to do with digestive enzyme efficiency. Different types of enzymes digest proteins (proteases), fats (lipase), starches (amylase) and sugars (disaccharidases). Each enzyme is known to function optimally at a specific pH. The optimal pH is 8.0 for proteases; 8.0 for lipase; 7.1 for amylase; 5.0-7.0 for sucrase; 5.8-6.2 for maltase; and 5.4-6.0 for lactase [296].

Starch and sugars are present in fruits. Starches are digested by amylase into maltose, 1:6 glucosides and maltotriose. Maltose is then acted on by maltase. Whereas maltase requires a pH from 5.8-6.2, proteases require a pH of 8.0. Conceivably, if fruits and proteins are consumed together, the starches may not be efficiently digested if the pH is more in the 8.0 range. This could result in the presentation of undigested carbohydrates into the colon, upon which colonic bacteria could begin the fermenting process. If this scenario occurs, various digestive symptoms might manifest. The pathophysiology associated with the condition known as carbohydrate malabsorption suggests that this scenario may occur to some degree.

Carbohydrate malabsorption is also referred to as disaccharide intolerance. Children with hereditary deficiencies in digestive enzymes often suffer from this condition in which carbohydrates are incompletely digested.

> "The failure to completely digest amylopectin, maltose, sucrose, or lactose, respectively, results in the bacterial decomposition of these carbohydrates in the lower intestine, with the production of glucose and other monosaccharides, organic acids, low pH (5.5 or less), and gases. This results in bloating, flatulence, and diarrhea from irritation to the lower bowel with ensuing increased motility [340-p.183]."

I have seen general GI distress, gas, and bloating disappear when patients stopped eating fruits with proteins at the same meal. It is possible that the enzyme theory may have some merit.

Another explanation has to do with the astringent nature of tannins and flavonoids which are found in fruits [215]. Polyphenols are a type of flavonoid and tannins are complex polyphenolic substances which can vary in molecular weight and structure. The most well-known property of tannins is their astringency, due to their ability to precipitate proteins [265,p.305]. When proteins are consumed, the stomach normally responds by producing hydrochloric acid (HCL) and pepsin. If fruits and fruit juices are then introduced to the stomach, the tannins may precipitate the proteins in the protective mucous layer in the stomach and small intestine. Now the mucosa's protective layer is disrupted and the HCL and pepsin may irritate

the GI mucosa resulting in digestive disturbances [215].

Whatever the precise explanation may be, clinical experience suggests that fruits should be eaten alone or with grains, yogurt, or cottage cheese. Many people derive great benefits when their meals consist of proteins and vegetables, and snacks consist of fruits and grains.

CONCLUSION

In the past, clinical nutrition has been an area of focus that received little attention in standard medical and chiropractic training. Fortunately, this is beginning to change. However, doctors are still often unprepared to effectively discriminate between sound nutritional and related diagnostic methods with those that are based in personal opinion and dogma.

In medicine, we can find many doctors who base their treatments soley on the recommendations of a drug salesman and reputable speakers who work for universities and drug companies. Not unlike medicine, in chiropractic we find many doctors who base their nutritional protocols soley on the recommendations of salesman and speakers who work for nutrition companies. While it is possible to obtain valuable information from drug and nutrition companies, one's practice should not be based solely upon this information.

The remainder of this text is designed to give chiropractors a working knowledge of nutritional biochemistry as it relates to the type of patient commonly seen in chiropractic practice. This patient is typically one who suffers with deconditioned musculoskeletal tissues, nociception, pain, and inflammation. Chapter 1 already discussed the biochemistry of nociception and Chapter 3 will focus on the details of the inflammatory process. The information in these two chapters provides the foundational information needed to better understand the practical use of nutrition in chiropractic practice.

Chapter 3

THE INFLAMMATORY PROCESS

INTRODUCTION

Inflammation in the healing process

Inflammation is the term given to describe the biological response that occurs as a result of tissue injury. Microbial infections, physical agents such as trauma, chemicals (i.e., toxins and caustic substances), necrotic tissue and all types of immunologic reactions can initiate the inflammatory process[92-p. 40].

We should not limit our understanding of inflammation to the point where we characterize it merely as the body's response to injury. The inflammatory process is actually the healing process. In this regard, we are told that, "the inflammatory response is closely intertwined with the process of repair. Inflammation serves to destroy, dilute, or wall off the injurious agent, but in turn sets into motion a series of events that, as far as possible, heal and reconstitute the damaged tissue"[92-p.39].

Without inflammation, tissue healing could not take place. In fact, based upon the above description, perhaps it would be best to describe the body's response to injury as the healing process rather than the inflammatory process. In this manner, instead of trying to treat inflammation [which implies that it is a bad process], our treatment approach would be to assist in the healing process, which mandates that we help the body to resolve the acute inflammatory reaction before it passes into a state of chronic inflammation.

It is chronic inflammation that is always destructive to tissues and is equated with disease[92]. Based upon this information, it seems appropriate that we should view acute inflammation as part of the healing process, and that chronic inflammation should be viewed as a disease.

The nature of inflammation

Inflammation is generally characterized as being either acute or chronic. Chronic inflammation may be a sequel to unresolved acute inflammation, or it may develop as such from the beginning[216]. In recent years, many articles and texts have described the inflammatory process[10, 15, 54, 66, 77, 87, 92, 93, 99, 131, 139, 160, 172, 216, 229, 235, 258, 262, 305, 337, 338, 362, 376, 377, 405, 422, 458, 503]. It should be understood that the inflammatory process is a physiological continuum and thus, it is not possible to definitively separate it into stages in real life situations[131, 237, 355]. However, for the purpose of investigation and explanation, Oakes[338] helped to classify the inflammatory process by dividing it into three general phases. Although there is some variation in the names assigned to the three phases, most authors agree with Oakes' classification. Phase I is the acute inflammatory phase, phase II is the repair phase, and phase III is the remodeling phase. Each phase will be discussed individually.

The outcome of acute inflammation should be the repair and remodeling of the injured tissues. In certain situations, acute inflammation does not resolve and a state of chronic inflammation develops. Several factors can promote the

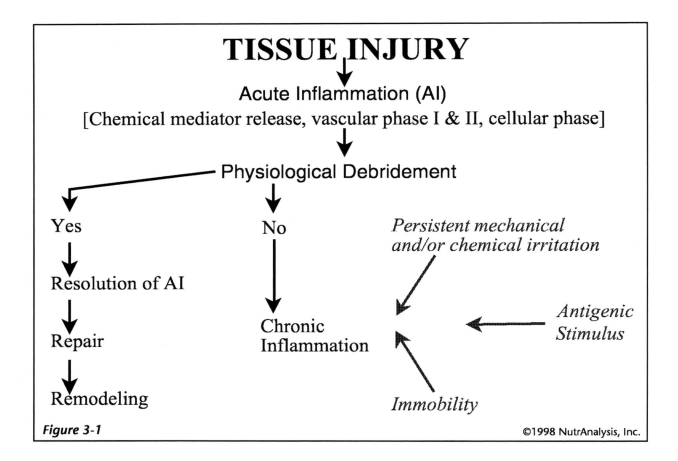

Figure 3-1   ©1998 NutrAnalysis, Inc.

development of chronic inflammation, many of which are discussed throughout the discussion of acute inflammation and repair (see *Figure 3-1*).

THE ACUTE INFLAMMATORY PHASE (FIRST 72 HOURS)

Regarding muscles, fascia, ligaments and tendons, the neuromusculoskeletal tissues at which chiropractors generally direct their corrective measures, we are told that :

"Biologic tissue experiences mechanical trauma in the form of tension, compression, or shearing forces. Muscle, nerve, connective tissue, and bone resist these mechanical stressors to differing degrees, depending on the specific components of the tissue, the physiologic state of these tissues, and the magnitude, velocity, and direction of the force. Whatever the

trauma, once mechanical damage has occurred, the initial biologic response is a generalized non-tissue-specific inflammatory response."[131]

The information in this quote demonstrates the need to fully understand the inflammatory process. In this section devoted to the acute inflammatory phase, several different components will be described. Acute inflammation consists of a vascular response and a cellular response. Both of these are modulated by cytokine activity, the complement system, and proteolytic enzyme release from damaged tissues.

Vascular response

The vascular response is characterized by three main processes, including platelet activation, vasodilation, and increased vascular permeability. Each will be described separately under its own heading.

Platelet activation

Platelet activation initiates the repair process. After vascular disruption, platelets are activated by two general mechanisms: adhesion to disrupted vascular surfaces and direct activation by so-called soluble factors. Some of the factors which cause platelets to become activated include collagen, microfilaments, fibronectin, thrombin, epinephrine, prostaglandins, thromboxane A_2, serotonin, PAF, immune complexes, and substance P[455]. After activation, platelets aggregate and release their contents which act throughout Phase 1 and into Phase 2 of the inflammatory process[281, 455, 505].

Platelets are only 2 microns in diameter, yet they house numerous types of mediators that influence the inflammatory response. Platelets contain growth factors, chemotactic factors, proteolytic enzymes, enzyme inhibitors, several clotting factors, serotonin, thromboxane A_2, platelet activating factor, platelet factor-4 (PF-4), interleukin-1 (IL-1), and thromboglobulin-beta (TG-β). Each mediator will be described individually under their respective headings. Like all other mediators of inflammation, platelet-derived mediators are involved in tissue repair; however, they can also promote the development of disease when they are produced in excess.

Growth factors: Platelet derived growth factor (PDGF) and transforming growth factor-beta (TGF-β) are important mediators to be aware of.

PDGF is derived from platelets, macrophages and endothelial cells[19]. PDGF is a potent growth factor for fibroblasts[281] and is chemotactic for fibroblasts, neutrophils and macrophages[470]. PDGF also stimulates the production of collagenase by fibroblasts, an essential part of tissue remodeling during the resolution of inflammation[19]. However, excessive release of PDGF may promote increased tissue fibrosis and various diseases.

Research suggests that PDGF may turn out to be the driving force behind atherogenesis[333, 374, 375, 465], and it may also be involved in promoting metastatic activity[11-p.754-58, 70, 92-p.77, 333, 455]. The fact that platelets measure only 2 microns in diameter indicates that they have access to nearly every tissue in the body. Clearly, inappropriate release of PDGF is pathological.

TGF-β is produced by platelets and macrophages and is a chemotactic agent for monocytes[19]. TGF-β is fibrogenic via its ability to induce the production of type I collagen and fibronectin, and by simultaneously decreasing neutral proteinase production and by enhancing production of enzyme inhibitors[19]. Research suggests that TGF-β may play a role in numerous inflammatory diseases, including inflammatory joint disease (particularly rheumatoid arthritis), scleroderma, glomerulonephritis, and pulmonary fibrosis[19].

Chemotactic agents for neutrophils: Platelets release 12-hydroxy-eicosatetraenoic acid (12-HETE), platelet factor-4 (PF-4), and platelet activating factor (PAF), all of which are thought to attract neutrophils[455].

Proteolytic enzymes: Platelets release both elastase and collagenase which can promote remodeling and tissue damage[455].

Enzyme inhibitors: Platelets release a variety of protease inhibitors including α-1-antitrypsin and α-2-macroglobulin. Protease or proteinase inhibitors serve to de-activate proteolytic enzymes such as trypsin, chymotrypsin, plasmin, elastase, collagenase and cathepsins[455, 476]. Platelets also release specific plasmin inhibitors, such as α-2-antiplasmin and plasminogen activator inhibitor-1 (PAI-1)[455]. It is important to have a mechanism to inhibit the various proteolytic enzymes because excessive activity of these enzymes can be destructive to tissues[476]. Thus, it appears that a major function of enzyme inhibitors is to limit tissue damage. However, at the same time, adequate activity of the proteolytic enzymes is required to inhibit pathological fibrosis.

Clotting factors: Platelets contain fibrinogen and von Willedbrand factor. Fibrinogen is converted into fibrin through the action of thrombin. Fibrin production is very important in the initial phases of repair because it functions to create a lattice framework for the laying down of new collagen to heal injured soft tissues[246]. However, for soft tissue integrity to be restored there must be a balance between the deposition and degradation of fibrin and collagen. For this reason, it is important to have adequate proteolytic enzyme activity, particularly plasmin as it specifically degrades fibrin. In other words, a deficiency in proteolytic enzyme activity could lead to insufficiencies in the degradation of fibrin and therefore, excessive fibrin and fibrous tissue deposition [which could lead to pathological changes in muscles, ligaments, joint capsules, and tendons].

A number of investigators have shown that fibrinolytic defects exist (usually manifesting as excessive levels of anti-enzymes) in certain patients with chronic low back pain[90, 190, 213, 221, 222, 352]. In these situations, supplemental use of proteolytic enzymes, such as bromelain, may be helpful. My clinical experience has demonstrated that, for certain patients, proteolytic enzyme supplements are the missing link.

Serotonin: Platelet serotonin, also referred to as 5-hydroxytryptamine, causes vasoconstriction, increases vascular permeability, and acts as a fibrogenic agent[455]. Serotonin is also a nociceptor irritant (see Chapter 8).

Thromboxane A-2: The precursor for thromboxane A-2 (TXA-2) is arachidonic acid. Arachidonic acid is the precursor for a group of eicosanoids including TXA-2, prostaglandin E-2, leukotriene B-4, prostacyclin and prostaglandin F-2a. TXA-2 promotes vasoconstriction, platelet aggregation, neutrophil adherence, and it works in concert with serotonin to exert a fibrogenic effect[455].

Platelet activating factor (PAF): PAF, TXA-2 and adenosine diphosphate (ADP) are among the many factors released by aggregating platelets [470]. Each of these mediators acts to further promote the aggregation and release phenomena. PAF is also synthesized by neutrophils and monocytes. PAF is thought to participate in prolonging the inflammatory process[455].

PAF stimulates neutrophil chemotaxis, adherence, and release of inflammatory mediators[455]. PAF also primes neutrophils for free radical release via respiratory burst (hydrogen peroxide, superoxide, and hydroxyl radicals).

In monocytes, PAF stimulates monocyte chemotaxis, cytotoxicity, and release of inflammatory cytokines including interleukin-1 (IL-1) and tumor necrosis factor (TNF). Once released,

IL-1 and TNF stimulate monocytes and macrophages to produce more PAF, which promotes a vicious circle of tissue damage[455].

IL-1 and TNF have been shown to contribute to joint injury and bone resorption[455]. IL-1, TNF and prostaglandins are also known to act as pyrogens[92-p.60].

Platelet factor-4 (PF-4): PF-4 increases vascular permeability, it is chemotactic for neutrophils and monocytes, and induces basophil histamine release[455].

Interleukin-1-beta (IL-1): IL-1 promotes inflammation, acts as a pyrogen, and it modulates fibroblast proliferation[455]. IL-1 is also thought to be involved in nociception (see Chapter 8).

Thromboglobulin-beta (TG-β): TG-β activates neutrophils and monocytes and stimulates fibroblast proliferation[455].

It is the rare doctor who thinks about platelet activity when it comes to patient care. After reading this material about platelets, it should be clear that we do not want excessive platelet activation and aggregation in our patients. A discussion of the nutritional factors associated with platelet function can be found in Chapter 8.

Vasodilation of local arterioles

Vasodilation is caused by the release of chemical mediators of inflammation from a variety of cells in the damaged tissues. The mediators involved in vasodilation include bradykinin, histamine and prostaglandins[92, 369]. Some authors say serotonin is a vasoconstrictor[455] and others say it is a vasodilator[470]. Endothelial cells themselves participate in injury-induced vasodilation by releasing prostacyclin (PGI-2), PAF, and endothelial-derived growth factor (EDGF) which is also called nitric oxide[94].

Vasodilation causes increased blood flow to the injured area, which causes redness and heat to develop. Vasodilated vessels cause an increase in hydrostatic pressure to cause fleeting transudation of protein-poor fluid into the extravascular space. Blood viscosity increases as red blood cells concentrate in small vessels and blood stasis develops[92].

Increased vascular permeability

Originally, increased permeability was thought to occur only in post-capillary venules[92, 93]. Increased permeability results from contraction of venular endothelial cells, which is induced by various chemical mediators including histamine, serotonin, bradykinin, complement (C3a & C5a), PAF, and leukotriene C-4, D-4, and E-4[92, 94]. Prostaglandin E-2 potentiates the permeability effects of other mediators[92]. Recall from Chapter 1 that mediators released by nociceptors and sympathetic terminals can also promote vasodilation and changes in vascular permeability, i.e., neurogenic inflammation.

In recent years, research has demonstrated that arterioles, capillaries and venules leak fluids during inflammation. Researchers suggest that, 1) direct injury will cause immediate leakage in arterioles, capillaries and venules, 2) shortly after injury, there is a phase of venular leakage that is caused by chemical mediators [as described above], and 3) any agent capable of inducing persistent inflammation is probably capable of inducing a late phase of capillary leakage[226]. Unfortunately, this particular paper does not discuss the clinical ramifications of these three aspects of increased permeability.

Increased vascular permeability permits an exudate of plasma proteins (i.e., albumin, fibrinogen, fibronectin and coagulation proteins) to enter the injured interstitial area. The exudate is temporarily sealed in the interstitial space by a combination of fibrinogen/fibrin clots. In this manner the exudate is blocked from entering blood and lymphatic vessels. This is termed as the "walling off" effect and is responsible for the clinical presentation of edema.

At the same time the various aspects of the platelet and vascular responses are occurring, leukocytes and fibroblasts enter the injured area. The term cellular response is used to characterize leukocyte involvement in the acute inflammatory phase.

Cellular response

As demonstrated thus far, many physiologic events take place in the first half of the acute inflammatory phase. Platelets and local tissue cells release a host of chemical mediators, many of which promote the *vascular response*. Many of the same mediators, as well as others, act as chemotactic agents for leukocytes and fibroblasts. Leukocyte and fibroblast entry into the area of tissue injury has been termed as the *cellular response*. Although fibroblasts enter the injured area during the acute inflammatory phase, they predominately exert their effects during the repair phase.

Guyton succinctly outlines the cells involved in the cellular response system. Tissue macrophages are first line responders, the second line are neutrophils, the third line are the circulating mononuclear cells, and the fourth line responders are newly formed granulocytes and monocytes by the bone marrow[177-p.369-70].

Before beginning this section on the various aspects of the cellular response, the reader should be aware of the fact that not too much information exists regarding soft tissue injuries. Most of the research discusses microbial invasion. Thus, we are forced to extrapolate and hypothesize about how the cellular response manifests in soft tissue injury.

Tissue macrophages

A certain population of circulating monocytes enter various tissues and assume the role of resident or tissue macrophages. Those housed in the liver are Kupffer cells; those in the central nervous system are microglial cells; and those in connective tissue are called histiocytes. Macrophages called type A and type C cells line the synovium. Tissue macrophages can survive for months and some are even known to survive for years[447]. Their main function is phagocytosis of damaged tissues. More about macrophage function will be discussed in the upcoming section devoted to circulating mononuclear cells.

Neutrophils

General information: Practically any type of tissue injury evokes an initial accumulation of neutrophils[285]. In most types of acute inflammation, neutrophils are the predominant cells in the first 24 to 48 hours. Macrophages begin to accumulate during the 2nd to 4th day[281].

Please understand that, when describing leukocyte function, authors rarely distinguish between neutrophil responses to microbial invasion and soft tissue injury. However, for the most part, research has demonstrated that in the absence of infection, "wound healing proceeded normally in guinea pigs rendered neutropenic," but on the other hand, "it was demonstrated that the presence of macrophage-monocytes in the wound was essential for effective healing[281]." So, it appears that macrophages are the main leukocyte involved in the variety of soft tissue injuries that chiropractors most commonly treat.

The process by which both neutrophils and monocytes respond to an inflammatory locus involves margination, adhesion, and emigration. The emigration of such leukocytes through the walls of venules into the adjacent tissues is thought to represent the main cellular phase of acute inflammation[281].

Margination: As a consequence of the slowing and stagnation of blood flow that occurs after injury, leukocytes fall out of the central column of vessels and assume positions in contact with the endothelium, a phenomenon called margination. In time, neutrophils virtually line the entire surface of the endothelium, which is termed pavementing[92-p. 45].

Cell adhesion: Adhesion of blood leukocytes and vascular endothelium to each other is one of the earliest events in acute immunogenic inflammation and nonimmunogenic inflammation, and it is a prelude to the process of leukocyte emigration[94]. The plasma membranes of both endothelium and leukocytes contain cell adhesion molecules (CAM). The adhesion molecules belong to three molecular families—the selectins and immunoglobulins are found on endothelial cells, and the integrins are found on leukocytes. If cell adhesion molecules are not produced, individuals can develop recurrent bacterial infections[92-p.46].

Specific adhesion molecules (selectins): Endothelial leukocyte adhesion molecule-1 (ELAM-1, or E-selectin) and GMP-140 (P-selectin) are both selectins. ELAM-1 is generally thought to be specific for neutrophils. ELAM-1 is largely confined to postcapillary venular endothelium, the anatomic

site of neutrophil adhesion and extravasation. ELAM-1 is induced by TNF and IL-1[94]. GMP-140 is thought to mediate adhesion of both neutrophils and monocytes. GMP-140 is translocated to the endothelial cell surface in the presence of thrombin and histamine. Thrombin, histamine, and free radicals stimulate endothelial cell production of platelet activating factor (PAF) which induces upregulation of Leu-CAMS (integrins) on neutrophils. GMP-140 and PAF work together to cause maximum adhesion of neutrophils[94]. Leu-CAMS are found on both neutrophils and monocytes and are needed for leukocyte adhesion and extravasation[2].

Specific adhesion molecules (immunoglobulins): Intracellular adhesion molecule-1 (ICAM-1) and vascular cell adhesion molecule-1 (VCAM-1) are members of the immunoglobulin family. ICAM-1 is expressed on endothelial cells and interact with LFA-1 and MAC-1 integrins on neutrophils and lymphocytes. ICAM-1 expression is markedly increased by IL-1 and TNF[94]. VCAM-1 is expressed on endothelial cells and interacts with VLA-4 integrin located on monocytes, lymphocytes, eosinophils and basophils. VCAM-1 expression is enhanced by IL-1, IL-4 and TNF. VCAM-1 does not play a role in neutrophil adhesion[94].

Emigration: Emigration refers to the process by which motile leukocytes (neutrophils, monocytes, lymphocytes, eosinophils and basophils) exit from blood vessels and enter injured tissues[92-p.46]. Various chemotactic agents stimulate specific receptors on the plasma membrane of the neutrophil, to which the leukocyte responds by migrating to the site of injury by squeezing between the endothelial cells and crawling across the basal lamina with aid of its own lysosomal enzyme system[11-p.974].

Chemotactic agents: Skover indicates that stimuli which attract neutrophils to injured tissues "are not limited to the classic neutrophil chemotactic factors such as complement C5a or f-met peptides from the bacterial cell wall. PF-4, IL-1, TNF and collagen polypeptides have been shown to elicit neutrophil migration with similar potency.[422]" Other chemotactic agents of non-bacterial origin include PDGF, 12-HETE, PF-4, PAF, cationic permeability factor[455], collagen fragments, fibrinopeptides, thrombin, kallikrein, and LTB-4[463]. It should be mentioned that many cell types can produce LTB-4, including neutrophils, eosinophils, basophils, mast cells, monocytes and macrophages[2, 170, 253, 370, 401].

Basics of neutrophil function: The three main functions of neutrophils include phagocytosis, degranulation and free radical generation[463, 470].

Phagocytosis: Phagocytosis occurs only when antigenic molecules are first recognized by the neutrophil. Recognition occurs in the presence of opsonins, including complement (C3b) and IgG, which attach themselves to a microbe and then to the neutrophil for phagocytosis[463, 489]. Thus, it appears that the process of phagocytosis is reserved for those situations where antigens are presented to neutrophils, such as microbial invasion and rheumatoid arthritis (RA)[236]. In the case of rheumatoid arthritis, the antigenic stimulus is still not known. Possible agents include bacteria, viruses and collagen[88, 102, 192]. Evidence exists to support the hypothesis that physical trauma to joints may result in the release of cartilage breakdown products that are antigenic in nature[164, 165]. The time course required for such breakdown to initiate a chronic immune response is not known. At this point, it appears safe to say that antigen presentation to neutrophils, and subsequent phagocytosis, does not appear to be a component of uncomplicated soft tissue injuries. However, it does appear that degranulation and free radical release may be involved in soft tissue injuries.

Degranulation: Neutrophils contain primary and secondary granules. Primary granules contain proteolytic enzymes such as cathepsin and elastase, and secondary granules contain collagenase, all of which can damage local tissues. Each granule also contains bactericidal chemicals as well as factors responsible for free radical generation. The cytokine GM-CSF is known to enhance secretion of primary (azurophil) and secondary (specific) granules. The degranulation patterns of each type of granule is different. Primary granules mainly release their contents into the phagocytic vacuole, and secondary granules mainly fuse with the plasma membrane and release their contents to the exterior. It appears that degranulation occurs at

cell death, in conjunction with phagocytosis and via an active secretion process that occurs during chemotactic migration. Two of the many neutrophil degranulation stimuli are LTB-4 and IL-8[463].

Free radical generation: Free radical generation by leukocytes is called the oxidative burst. Neutrophils are primed for enhanced oxygen radical generation in the presence of GM-CSF, TNF-α, LTB-4 and PAF. Both LTB-4 and PAF can function as activators of the NADPH oxidase system[463], which results in the production of O_2^-, H_2O_2, $\cdot OH$ and $-OCL$[470]. If these free radicals are not quenched, they can severely damage the surrounding tissues and perpetuate inflammation.

Summary: The key point to keep in mind is that some of the activators of degranulation and free radical production include LTB-4, PAF and various cytokines, all of which are generated during the initial steps of the inflammatory process involving mast cells and platelets. TG-β, released from aggregated platelets, is also thought to be an activator of neutrophils[455]. This information is critical to appreciate because mast cell and platelet function are modulated by certain nutritional factors (see Chapter 8). For example, several papers suggest that bioflavonoids can help reduce the inflammatory activity of neutrophils[32, 67, 291, 396].

The information presented thus far, regarding the basics of neutrophil function, suggests that neutrophils may be involved in soft tissue injuries. It does not appear that phagocytosis plays a major role. However, degranulation and free radical release may occur in soft tissue injuries.

A final point that should be mentioned before proceeding, is the fact that substance P and CRGP are thought to influence neutrophilic phagocytosis and infiltration[6]. Recall that substance P and CGRP are released from sensitized nociceptors.

Function of neutrophils in soft tissue injuries: It should be emphasized that standard texts on pathology and inflammation do not precisely address the topic of soft tissue injuries. As a consequence, the function of neutrophils in soft tissue injuries is not made clear. In the case of authors who discuss soft tissue injuries, most provide vague descriptions of neutrophil function[54, 99, 139, 211, 216, 229, 258, 376, 422], while others do not mention neutrophils at all[131, 235, 305, 337, 451].

Hettinga describes an additional manner in which neutrophils may be involved in soft tissue injuries. She states that, "the first motile white cell to arrive are neutrophils, which have a predilection for destroying bacteria. Since there are usually no bacteria with most traumatic injuries, many of the neutrophils actually act as a deterrent to healing and die without assisting the process." Hettinga explains that when macrophages enter the area of tissue injury, they phagocytize tissue debris and neutrophil carcasses in preparation for the repair phase. When neutrophils are destroyed by macrophages, they release their proteolytic enzymes which can damage and irritate local tissues and prolong acute inflammation[199].

Thus, it appears that neutrophils may promote inflammation in soft tissue injuries in at least three ways: 1) degranulation, 2) free radical release, and 3) proteolytic enzyme release when neutrophils are phagocytized by macrophages. Keep in mind that it does not appear that neutrophils assist in the resolution of acute inflammation, and it does not appear that neutrophils are involved in the phagocytosis of tissue debris.

Circulating mononuclear cells

General information: As mentioned earlier, there are tissue macrophages in addition to those that circulate in the blood as monocytes. Circulating monocytes are low in number compared to neutrophils and lymphocytes. Whereas neutrophils average 60% and lymphocytes average 30% of all circulating white blood cells respectively, monocytes comprise less than 10% of white cells. The storage pool of monocytes in bone marrow is also much less than that of neutrophils[177-p.370]. By virtue of these facts, monocyte entry into the injured area is slower than neutrophils and upon arrival, it takes some 8 hours for a monocyte to mature into a macrophage of full potential. Ultimately, in the later aspects of the acute response and in the repair phase, macrophages dominate the phagocytic cells in the area[177-p.370].

Macrophages are required in tissue healing: Experiments have demonstrated that the elimination of macrophages from wounds will inhibit healing and the addition of macrophages to age-compromised wounds augments wound repair[422].

Ultimately, tissue repair cannot take place unless the acute inflammatory phase has resolved, which occurs as a consequence of macrophage debridement of the injured area[229, 131-p.18]. Macrophages also stimulate collagen formation and generate endothelial cell growth which lays the groundwork for cell proliferation[211]. An important point to note is that the presence of the confluence of mediators released by macrophages increases wound strength in the early stages of healing (day 4) by a mechanism unrelated to collagen synthesis[422] [the type of mechanism is not mentioned].

Chemotactic agents: A number of factors have been shown to be chemotactic for monocytes including bacterial products, thrombin, denatured albumin, fibronectin fragments, elastin fragments, collagen fragments, and collagenase-digested collagen[447]. In addition, several monocyte- and lymphocyte-derived cytokines (IL-8) and factors produced by erythrocytes, tumor cells, and platelets, such as PDGF, TGF-β[93, 94-p.77, 447], and PF-4 and PAF[455] are also known to be chemotactic for monocytes.

Once monocytes leave circulation and enter the area of injury, they mature into macrophages which can then be activated to perform various functions. We should be aware that macrophage function is quite complex and there is disagreement as to the precise mechanism by which macrophages function during inflammation.

Basics of macrophage function: Not all macrophages function in the same fashion. Van Furth classifies macrophages with such descriptors as resident/tissue, exudate, exudate-resident, activated, and elicited[459]. Unfortunately, van Furth does not discuss their various functions and mechanisms of stimulation.

Werb states that macrophages should be classified as either activated, elicited or inflammatory, or resting[476]. Unfortunately, Werb provides an explanation that is overly simplified and not helpful in gaining an effective understanding of macrophage function.

As it turns out, the best way to categorize macrophages is according to situation-specific functions. Thomas[447] delineates macrophage activities into two categories, those being simple functions and complex functions. Simple functions include migration, pinocytosis, phagocytosis, and intracellular digestion. Complex functions include tissue remodeling, wound repair, senescent or dead cell removal, lipid and lipoprotein metabolism, immunoregulation, antimicrobial activity, antiviral activity, antineoplastic activity, and antibody-dependent cell-mediated cytotoxicity.

The various complex functions of macrophages can be very tightly controlled because their plasma membranes are endowed with over 100 different receptors. In response to the needs of the tissue environment, macrophages can release over 100 secretory products[2].

Adams indicates that all complex functions require that the macrophage be fully activated. Once activated, an additional signal is provided to initiate the specific function[2]. Recall that tissue repair is characterized as a complex function.

Activation of macrophages for complex functions: In general, macrophages can be activated by lymphokine presentation from sensitized T lymphocytes and by direct exposure to various antigens[92-p.62]. The lymphokines which activate macrophages include interferon-gamma (IFN-gamma) and the interleukins IL-2 and IL-4[19, 447]. Also capable of activating macrophages are the cytokines IL-1, TNF-a, and IL-6, the growth factor TGF-β, and a colony stimulating factor known as GM-CSF[2].

Some of the same ligands that activate macrophages are also capable of suppressing activation, including IL-4, TGF-β and TNF-a. Prostaglandin E-2 and serotonin are also capable of exerting a suppressing effect[2]. This is only an example of the intricacies involved in the body's modulation of cell function, and demonstrates the potential danger of drugs that stimulate or inhibit specific molecules.

In addition to having receptors for the factors that activate complex functions, macrophages also have surface receptors for fibrin, fibrinogen products, fibronectin and coagulation factors VII

and VIIa[2]. It is not stated how these various molecules influence macrophage function. It appears that at least fibrinogen may play a role in signaling macrophages to clean up the injured area. The *Cecil Textbook of Medicine* indicates that dead cells and tissue fragments at sites of infection or injury are disposed of by macrophages recruited to the damaged area. Ingestion may be aided by circulating fibronectin, which opsonizes denatured collagen for phagocytosis by macrophages. The activated macrophages also secrete neutral proteases (collagenase, elastase) that break down damaged connective tissue and fibrin mesh (plasminogen activator), clearing the way for the reconstitution of injured tissues[23].

Chronic inflammation: Although macro-phage activity is critical for tissue healing, unregulated macrophage activation may have deleterious effects, such as participating in the pathogenesis of certain chronic diseases such as rheumatoid arthritis and atherosclerosis[92-p.62]. The latest edition of *Robbins Pathologic Basis of Disease* states that the, "macrophage is the prima donna of chronic inflammation"[92-p.77].

Macrophages eventually die off or leave the area of injury; however, this occurs only if the irritant is eliminated. If the irritant persists, then macrophages will continue to accumulate[92-p.77]. In the presence of chemotactic and activating factors, macrophages can be driven into a state of hyperfunction in which they release numerous pro-inflammatory mediators.

Cotran[92-p.77] divides macrophage mediators into two categories; those involved in tissue injury and fibrosis. Some of the mediators involved in tissue injury include free radicals, neutral proteases (elastase, collagenase), acid hydrolases, neutrophil chemotactic factors, complement components, coagulation factors, eicosanoid (leukotriene B-4, etc.), and nitric oxide. Mediators involved in tissue fibrosis include cytokines (IL-1, IL-8, TNF-a) and growth factors (PDGF, TGF-β).

In total, macrophages have over 100 receptors and can secrete over 100 substances. Any number of possible interactions might lead to an inappropriately activated macrophage. As an example, PAF from aggregating platelets induces

IL-1 production by macrophages[455]. The biological effects of IL-1 can promote degradation of damaged tissues at a site of tissue injury and subsequently help regulate the repair of such tissue. However, overproduction of IL-1, as a result of continued stimulation of a macrophage, may result in the exaggerated destruction of normal tissue and/or excessive fibrosis responsible for the histopathology associated with certain chronic inflammatory conditions[470].

A final point that should be mentioned before proceeding is the fact that substance P releases from nociceptive receptors can also influence macrophage activity. Research demonstrates that substance P may promote monocyte chemotaxis and increase macrophage activation, phagocytosis, and the production of inflammatory mediators, such as free radicals and thromboxane A_2[6].

Newly formed granulocytes and monocytes

Newly formed granulocytes (neutrophils) and monocytes are produced by bone marrow cells. It appears that this fourth line of defense is more applicable to serious injuries, infections and cancers. As chiropractors do not typically treat these conditions, this aspect of immune function will not be discussed.

The Complement System

The complement system consists of 20 component proteins found in plasma. Complement is one of three plasma-derived systems which are involved in different and overlapping aspects of the inflammatory process. The other two systems include the kinin and clotting systems.

It is not clear what role the complement system plays in the inflammatory process when associated with soft tissue injuries. Papers devoted to wound healing usually discuss the complement cascade; however, such papers do not differentiate between open and closed wounds and their relationship to bacterial invasion. Below are quotes from various authors that discuss soft tissue injuries:

- "Cleavage fractions of complement (C3 and C5) indirectly contribute to the overall process of inflammation by inducing mast cells to release histamine"[99-p.299].

- In response to traumatic injury, "the complement system comprises a series of reactions initiated by an antigen-antibody complex which stimulates the processes of phagocytosis (removal of cellular debris) and chemotaxis (attraction of inflammatory cells)"[229].

- "The complement system, which consists of a number of serum proteins circulating in an inactive form, is switched on and has a direct effect on the cell membrane as well as helping to maintain vasodilation. Various complement products are involved and these are activated in sequence"[337-p.22].

Unfortunately, these quotes do not illustrate the mechanism by which the complement system participates in soft tissue injuries. The following quote comes from a paper on wound healing that sheds light on how the complement system may be involved in soft tissue injury:

"The complement system is another protein amplification cascade. It circulates as functionally inactive molecules that assist the polymorphonucleocyte (PMN) in its microbicidal task. Activation is a dynamic process involving two parallel but independent mechanisms that generate proteins with biologic activities including cytolysis of bacteria, induction of mast cell degranulation, and chemotactic recruitment and phagocytic activation of leukocytes."[422]

From this quote, we are led to believe that complement and neutrophils would be involved in injuries only if bacterial invasion has occurred. The following quote from *Robbins Textbook of Pathology* appears to confirm this conclusion about the complement system: "This system functions in immunity for defense against microbial agents, culminating in lysing microbes by the so-called membrane attack complex (MAC)"[93-p.66-67].

Several steps are thought to be involved in the process of membrane damage by complement[89]: Accumulation of a bulk of complement proteins; changes in membrane environment and charge;

modification of membrane properties and functions; stimulation of cellular functions; membrane lesions and swelling; and finally, membrane damage or disruption. We are also told that, "complement has been shown to be capable of mediating the lytic destruction of many kinds of cells including erythrocytes, platelets, bacteria, viruses possessing a lipoprotein envelop, and lymphocytes, although with greatly varying degrees of efficiency in each instance"[89]. Because complement can destroy body cells, as well as microbes, it now appears as if complement may be involved in soft tissue injuries after all.

Like several of the other aspects of inflammation discussed thus far, it is clear that blanket statements about complement will not suffice. As an example, elevated serum complement concentrations are associated with the following diseases: obstructive jaundice, thyroiditis, acute rheumatic fever, rheumatoid arthritis, polyarteritis nodosa, dermatomyositis, acute myocardial infarction, ulcerative colitis, typhoid fever, diabetes, gout and Reiter's syndrome[435]. Some of these conditions are associated with microbial invasion and some are not. Clearly, a better understanding of the complement system is necessary if we are to understand any potential relationships between complement and soft tissues injuries/joint complex dysfunction.

The activation of the complement system can occur through both the so-called alternative and classical pathways. Activators of the alternative pathway of complement include polysaccharides, fungi, bacteria, viruses, certain mammalian cells, and aggregates of immunoglobulins. It is not known which structures are common in activators that are recognized by the alternative pathway. It is clear, however, that recognition involves a complement molecule known as C3b[322].

Activators of the classical pathway differ from those of the alternative route. Antibodies are involved in the activation of the classical pathway of complement. Recall that the family of immunoglobulins function as antibodies, which bind to specific sites on antigen molecules to form immune complexes which are ultimately phagocytized. Antigens can be toxins, foreign proteins, or particulate matter such as bacteria and

tissue cells[312-p.74]. The complement molecule referred to as C1q binds to the Fc region of IgG and IgM[322] which facilitates immune complex delivery to phagocytic cells[321].

I have yet to read that complement can be activated by the presence of debris from tissue injury. It seems likely that this may take place in certain patients, as not all of the conditions associated with elevated complement [mentioned earlier] are microbial-induced. In certain patients, food antigens may also play a role in activating complement. It seems that patients with food allergies have increased levels of circulating food-specific IgG4. Although IgG4 itself is incapable of activating the classical complement pathway, its involvement in immune complex formation with the complement fixing IgM antiglobulin may indirectly initiate complement mediated tissue injury[410] [Unfortunately, this paper did not discuss the likelihood of this relationship].

Perhaps there may be a relationship between the antigens produced by tissue injury and food antigens, such that the probability of complement activation may increase. Concerning this, we can only speculate.

Before closing this section on complement, some of its other pro-inflammatory activities should be mentioned. For example, anaphylatoxins are split products of the corresponding complement components and are referred to as C3a, C5a, and C4a respectively. These products can increase vascular permeability and cause vasodilation mainly by releasing histamine from mast cells. C5a also activates the lipoxygenase pathway in neutrophils and macrophages, causing the release of leukotrienes. C5a is also a powerful chemotactic agent for neutrophils, monocytes, eosinophils, and basophils[93-p.66-67].

Proteolytic enzyme release from damaged tissues

Very much like the complement scenario, the relationship between proteolytic enzyme release and soft tissue injuries is not clear. Several authors state that injured cells release proteolytic enzymes which participate in the inflammatory response and may also damage healthy cells:

- Cells that are damaged during tissue injury release proteolytic enzymes[177-p.849].

- "Enzymes from the damaged cells can cause an inflammatory response in the tissues on the margin of the central injured area"[199].

- "The physical trauma and reduced oxygen supply to cells and blood vessels ruptures intracellular lysosomes enzymes that initiate a cascade of events. Disruption of blood vessels also leads to local cell death via lack of oxygen delivery, with the same effect of lysosomal enzyme release. Lytic enzymes release potent chemical mediators: histamine and bradykinin"[51-p.15].

- "Lysosomal enzymes and proteases released from injured cells as well as from neutrophils participate by direct enzymatic catabolic damage to healthy tissues"[99-p.299].

I was unable to find any other authors who discussed proteolytic enzyme release as a consequence of soft tissue injury. Unfortunately, the above quotes are general in nature. Other than neutrophils, these authors do not mention other cells which release proteolytic enzymes.

Most of us will recall that lysosomes are cell components which contain enzymes. A recent edition of a noted histology text states[166]: "Most cells contain lysosomes. Hepatocytes and macrophages, cell types rich in lysosomes, contain approximately 200." This information does not necessarily help us if we are interested in the pathogenesis of soft tissue injuries because, at this point, we still do not know which cells associated with the musculoskeletal system contain lysosomes. I spent a significant amount of time searching through books and making phone calls, trying to figure this out.

The confluence of material I came across indicates that lysosomes are most densely concentrated in cells that turnover rapidly, such as fibroblasts and endothelial cells, while muscle cells and nerve cells are not well endowed with lysosomes. In response to tissue injury, lysosomal enzyme release probably occurs from local fibroblasts and endothelial cells. Tissue basophils, more commonly known as mast cells, contain proteases[157, 401] which are probably released during injury. Neutrophils, monocytes and macrophages all possess lysosomes.

Depending on the cell type, lysosomes may contain a variety of enzymes. Two common varieties include acid proteases and neutral proteases. Acid proteases are only active in an acidic pH, and thus, it is thought that they may be active during ischemic and hypoxic conditions[92-p.6]. Acid proteases are also known to be involved in the degradation of bacteria or debris by phagocytic cells[92-p.72]. The neutral proteases function at neutral and slightly alkaline pH. Neutral proteases are categorized as either serine proteases or metalloproteases[477]. Compared with acid proteases, neutral proteases are capable of degrading extracellular components such as collagen, basement membranes, fibrin, elastin and cartilage through which they participate in purulent and tissue deforming inflammatory processes[92-p.72].

It appears that proteolytic enzyme activity is a problem in the case of immune-mediated inflammatory conditions, such as rheumatoid arthritis. Van den Berg states that, "there is no doubt that PMNs can be highly destructive for articular cartilage in vitro, by the release of its enzymes cathepsin G and elastase"[456]. Research efforts have been directed at developing drugs that can act as inhibitors of serine proteases and metalloproteases[141, 133].

Regarding soft tissue injuries and joint complex dysfunction, it is likely that proteolytic enzymes participate in the inflammatory process; however, the degree to which they are involved is not clear. In fact, there is actually more evidence suggesting that a *deficiency* in proteolytic enzyme activity might be the real problem in non-immune mediated inflammation associated with soft tissue injuries and joint complex dysfunction. This topic will be discussed in Chapter 8.

THE REPAIR PHASE (48 HOURS TO 6 WEEKS)

The repair phase occurs in the wake of acute inflammation. Tissue repair is a much more detailed process than we are led to believe. Most general texts and review articles do not discuss clinically important details that may influence the healing process. I should admit that this explanation of the repair phase should also be viewed as deficient. My background does not permit me to review this field as a physiologist or biochemist. Despite this fact, I do think that you will find that there is a great deal of helpful clinical information contained in this section.

Our discussion of the repair phase is divided into seven sections:

   a.   Repair versus regeneration

   b.   Injured area must be clean before effective repair can occur

   c.   Ebb and Flow phases of healing

   d.   Factors other than cortisol that affect tissue healing and repair

   e.   Granulation tissue

   f.   Angiogenesis

   g.   CT Scar - Fibroblasts

Repair vs. Regeneration

Almost all tissues of the body are capable of repairing injuries, the teeth being the only exception. The repair process restores continuity to interrupted tissues. In other words, "tissue forms only between the severed parts, without differentiating totally new elements"[171]. Epimorphic regeneration refers to the "replacement of an amputated appendage by a direct outgrowth from the severed cross section"[171]. Whereas mammals lack epimorphic regeneration, certain tissues do have an ability to regenerate. Regeneration is possible if the cells

that are lost due to injury are labile or stable[503]. Examples of labile cells include epithelial cells, red blood cells, bone and peripheral nerves. Some stable cells include skeletal and smooth muscle, renal glomeruli and endocrine glands. In contrast, it is not possible for permanent cells to regenerate, such as cardiac muscle and neurons of the central nervous system[503].

Each tissue has a different repair capability[104]. Bone, for example, has a high regenerative capacity and can actually heal without a scar[382].

Muscle has high reparative capacity, but extensive damage results in scarring and atrophy of muscle fiber bundles. Regenerated muscle fibers can arise from growth of preexisting myofibrils[104].

Tendons and ligaments are notably slow to heal[104]. This is probably because even after forty weeks, collagen may still not be present in normal concentration and organization[131].

Articular cartilage has a notoriously limited potential for either healing or regeneration. The ability of articular cartilage to heal seems to depend upon the severity of the injury[382]. Patients requiring surgery are least likely to heal. In the case of chiropractic patients, immobility seems to be a factor that promotes degeneration and restoring mobility seems to curtail degeneration (see Chapter 9). Research has shown that improving mobility can even enhance cartilage healing after traumatic injuries[382].

Physiological debridement

As mentioned earlier, tissue repair cannot take place unless the acute inflammatory phase has resolved, which occurs as a consequence of macrophage debridement of the injured area[229, 131]. "Macrophages are the most vital cell in the healing process because they not only clean the wound, but also stimulate collagen formation and generate endothelial cell growth. Collagen formation and endothelial cell growth lay the groundwork for cell proliferation[211]." The *Cecil Textbook of Medicine* indicates that dead cells and tissue fragments at sites of infection or injury are disposed of by macrophages recruited to the damaged area.

Ingestion may be aided by circulating fibronectin, which opsonizes denatured collagen for phagocytosis by macrophages. The activated macrophages also secrete neutral proteases (collagenase, elastase) that break down damaged connective tissue and fibrin mesh (plasminogen activator), clearing the way for the reconstitution of injured tissues[23].

Ebb and flow phases of healing (cortisol connection)

In 1932, Dr. David Cuthbertson published a paper in which he discussed his observations of patients with long bone fractures. His work is discussed in *Modern Nutrition in Health and Disease* where the authors state that, "he noticed that these patients lost large quantities of nitrogen, potassium, and phosphorus in their urine following injury, and this accelerated excretion rate could not be reversed by vigorous oral feedings"[427]. Cuthbertson divided the post-traumatic responses into the "ebb" and the "flow" phase.

The ebb-phase, or shock phase, is usually brief and lasts from 12 to 24 hours. It is generally characterized as a period of hypometabolism that is typified by a reduction in blood pressure, cardiac output, body temperature and oxygen consumption. On the contrary, the flow-phase is characterized as a protracted period of hypermetabolism that is typified by an elevation in cardiac output, increased urinary nitrogen losses, altered glucose metabolism and accelerated tissue catabolism. It is implied that these changes are due to chronic hypercortisolism[427].

In a text devoted specifically to wound healing, Goodson explains that, "cortisol is the only one of the stress hormones known to have a direct influence on healing. However, after an initial sharp rise, it is only mildly elevated relatively soon after injury, and is probably not in the pharmacological range known to inhibit healing. This is an area for further research."[168] Dinarello concurs and states that measuring cortisol values is not particularly useful[117]. Despite these assertions, it does appear that hypercortisolemia may play a significant role.

Berne[31] states that excessive endogenous cortisol output can occur in many situations. For example, plasma cortisol levels are increased by surgery, burns, infection, fever, psychosis, electroconvulsive therapy, acute anxiety, prolonged and strenuous exercise, hypoglycemia, and pain. In normal situations, the cortisol response should be blunted by a negative feedback mechanism controlled by the hypothalamus. However, during prolonged periods of stress, "the normal diurnal pattern of cortisol secretion may be lost, and feedback suppressibility may be impaired"[31]. As alluded to in the previous sentence, cortisol secretion occurs in a circadian rhythm. Levels are highest in the morning and lowest at midnight.

It is, in fact, very common to find abnormalities in the circadian release of cortisol without traumatic injuries or apparent pathologies. Indeed, the normal aging process is associated with excessive release of cortisol. Increased cortisol levels are a predisposing factor for many age-related diseases including obesity, pre-diabetes, latent type II diabetes, atherosclerosis, hypertension, cancer and depression[115-p.27]. Clearly, many people have high cortisol levels prior to experiencing a soft-tissue injury. Such individuals may already be plagued with reduced healing capabilities to varying degrees.

The reason why confusion exists regarding cortisol and the catabolic state is that routine cortisol testing utilizes blood or urine specimens. First, neither blood or urine is an appropriate body fluid for checking the cortisol circadian rhythm. Second, both blood and urine samples are used to test total cortisol, and neither appropriately reflects the free bioactive fraction. Saliva appears to be the only body fluid that provides for a noninvasive assessment of free cortisol. Many varieties of adrenal dysfunction including problems with feedback control are quite common and can be accurately assessed with a saliva test known as the Adrenal Stress Index (ASI)[603]. In actual fact, a great deal of research has verified the utility of salivary testing for cortisol[561, 639, 676, 697, 839, 845].

Apparently, Goodson and Dinarello are not aware that there is a significant difference between saliva testing for free cortisol versus urine and blood testing for total cortisol, which explains why they see little value in testing cortisol levels. Because cortisol testing is still traditionally viewed as ineffectual, much confusion exists regarding the nature of the catabolic state associated with traumatic injury. Consequently, much time is wasted on evaluating acute phase proteins.

Consider the following information presented by Goodson. "Although wound healing may commence during the flow-phase, general anabolism and true recovery do not begin until it has subsided"[168]. The nitrogen loss mentioned above is due to muscle protein breakdown, which reaches a peak after injury and remains high for an extended period of time. Goodson indicates that the reason for this "is not clear since most acute phase hormones approach normal levels within a day or two"[168]. As alluded to earlier, without knowledge of salivary cortisol testing, this is the only possible conclusion. To help the reader develop a better understanding about acute phase proteins, the topic will be discussed in the next two paragraphs.

In general, we would not consider the acute phase response to be of concern in the average population of chiropractic and medical patients. Approximately 8 to 12 hours after the onset of infection or trauma, the liver upregulates its synthesis of acute phase proteins. This acute phase response is thought to be initiated by various cytokines, such as interleukin-1 and tumor necrosis factor, which induce the production of interleukin-6 (IL-6)[117]. IL-6 is the principle hepatocyte-stimulating factor for acute protein synthesis[19]. In response, true acute phase reactants increase several hundred fold, those being serum amyloid A (SAA) and C reactive protein (CRP). A variety of normal plasma proteins also increase several-fold during the acute phase response. These include haptoglobin, certain protease inhibitors, complement components, ceruloplasmin, and fibrinogen[117].

Unfortunately, the presence of the various acute phase reactants has very little diagnostic value, other than to indicate the presence of an inflammatory process that is already clinically apparent[24]. As an example, moderate elevations in CRP can be found in myocardial infarction, malignancies, pancreatitis, mucosal infections, and most connective diseases. Insignificant elevations are found in angina, seizures, common cold,

gingivitis, and cerebrovascular accidents. SAA elevations have been found in rheumatoid arthritis, acute gout, inflammatory bowel disease, and myocardial infarction[24]. In the future, testing for salivary cortisol levels will probably become mainstream.

Additional factors that affect tissue healing and repair

Several factors can inhibit resolution of the acute inflammatory response and promote a state of chronic inflammation. Remember that chronic inflammation does not permit appropriate tissue repair.

- Ineffective healing can also occur if damaged soft tissues are re-injured. "Collagen is the basic framework of all soft tissues. Once a tear occurs within the collagen bundles, the defect is replaced by haphazard, loose connective tissue formed in the blood clot which initially fills the torn area. Thus, intrinsic structural strength may be reduced significantly, leading to impaired power, mobility, skill and eventually to further damage."[3] Increased mobility after injury must be carefully graded per individual patient. Immobilization can result in debilitating tissue fibrosis while aggressive early mobilization can severely re-injure tissues[181].

- "The repair rate is influenced by the blood supply and temperature of the damaged tissue; tissues with a poor blood supply and temperature of the damaged tissue; tissues with a poor blood supply heal slowly. Deficiencies of nutrients (especially protein and vitamin C), old age, corticosteroid medications, and the presence of debilitating illness also interfere with healing."[503]

- In a recent article, Fick[139] states that, "pharmacologic control of inflammation is a mainstay of medical treatment. NSAIDs are the most widely prescribed drugs for routine management." He goes on to describe NSAID therapy in the following manner:

"The popularity of NSAIDs will undoubtedly continue. However, it is very difficult for most physicians to assess the benefits of NSAIDs for athletes. The entire process of trauma, inflammation, pain, rehabilitation, and return to competition is very subjective. A recent meta-analysis concluded that NSAIDs do not seriously delay the healing process, have modest benefits over placebo when given after an injury, and may enhance performance."

Regarding this quote, we need to ascertain the meaning of, "NSAIDs do not seriously delay the healing process." Does this mean that NSAIDs moderately delay healing? It appears that they would be, based on the information presented in Chapter 4. Unfortunately, Fick does not conclude his discussion on NSAIDs by providing parameters for their use. Kellet[229] suggests that NSAIDs should not be used beyond the 72 hour point because "any anti-inflammatory activity lasting beyond this period would, theoretically, at least be detrimental since the repair mechanism (phase 2) is itself an inflammatory process."

- The following medications detrimentally affect wound healing: Glucocorticoids, cytotoxic agents, antineoplastic agents, anticoagulants, immunosuppressive agents, penicillamine, NSAIDs, female sex hormones, and broad spectrum antibiotics[12].

- Systemic factors that compromise wound healing include[12]: Immunocompromised patient, diabetes, peripheral vascular disease, aging, malignancy, genetic defects, coagulation disorders, collagen disease, hypovolemia, shock, and nutritional status (hypoproteinemia, hypoxia and deficiencies in ascorbate, vitamin E, zinc, and vitamin A).

Granulation tissue

Granulation tissue is the term used to describe the entire complex of inflammatory cells, proliferating fibroblasts, endothelia, new capillaries, and secreted glycoproteins and proteoglycans[166]. Important features of granulation tissue include its resistance to infection, lack of innervation (no sensibility to pain), and rich blood supply. At the histological level, all wounds contain varying proportions of granulation tissue during repair[104]. It is thought that "macrophages orchestrate the formation of granulation tissue and are capable of doing this in an ischemic environment. In fact, hypoxia and lactate stimulate macrophages to synthesize and secrete angiogenic factor(s) responsible for the growth of capillaries into the repair zone"[422].

Granulation tissue is what one sees as an open wound begins to heal. Chiropractors do not typically observe granulation tissue, although it may be present in the injured musculoskeletal structures that DCs address. The degree to which tissue tearing/damage exists would most likely reflect the quantity of granulation tissue that is produced.

Angiogenesis

Angiogenesis refers to new vessel formation. "Angiogenesis is a process that represents an integrated series of endothelial responses—endothelial cell migration, proliferation, and maturation—that is characteristic of the healing phase of inflammation and chronic inflammation"[94]. As mentioned earlier, new vessels are a component of granulation tissue. Consider the following information regarding angiogenesis:

"The vascular growth that occurs in wound healing requires endothelial cell migration and proliferation, events that occur rarely in the normal adult...Capillaries normally proliferate only during embryonic development, ovulation, menstruation, inflammation, and tissue repair. New vessels generally do not grow in adults except in those situations, and in some pathological ones...The angiogenic cascade in wound healing parallels that seen in development and, to a lesser extent, in tumors."[480] "From the vantage point of the proliferation of new blood vessels in the synovium, synovitis in RA resembles both tumor growth and wound healing."[192]

Various biochemicals act as angiogenic factors which can promote or inhibit angiogenesis. From what I have read and understand, it appears that too much or too little angiogenesis is pathological.

Bucci[51-p.16]. states that, "hypoxia and cytokines, released during inflammation, program fibroblasts and endothelial cells to reproduce and form new blood vessels (angiogenesis), respectively." West et al. suggest that the degradation of hyaluronic acid in remodeling tissues may produce fragments that are angiogenic[478]. Prostaglandin E-1 and E-2 are able to induce capillary growth by either stimulating macrophages or by some unknown mechanism. Prostaglandin levels are elevated in tumors, activated macrophages, wounds and inflammatory exudates[150].

In general, it seems like injured tissues, endothelial cells, macrophages, mast cells and platelets collectively release a pool of angiogenic factors including transforming growth factor-β, tumor necrosis factor, and fibroblast growth factor (PDGF). Platelets release platelet-derived growth factor and enzymes that potentiate the activity of other angiogenic factors[480].

From a pathogenic perspective, it appears that angiogenesis is driven by the presence of inflammatory cells. Thus, from a treatment perspective, a potential approach might be the nutritional reduction of the pro-inflammatory state that predisposes tissues to injury and inflammation. There is also some evidence suggesting that consuming shark cartilage may help to reduce the angiogenesis associated with tumor growth[261], and thus, perhaps shark cartilage can help other conditions associated with angiogenesis, such as arthritis. We should also consider the fact that vitamin C deficiency decreases angiogenesis, resulting in the formation of abnormal capillaries that rupture easily[266]

[again, biochemical balance is the key].

From the chiropractic perspective, angiogenesis should be considered as a factor that may perpetuate joint complex dysfunction as angiogenesis is also known to play a role in osteoarthritis[59, 60].

Fibroblasts

General information

The cell that is central in the repair phase is the fibroblast. The deposition of repair tissue by fibroblasts, which occurs from the 2nd day of the inflammatory process until the 21st day[281], cannot lead to resolution of inflammation unless acute inflammation has resolved.

When fibroblasts arrive at a site of injury, they anchor to the surrounding extracellular matrix and begin to synthesize collagen, elastin, fibronectin and proteoglycan. Fibroblasts also adhere to inflammatory phagocytes. This process is thought to play a role in the cell-cell communication that occurs during inflammation[281]. Various cell adhesion molecules, which were mentioned earlier, are thought to mediate fibroblast adherence. The details of fibroblast adherence are quite involved and not completely understood by investigators at this time.

Chemotaxis

Chemotactic factors for fibroblasts include: PDGF and TGF-β from platelets and macrophages; TNF and fibronectin from macrophages; peptides derived from proteins (collagen, elastin, & fibronectin); LTB-4, 5-HETE, 12-HETE from leukocytes; and serum-derived chemotactic factor for fibroblasts from the complement component C5[281]. "PDGF appears to induce not only the migration of inflammatory cells and fibroblasts into the wound, but also the production of TGF-β, which seems to have a more profound effect on the stimulation of mature collagen fibers and matrix production"[281].

The fibrin-collagen connection

Fibrin is the end product of the coagulation cascade that is formed from fibrinogen. Thrombin converts fibrinogen to fibrin. Fibrin serves as scaffolding on which collagen can be deposited. Kottke[246] states that there is a direct relationship between the fibrin coagulum and collagen deposition. For example, normal tendon repair occurs as a consequence of tension exerted on the fibrin coagulum to produce a linear pattern and then collagen is organized on this matrix[246]. The end of the repair phase is marked by a reduction in the number of fibroblasts.

Unfortunately, the healing process does not always proceed in a normal fashion. It turns out that excessive accumulation of fibrin and collagen can lead to chronic hypomobility and pain. For example, "the accumulation of fibrin is one of the most striking pathologic features of rheumatoid synovitis"[192]. In recent years, research has also suggested that fibrin deposition may play a role in the pathogenesis of chronic low back pain in certain patients[90, 178, 213, 221, 352]. The following quotes allude to possible mechanisms that may be involved in the pathogenesis of abnormal fibrin deposition in neuromusculoskeletal structures after injury:

- "The proliferation of collagenous scar tissue is seen in virtually all soft tissue injuries and may be influenced in several ways. Initially, the greater the amount of exudate released during the post-traumatic inflammatory period, the greater the amount of fibrin released to the tissues. As inflammation may persist for several days, it is important to minimize this exudate process of some time."[99-p.301]

- "Proteoglycans and GAGs are also important in wound healing. The earliest matrix in these wounds results from the deposition of fibrin as a hemostatic response. It has been proposed that an interaction between hyaluronic acid and fibrin creates an initial scaffold on which cells involved in healing may migrate into the wound site."[475]

- "Fibrin is the major coagulation-promoting component of the initial matrix. This primary responsibility is coupled with ancillary roles that potentiate the

healing sequence...The original hemostatic clot during the replacement phase must be transformed from the initial glue into a connective tissue replacement with structural integrity. This is accomplished by activation of the fibrinolytic cascade. Plasmin is a serine protease responsible for the degradation of the fibrin clot...Plasmin cleaves the arg-lys peptide bond of fibrin and produces soluble fibrin degradation products...These fragments are potent chemoattractants that induce migration of endothelial cells as other mesenchymal cells and also stimulate collagen synthesis and increase prolyl hydroxylase activity."[422]

Many of the chemotactic factors mentioned earlier also act as stimuli for fibroblasts to synthesize and deposit collagen. The following quote provides a concise explanation:

"Transforming growth factor-β and many of the other growth factors, in addition to regulating growth, stimulate formation of collagen, fibronectin and other matrix components by fibroblasts and have potent angiogenic activity. Further stimulation of fibroblast matrix synthesis by IL-1, TNF, and PDGF leads to scar formation and repair of the tissue injury. Remodeling of scar tissue depends on collagenase produced by fibroblasts and macrophages, and normally this is accomplished with minimal or no scarring. In a chronic inflammatory response this healing process can become excessive due to continued secretion of fibroblast-active cytokines with the potential for tissue pathology."[470]

In certain patients with joint complex dysfunction and soft tissue injuries, it is likely that chronic joint and muscle pain are associated with excessive fibrin and collagen deposition. Clearly, the biochemical factors described above may be involved. Histological studies of tender muscles demonstrate the presence of platelet clots and degranulating mast cells[22]. Both of these cell types, particularly platelets, release pro-inflammatory and fibrogenic mediators. This information requires that chiropractors consider inflammation, fibrosis and hypomobility from more than just a biomechanical perspective. Chapter 8 will discuss nutritional factors associated with platelets, mast cells, and fibrin deposition.

Many patients also need nutritional support to enhance collagen synthesis. We should keep in mind the following facts about collagen:

"Of all animal proteins, collagen is the most abundant and ubiquitous. In humans and most other vertebrates, it accounts for approximately one third of the total body proteins. It is the major structural protein that holds cells together to give organs their characteristic architecture."[351]

"Deficiencies of protein, vitamin C, and zinc can cause impaired collagen synthesis and delayed healing"[211]. Reid[362-p.75]. states that, "hypoxia and acidosis turn on the fibroblast, but oxygen is necessary for the production of collagen." Reid also mentions that glycine, vitamin C, iron and alpha-ketoglutarate are needed for collagen synthesis. This topic will be discussed in greater detail in Chapter 9.

Scar Tissue

Scar tissue refers to the randomly deposited connective tissue matrix (fibrin, collagen and proteoglycan) that occurs during the repair phase. The previous section detailed some of the biochemical factors associated with scar tissue formation. As alluded to earlier, scar tissue itself is not pathological; however, with chronic inflammation and hypomobility, scar tissue deposition can be excessive, and this is pathological. The following quotes describe clinical factors associated with pathological scar tissue formation:

"If the initial inflammation is rested and allowed to heal, a normal scar along normal lines of stress will result. If excessive overuse or immobilization occurs, increased fibrous scar tissue will result, which may spread and become tethered to surrounding normal tissue. Increased fibrous

tissue results in a loss of mobility and extensibility of the tissue. Loss of extensibility means loss of function. Loss of function results in reaggravation of the tissue during normal use and a vicious cycle of microtearing-inflammation-scarring. The scar itself may become a source of nociceptive stimulation."[184]

"Scar tissue is less elastic, less resilient, less pliable, and less resistant to shear and tensile forces than is original tissue. It can adversely affect mobility and extensibility and, therefore, may play a part in altered biomechanics. An example would be the thickened fibrous scar of the zygapophyseal joint, which is less elastic than the original tissue and functionally restricts local intervertebral kinetics. The lack of motion at one level will be compensated for by hypermobility at adjacent levels, which in turn will usually result in degenerative disc disease and osteoarthritis some time in the future."[99-p.301]

Kirkaldy-Willis[234] indicates that restricted joint movement and disuse can lead to tissue fibrosis. Kottke states that histological evidence of fibrosis can occur in *as little as four days of joint immobilization*[246]. Clearly, proper joint mobility is critical if appropriate remodeling and optimal healing of scar tissue is to occur.

THE REMODELING PHASE

Connective tissue is the slowest of the various musculoskeletal tissues to return to normal function after immobilization or injury[131]. "Poorly vascularized sites, such as tendons and ligaments, are notably slow to heal. Retarded healing is compounded by the fact that these tissues especially depend on a precise and compact organization of collagen fiber bundles"[104]. "A healing ligament may have about 50% of its strength by 6 months after injury, 80% after 1 year, and 100% after only 1 to 3 years, depending on the type of stresses placed on it and the prevention of a repeated injury"[131].

As mentioned in the Repair Phase section (see Repair vs Regeneration), unlike connective tissue elements, muscles have good regenerative capacity which is most likely due to their superior vascular supply[131]. "Regardless of the mode of destruction, whether by trauma, ischemia, or toxic degeneration, regeneration of muscle can occur"[451]. Six weeks after injury, injured muscle appears grossly and microscopically normal except for occasional small areas of fibrosis[451]. At six weeks muscle weight is not normal, but by three months muscle is thought to be normal in weight and structure[131].

The precise mechanism of remodeling is unknown. A balance is somehow achieved between collagen deposition versus the degradation, produced by the collagenase that is released by fibroblasts and macrophages[470]. A key factor in the remodeling process is the restoration of a normal range of movement. It is agreed that healing musculoskeletal tissues will realign themselves along the lines of stress imposed by movement[62, 63, 246, 229, 131, 362-p.76]. Kottke[246] provides an interesting description of the types of connective tissue that develop with and without motion:

> "Loose or areolar connective tissue forms between organs and other structures, such as joint capsules, fascia, intermuscular layers, and subcutaneous tissue, where movement occurs repeatedly. It will allow movement through limited distances, adapt by shortening and fixation, if there is no motion, or elongate slowly under prolonged or repeated tension...In areas where motion does not occur, such as in fascia planes and capsules of muscles or organs, collagen is laid down as dense meshwork, sheets, or bands. This type of connective tissue is also laid down in scars. If motion is maintained during healing of a wound, connective tissue of the areolar type develops. If the wound is immobilized, a dense contracted scar forms."

Based on this information, rehabilitation exercises can play a dramatic role in the remodeling of injured tissues. A great deal of information is available that describes rehabilitation protocols for the spine. Unfortunately, spinal rehabilitation has been neglected by both chiropractic and medical doctors. As this book is devoted to nutrition, specific rehabilitation procedures will not be discussed. However, I would like to point out that the best approach to any rehabilitation program is to start a program before injury occurs. In other words, we should all exercise our spinal muscles as an injury prevention measure. The logic in such an approach is clear for the following reasons:

- Back pain is the second leading reason reported by patients for visiting physicians[101].

- Back pain is the second leading cause of absenteeism in the work place[101].

- 80% of adults will experience low back pain at least once in their lives[81].

- At any given moment, 15% to 20% of the adult population have low back pain[363].

- Tens of billions is spent annually to care for those with back pain. The annual cost reaches $100 billion if we include those who are disabled with chronic pain[363].

These figures could probably be reduced drastically if we all performed prophylactic rehabilitation exercises in our homes/gyms and if doctors routinely utilized rehabilitation in their practices. Indeed, research has demonstrated that degenerated and atrophied muscles are present in so-called healthy asymptomatic subjects[344, 360]. Consider the following description of the spinal deconditioning syndrome provided by Mayer and Gatchel[293-p.208]:

> "Although deconditioning is likely to be induced more slowly in the spine than in an immobilized extremity, extended periods of inactivity and restricted motion take

their toll on function. The effects can include stiff hypomobile joints, muscle atrophy, loss of endurance, tightening of connective tissues, inhibition of neural outflow, and eventual loss of cardiovascular fitness. Because atrophic muscles are more irritable and subject to overload, recurrent spasm or deformities are often produced. These symptoms may then be misinterpreted as 'new injuries,' with continued bed rest following, which perpetuates the disuse phenomenon."

A basic approach to rehabilitating the spine follows shortly. The purpose of such a program is to recondition neuromusculoskeletal structures, aide in the remodeling of injured tissues, and prevent the onset of the deconditioning syndrome. Fitz-Ritson[145] suggests a 4-phase approach to rehabilitation based on the following treatment objectives: 1) alleviate pain as quickly as possible; 2) shorten the treatment time; 3) prevent chronic pain patterns from developing; and 4) rehabilitate the injured area/individual to normal, or close to normal as quickly as possible. A brief introduction to the recommended phases follows:

Phase I
- Operational endpoint - "no pain at rest"
- A series of range of motion exercises performed to pain tolerance

Phase II
- Operational endpoint - "capacity to perform unstressed basic daily activities"
- Active exercises for stretching and range of motion which involve self imposed resistance

Phase III
- Operational endpoint - "capacity to perform normal activities under some constraints and conditions"
- Isometric strengthening exercises

Phase IV
- Operational endpoint - "recovery of full, normal and uncontrolled activities, and release from active care"
- Isokinetic/isotonic exercises for strengthening

The four phases demonstrate that exercise should be performed in a graded fashion so as to not re-injure the healing tissues and subsequently re-ignite the inflammatory process. For basic exercise protocols see the following references[20, 145, 198, 205, 272a, 283, 293, 302, 315, 380], and for detailed protocols and programs see Liebenson[272, 272a].

At this point, it should be clear that nociception and inflammation are serious concerns. In fact, much of medicine is devoted to reducing chronic inflammation with pharmacologic agents. The following chapter discusses the various medications that are used to treat pain and inflammation. Thereafter, the remainder of the text, i.e., Chapters 5-10, is devoted to the nutritional modulation of inflammation, nociception, pain and tissue healing.

Chapter 4

Pharmacological Therapy of Pain and Joint Dysfunction

PHARMACOLOGICAL ADJUSTMENTS

Consider the following quote which came from an issue of *Drug Therapy* :

"The combination of cyclobenzaprine (Flexoril, a muscle relaxant) and naproxen (an NSAID) was better than naproxen alone in reducing objective muscle spasm and tenderness and *increasing motion of the lumbosacral spine.*" (1992;(Oct):p.101)

From this information we can see that medical research indicates that it is indeed possible to pharmacologically adjust the spine and improve joint motion.

Advertisements for NSAIDs also claim that these medications improve joint motion. The makers of Naprosyn (naproxen) state that,

"For chronic arthritis expect nothing less: Reduction of morning stiffness, reduction of joint pain and tenderness, *increased range of motion* and favorable safety profile." (*Hospital Medicine* 1992(Oct):p.6-7)

The makers of Tylenol (acetaminophen) currently advertise it as the medication "For the Mechanical Pain of Osteoarthritis" The copy reads:

"The pain of osteoarthritis is primarily non-inflammatory, characterized by structural changes within the joint space. These changes can cause occasional pain on motion, which can be treated with a pure analgesic, like Extra Strength TYLENOL." (*Postgraduate Medicine* 1993(Jan):p.142)

Because various drugs pharmacologicaly adjust the spine, it behooves us to understand the mechanisms by which these drugs work. Additionally, by having a better understanding of pharmacology, we will be able to effectively speak with our medical colleagues about their approach to patient care. Why is this important? Very simply, who would you feel more comfortable developing a relationship with; a medical doctor who understands joint oreceptor physiology and thus, appreciates the need for certain patients to be adjusted, or a medical doctor who thinks all chiropractors are unscientific quacks and the adjustment is just a part of a therapeutic psychosomatic horse and pony show? In the same way, who do you think a medical doctor/group would feel more comfortable referring patients to; a chiropractor who understands that NSAIDs act to inhibit prostaglandins and muscle relaxants influence inhibitory interneurons in the spinal cord, or a chiropractor who thinks that drugs should never be taken and all medical doctors are dangerous and do not care about their patients?

The drugs to be discussed in this chapter include: aspirin and nonsteroidal anti-inflammatory drugs (NSAIDs), acetaminophen, corticosteroids, muscle relaxants, opiate analgesics, MAO inhibitors and tricyclic antidepressants. The mechanism of action and the side-effects of the various pharmacological agents will be described.

This chapter is in no way meant to stand as a treatise on pharmacology for chiropractors. What DCs should take away from this section is the fact that joint motion can be improved by means other than the adjustment.

ANTI-INFLAMMATORY AGENTS

Aspirin and NSAIDs

Aspirin, Advil (ibuprofen), Motrin (ibuprofen), Nuprin (ibuprofen), ibuprofen, Butazolidin, Feldene, Naprosyn, Anaprox, Indocin, Clinoril, Ansaid, Tolectin and Dolobid are all nonsteroidal anti-inflammatory drugs (NSAIDs). NSAIDs are the most commonly used medications in the treatment of pain, the next most common being acetaminophen[137-p.272].

Aspirin/NSAIDs (A/N) are known to have analgesic effects, anti-inflammatory effects, antipyretic effects and anti-aggregating effects on platelets. All of these activities are thought to occur because NSAIDs act to inhibit the cyclo-oxygenase (CO) enzyme. CO functions to convert cell membrane-bound arachidonic acid into prostaglandins, thromboxanes and prostacyclin, which are collectively referred to as prostanoids. Ultimately, the beneficial effects of A/Ns are thought to be due to the inhibition of prostaglandin and thromboxane production. One of the prostaglandins formed from arachidonic acid is prostaglandin E-2 (PGE-2), which has the ability to sensitize nociceptors and ultimately result in the experience of pain[528].

A/Ns are thought to work both systemically and within the central nervous system (CNS). The analgesic effect is thought to be due to the inhibition of prostanoid activity at the spinal cord level[520, 528]. The anti-inflammatory effect is thought to be due to PGE-2 inhibition at the site of inflammation, which also contributes to their analgesic effect[528]. The antipyretic effect is thought to be due to their ability to inhibit CO activity in the CNS which allows for proper hypothalamic temperature regulation[528]. The anti-aggregation effect on platelets is thought to be due to inhibition of thromboxane synthesis[23].

Shearn describes additional effects for both aspirin and NSAIDs[528].

"Aspirin also interferes with the chemical mediators of the kallikrein system. Aspirin inhibits granulocyte adherence to damaged vasculature, stabilizes lysosomes, and inhibits the migration of polymorpho-nuclearleukocytes and macrophages into the site of inflammation...The NSAIDs decrease the sensitivity of vessels to bradykinin and histamine, affect lymphokine production from T lymphocytes, and reverse vasodilation," and to varying degrees, all NSAIDs inhibit prothrombin synthesis.

Many people still have the misconception that the main mechanism of action of NSAIDs is unknown. The fact of the matter is that it has been known since 1971 that NSAIDs inhibit prostaglandin production[514-p.663].

Side-effects:

The side-effects of NSAID use is also due to the inhibition of prostaglandin synthesis. This is because prostaglandins have detrimental and beneficial effects, both of which are inhibited by NSAIDs.

It is important to understand that the therapeutic dose, which varies among individuals, is also the dose which produces detrimental side-effects. The therapeutic dose for NSAIDs varies among the respective medications. For example, to achieve pain relief, the therapeutic dose for aspirin is 2,600-4,000mg/d; 800-3,200 mg/d for ibuprofen and 550-1650 mg/d for Naprosyn[511].

About 10,000 to 20,000 deaths occur each year from NSAID-induced ulcer complications[522]. Clearly, a better method of pain therapy is needed. Perhaps chiropractic can play a large role in this field.

As early as 1967, indomethacin was thought to accelerate bone destruction in osteoarthritis of the hip. Subsequent reports have provided further clinical evidence of harmful effects of NSAIDs on osteoarthritic hips. Research also demonstrates that NSAIDs interfere with metabolism of articular cartilage and repair of bone[525].

The administration of NSAIDs may also lead to loss of intestinal integrity. This increases gastrointestinal permeability to antigenic molecules which can translocate across the GI mucosa and showed that permeability abnormalities were in fact due to an effect of NSAID therapy in both the proximal and distal intestine, and the effect was systemically mediated. It is believed that the absorption of macromolecular-antigenic molecules contributes to the persistence of arthritis[35].

Not only do NSAIDs damage the stomach and small intestine, as described above, they also damage the colon. Thus, the entire GI tract is susceptible to NSAID-induced injury. Research demonstrates that four distinct types of ulcerative colitis can result from NSAID therapy[513].

NSAID-induced hypersensitivity affects a substantial number of people, including 20% or more of asthmatic patients. Research indicates that peripheral monocytes of aspirin-sensitive asthmatics synthesize more arachidonate products than in normal persons or asthmatic control groups. Aspirin induced reactions, such as asthmatic attacks, rhinitis, sinusitis and urticaria, are thought to be due to an increased production of leukotrienes from arachidonic acid. This is because the NSAIDs block cyclooxygenase and not the leukotriene-producing lipoxygenase pathway[521].

NSAIDs may also contribute to esophageal disease. This can occur because NSAIDs can get trapped in the esophagus in patients with reflux disease and may injure the epithelium[526].

Acetaminophen

Acetaminophen is the active ingredient in Tylenol and is reported to have analgesic and antipyretic effects which are equivalent to that of aspirin. The analgesic effect of acetaminophen is thought to occur in the central nervous system, much like aspirin, via the inhibition of prostaglandin synthesis[528].

To this date, many reputable textbooks in pharmacology still promote the notion that acetaminophen does not have anti-inflammatory or anti-platelet activities. Even advertisements for acetaminophen state that TYLENOL is a pure analgesic. Contrary to these assertions, a recent letter to the editor in PAIN explains that research has demonstrated that acetaminophen does indeed possess anti-inflammatory properties[531]. These researchers do not mention if these effects are due

to the inhibition of cyclooxygenase.

Side effects:

The most common side-effect ascribed to the use of acetaminophen is liver damage. Acetaminophen is detoxified by hepatic glutathione, a tripeptide consisting of glutamic acid, glycine and cysteine. Glutathione is one of the body's most important free radical scavengers. When hepatic glutathione is depleted, reactions between acetaminophen and hepatic proteins is increased and hepatic necrosis is the result[514-p.692-5]. If there is a low concentration of hepatic glutathione, the likelihood of acetaminophen-induced liver damage increases. In certain individuals, therapeutic doses can cause a mild increase in hepatic enzymes, which resolves when the drug is withdrawn[528]. With larger than therapeutic doses, dizziness, excitement and disorientation are seen. Therapeutic doses being approximately 325-500 mgs 4 times daily[528].

Corticosteroids

The adrenal cortex produces both mineralocorticoids and glucocorticoids. The major mineralocorticoid in humans is aldosterone and the major glucocorticoid is cortisol. Synthetic glucocorticoids, which have minimal mineralocorticoid activity, are the preparations of choice to treat inflammatory conditions, whereas natural preparations, such as cortisone or hydrocortisone, are the common choice when treating adrenocortical insufficiency[523].

Commonly prescribed synthetic glucocorticoids include methylprednisolone (Medrol), prednisolone (Cortalone), prednisone (Meticorten, Deltasone Cortan), paramethasone (Haldrone), triamcinolone (Aristocort), dexamethasone (Decadron) and betamethasone (Celestone). During this discussion, the various synthetic glucocorticoids will be collectively referred to as corticosteroids[523-p.1662-85].

Corticosteroids block all of the known pathways of eicosanoid (prostanoids and leukotrienes) metabolism by stimulating the synthesis of a protein called lipocortin, which in turn inhibits the activity of phospholipase A-2[516]. Phospholipase A-2 is found in cell membranes and when it is stimulated through mechanical or chemical means it liberates arachidonic acid from the cell membrane. Arachidonic acid, as described earlier, can then be acted upon by cyclo-oxygenase which produces prostanoids. When arachidonic acid is acted upon by another enzyme known as lipoxygenase, leukotrienes are produced. Leukotrienes, specifically leukotriene B-4, can act like PGE-2 to sensitize nociceptors. The lipoxygenase enzyme system is found predominantly in platelets, mast cells and leukocytes. Aspirin/NSAIDs only inhibit cyclo-oxygenase and not lipoxygenase (*see figure 4-1*).

Because corticosteroids inhibit phospholipase A-2, they are capable of inhibiting the production of both prostaglandins and leukotrienes. Despite these effects, NSAIDs are still the drugs of choice for most cases of pain and inflammation. The use of corticosteroids is usually reserved for autoimmune related conditions rather than pain and inflammation.

In addition to the above mentioned effects of corticosteroids, they can also dramatically reduce the manifestations of inflammation due to their ability to modulate the concentration, distribution and functions of peripheral leukocytes. Generally speaking, corticosteroids inhibit the functions of leukocytes and tissue macrophages[515]. Such inhibition reduces the release of collagenase and elastase, and reduces the production of free radicals.

Side effects:

The beneficial effects of corticosteroid use come from the inhibition of prostaglandins and leukotrienes, and from their immunosuppressive effects. The detrimental side-effects are a result of the same mechanisms and additional effects which steroids have on cell function.

The following quote came from page 6 of Dr. Warren Hammer's book entitled, *Functional Soft Tissue Examination and Treatment by Manual Methods*, which is published by Aspen Publishers of Gaithersburg, Maryland, 1991.

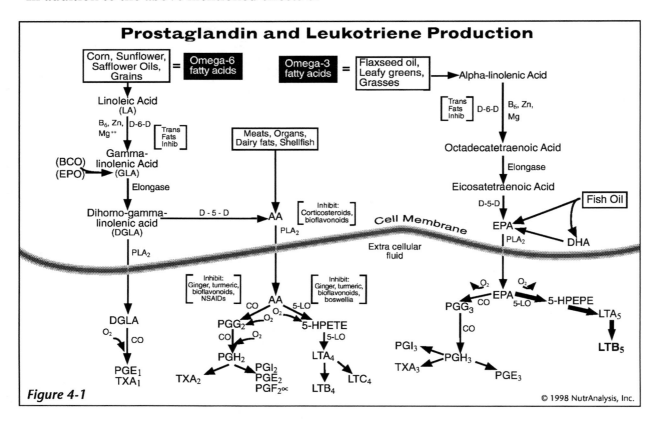

Figure 4-1

Gaithersburg, Maryland, 1991.

"Some side effects of corticosteroids are avascular necrosis, especially of the hip[512], which results from an adverse effect on lipid metabolism causing fatty emboli; tendon rupture due to the inhibition of the formation of healing adhesions, which results in weakening[521]; alteration of biomechanical ligamentous properties due to inhibition of the formation granulation and connective tissue[509]; arthropathy due to softening of the subchondral bone, delay in chondroitin sulfate synthesis, and inhibition of the formation ground substance in mesenchymal tissue [articular cartilage][510]; vertebral osteoporosis [530]; infectious arthritis and bursitis[517]; and depressed mental status due to decreased corticoadrenal function[518]. Some of the articular damage has been attributed to steroid analgesia, which results in microtrauma[517] due to painless overuse."

A negative nitrogen balance induced by corticosteroid therapy may play an important role in accelerating lean body mass (LBM) depletion in patients with chronic inflammatory diseases. This may, in turn, produce a decreased functional status and poorer outcome in the long term[527].

The premature withdrawal of corticosteroids may be associated with exacerbation of symptoms unless other agents are used concurrently. Nevertheless, the symptomatic relief offered by corticosteroids in most inflammatory conditions is so great that they are frequently used despite their adverse effects, including hyperglycemia, myopathy, ischemic necrosis of bone, cataracts, truncal obesity, Cushingoid habitus, and gastric ulcerations[527].

Prolonged exposure to systemic corticosteroids can cause bone loss, osteoporosis, and fractures. Corticosteroid-induced osteoporosis is increasingly recognized as a causative factor in the approximately 18 million patients who are undergoing treatment with exogenous corticosteroids[529].

MUSCLE RELAXANTS

Generally speaking muscle relaxants are used to treat spasticity due to descending pathway dysfunction (i.e., an upper motor neuron lesion), and acute muscle spasms due to a variety of insults.

Spasticity

An upper motor neuron (UMN) lesion is characterized by absent abdominal reflexes, an extensor toe sign, hyperreflexia and spasticity of physiological flexor muscles. Such signs are found whenever a UMN is damaged anywhere along its course from its origin to the alpha-motoneuron. Strokes, multiple sclerotic plaquing, tumors and cord transection are all possible causes of UMN damage. The spasticity is thought to develop because with a loss of the UMN's inhibitory input, the alpha-motoneuron becomes hyperexcitable which results in abnormal muscle contraction.

The drugs used to treat spasticity associated with UMNs include diazepam (Valium) and baclofen (Lioresal), which act within the CNS, and dantrolene (Dantrium), which acts directly on skeletal muscle.

Diazepam and baclofen are thought to facilitate the activity of interneurons which release gamma-aminobutyric acid (GABA). These interneurons are thought to cause presynaptic inhibition of Ia afferent fibers from muscle spindles. Such inhibition reduces the excitatory drive to the associated alpha-motoneuron and the result is decreased spasticity. Dantrolene is thought to reduce spasticity by decreasing the amount of calcium released from the sarcoplasmic reticulum[514-p.486-90]. This means that troponin C will be exposed to less calcium ions which serves to reduce crossbridge formation between actin and myosin.

Side-effects:

The side-effects associated with administration of diazepam and baclofen are related to their activity as CNS depressants. Diazepam, or Valium, is a member of the benzodiazepine family which includes other drugs such as Librium, Zanax, Ativan and Halcion. All of the benzodiazepines have similar side-effects which include symptoms such as drowsiness and ataxia[514-p.486-90]. Diazepam produces sedation in most patients at the doses required to significantly reduce muscle tone[524].

Baclofen is a derivative of GABA and its use is often limited by its untoward side-effects, which include symptoms such as drowsiness, insomnia, dizziness, weakness, ataxia, and mental confusion[514-p.486-90].

The side-effects of dantrolene are such that, although spasticity can be relieved, the associated weakness it produces may handicap the patient more than the spasticity it relieves[514-p.486-90].

Acute muscle spasms

A variety of conditions such as trauma, inflammation, anxiety and pain can be associated with acute muscle spasms. Medications designed to alleviate such spasms include: cyclobenzaprine hydrochloride (Flexeril), carisoprodol (Soma), chlorzoxazone (Paraflex), chlorphenesin carbamate (Maolate), metaxalone (Skelaxin) and methocarbamol (Robaxin).

The efficacy of these drugs has yet to be established. It is thought that, collectively, their limited efficacy may be due solely to general depression of the CNS[514-p.486-90].

It is known that these drugs are not useful in the treatment of spasticity associated with chronic neurological disease.

Side-effects:

The most common side-effects associated with the drugs used to treat acute muscle spasms are drowsiness and dizziness, presumably because of the depressant effect on the CNS. Other symptoms include nausea, ataxia, vertigo, confusion and headaches[523-p.672-82].

OPIATE ANALGESICS

Morphine, meperidine (Demerol), hydromorphine (Dilaudid), methadone (Dolophine), codeine, levorphanol (Levodrmoran) and Fentanyl are all considered members of the family of opiate analgesics, also called opiate agonists. These agents function to activate the descending pain modulating system within the central nervous system. They act upon a specific class of opiate receptors called a mu-receptor, which is highly concentrated in the periaqueductal gray (PAG) region of the midbrain[137].

The basic circuitry of the descending pain modulating system is such that opiate agonists will activate the PAG which will subsequently release transmitters (B-endorphin, enkephalin, GABA, and/or dynorphin) that travel to the rostral ventral medulla to stimulate the serotonin-rich nucleus raphe magnus (NRM). The NRM's serotonergic projections travel down the spinal cord within the reticulospinal pathways and synapse with interneurons in the superficial dorsal horn[137]. These interneurons release enkephalin which inhibits the nociceptive afferent system[176]. According to Wyke[493], these are the same inhibitory interneurons that are stimulated when joint mechanoreceptor afferents are depolarized during a chiropractic adjustment.

Side-effects:

The side-effects of opiate administration include: mood changes, nausea, vomiting, sedation, mental clouding, respiratory depression, cough suppression, decreased GI motility, increased biliary duct pressure, pruritus, histamine release and urinary retention[137].

Chapter 5

A DIET-INDUCED PRO-INFLAMMATORY STATE

Recall that Chapter 1 focussed on nociception and Chapter 3 focussed on the inflammatory process. Then, Chapter 4 briefly discussed the various drugs used to reduce inflammation, nociception and pain. It should be understood that pharmacologic agents are very effective in reducing these symptoms; however, drug therapy is associated with unwanted side-effects, and moreover, chiropractors are not licensed to prescribe drugs. Nonetheless, since inflammation and nociception are peripheral biochemical processes intimately related to spinal dysfunction, it is important to include a biochemistry component in patient care to provide a thorough treatment program. This is where nutritional biochemistry fits into chiropractic practice. In Chapter 5, we will begin our investigation into the nutritional factors related to inflammation.

Chapter 3 outlined the inflammatory process in some detail. Recall that the inflammatory process is driven by various chemical irritants, especially prostaglandin E-2, leukotriene B-4, histamine, 5-hydroxytryptamine, and bradykinin. Recall that these chemical mediators of inflammation are released during tissue injury. Various growth factors (i.e., PDGF, TGF-β) and cytokines (i.e., IL-1 and TNF) are also released. Collectively, these factors stimulate the vascular and cellular phases of acute inflammation. Recall that the cellular phase is characterized by macrophage and fibroblast migration into the injured area, as a consequence of the acute inflammatory response.

Without the initial release of the chemical mediators of inflammation, the inflammatory process would not occur and healing would not take place. At the other end of the spectrum, if the release of the chemical mediators does not resolve, then inflammation will rage on and become chronic...the end result will be persistent nociceptor depolarization, pathological tissue fibrosis and chronic pain.

In 1992, I suggested that the term "pro-inflammatory state" should be used to describe the general biochemical state, resulting from dietary habits that predispose the body to produce excessive chemical irritants[402]. Such a state could initiate and/or perpetuate inflammation and chronic pain. Several factors appear to be involved. Primarily, the problem appears to begin with a diet that contains excessive amounts of meat and desserts, and deficient quantities of vegetables and fruits. Over an unspecified time period, this imbalance may lead to increased tissue acidity, inadequate potassium intake, inadequate magnesium intake, free radical production, and fatty acid imbalances, all of which can promote inflammation and create a pro-inflammatory state. Each of these factors will be discussed separately on the following pages.

INTRODUCTION

In 1991, the results of a clinical trial demonstrated that a dietary focus on vegetables and fruits could dramatically reduce inflammation and pain in patients with rheumatoid arthritis[237]. In part, the researchers originally set out to test the utility of a vegetarian diet and then realized that many of their subjects needed to switch to a lactovegetarian diet to insure nutritional adequacy. The study revealed that a vegetable-based diet markedly improved all arthritis indices tested including the number of tender and swollen joints, Ritchie's articular index, pain score, duration of morning stiffness, grip strength, erythrocyte sedimentation rate, C-reactive protein, WBC count, and a health assessment questionnaire. These benefits were present after one year. Kjeldsen-Kragh et al. concluded that,

> "a switch to a vegetarian diet causes an extensive change of the profile of the fatty acids of the serum phospholipids. These changes may favor production of prostaglandins and leukotrienes with less inflammatory activity."[237]

While these researchers focussed on eicosanoid modulation, it is likely that increased vegetable and fruit consumption also increases the dietary intake of alkaline minerals, potassium, magnesium, antioxidants and various phytochemicals such as flavonoids, terpenoids and carotenoids. Irrespective of these authors' biochemical conclusions, the results of this study clearly demonstrated that vegetables and fruits have a significant anti-inflammatory effect. (It should be mentioned that the Kjeldsen-Kragh et al. article will be referred to several times in this chapter so remember the name Kjeldsen-Kragh)

Many papers have been published in recent years which explain that a fruit and vegetable-rich diet can offer protection against, and help treat, chronic diseases such as heart disease, cancer, diabetes, hypertension and other medical conditions[538, 560, 590, 652, 600, 770, 816, 838]. All of these chronic diseases are typically viewed as being inflammatory in nature. In other words, local inflammatory processes play a significant role in promoting these diseases. Leslie views most of these diseases as "undesirable inflammatory responses"[700]. Heart disease and cancer are the best examples of pro-inflammatory diseases.

Over 5 years ago, Ross made it clear that atherosclerosis was driven by inflammation. He focused on how pro-inflammatory cytokines, growth factors, free radicals and eicosanoids would be able to initiate and perpetuate atherogenesis[780]. Ross describes atherosclerosis as a disease process that is preceded and accompanied by inflammation, and in its advanced stages represents an excessive inflammatory-fibroproliferative response to many different insults[780]. For additional evidence to demonstrate that atherosclerosis is an inflammatory condition, one only needs to consider that aspirin, an anti-inflammatory drug, is used in the treatment and prevention of heart disease[773]. In fact, atherosclerotic heart disease is commonly viewed as an undesirable inflammatory response of the arteries[788].

It has become so common place to view heart disease and cancer as pro-inflammatory, even standard pathology books take this position. For example, regarding the pathogenesis of stomach cancer:

> "Acute gastritis is an acute mucosal inflammatory process, usually transient in nature...Chronic gastritis is defined as the presence of chronic mucosal inflammatory changes leading to mucosal atrophy and epithelial metaplasia, usually in the absence of eosins. The epithelial changes may become dysplastic and constitute a background for the development of carcinoma."[93-p.770-71]

As stated above, the nutrients in fruits and vegetables prevent the development and/or help to treat a variety of inflammatory diseases such as rheumatoid arthritis, heart disease and cancer. The exact components in fruits and vegetables which exert the anti-inflammatory effects are not precisely known. In this chapter, I will discuss various components which seem to be involved. More factors are probably involved and this information will become available to us as research moves forward.

INCREASED TISSUE ACIDITY

General information about tissue pH

Whereas normal arterial pH is 7.4, normal venous and interstitial fluid pH is about 7.35. It is very important to tightly regulate extracellular pH as the body cannot survive at a pH below 6.8 or above 8.0[177-p. 331].

Normal intracellular pH levels range between 6.0 and 7.4, and average about 7.0[177-p. 331]. The physiological reason for such a range is that there are many intracellular compartments, including the cytoplasm, mitochondria, endoplasmic reticulum, and nucleus[371]. The intracellular pH can also be altered and enter the acidic range when the cell is compromised, such as during states of rapid metabolism and poor blood flow to tissues[177-p. 331].

Pain, inflammation and pH

Research has demonstrated that the pH in inflamed and ischemic tissues can be as low as 5.4[186]. This is an important fact to be aware of as certain nutrition companies have promoted the incorrect notion that pain and inflammation are associated with an alkaline pH. Subsequently, many companies recommend supplements to acidify patients who suffer with pain and inflammation. This approach should be seriously questioned as most patients already appear to be too acidic.

Regarding nociceptor stimulation, it should be understood that an acidic pH can depolarize nociceptors[186]. There is also synergism between an acid pH and the other chemical irritants, which serves to enhance nociceptor responsiveness[186]. Furthermore, it is known that local tissue acidity is a powerful activator of bradykinin, which is the most potent nociceptor irritant. Local acidity also inactivates the enzyme kininase I, which deactivates bradykinin. This may then allow bradykinin concentration to increase even more rapidly[433]. In addition to its role as the most potent nociceptor irritant, bradykinin has many other pro-inflammatory effects[433]: 1) causes the four cardinal signs of inflammation (dolor, rubor, tumor, and calor), 2) activates phospholipase A-2 which results in the production of prostaglandins, leukotrienes, and thromboxanes, 3) causes arteriole vasodilation, venule vasoconstriction, and increased vascular permeability, and 4) acts a chemoattractant for leukocytes. Indeed, increased tissue acidity may result in a cascade of inflammatory changes that promote nociception.

Several papers have looked at the clinical significance of an acidic pH in local tissues. Nachemson[327] determined the pH of lumbar discs in patients with radiculopathy and found that "there as a significant negative correlation between pH and disc degeneration, pre-operative pain, and most significantly, the amount of connective tissue reaction around the nerve-root." In other words, with increased local acidity there was increased pain, disc degeneration and fibrous deposition. Of interest to note is that in Nachemson's sample of patients, the disc pH levels ranged from 5.7-7.5. Hambly[183] indicates that, "discs known to be painful at the time of surgery yielded pH levels below 7.0." Research has also demonstrated that when disc pH drops below 6.8, proteoglycan synthesis is impaired[339].

An important point to consider is that all of the above mentioned studies were observational in nature, i.e., an acidic pH was associated with pathophysiology. An intriguing aspect of these studies is the fact that different patients routinely had different pH levels. Unfortunately, none of the studies emphasized this fact nor sufficiently investigated why pH values would vary so widely among patients. The importance of this issue becomes apparent when we consider the fact that pain and degenerative changes were shown to increase in proportion to decreasing pH levels. Clearly, we can conclude that an acidic pH should be avoided, if possible. Unfortunately, unless a patient is hospitalized with overt metabolic acidosis, virtually no information exists that describes how to address the problem of local tissue acidity from a therapeutic perspective.

Dietary regulation of pH

It is very interesting to note that our dietary habits powerfully influence the modulation of body pH. This can be better appreciated after a brief review of acid-base physiology. A not-too-well-known fact is that the human body is an acid producing machine. Major factors which contribute the body's "fixed acid production" include intermediate and bacterial metabolism[80]. The metabolism of glucose, triglycerides and nucleoproteins yield hydrogen ions and/or carbon dioxide, both of which are acidic molecules. Gastrointestinal bacterial metabolism of unabsorbed carbohydrates, fats, and proteins also results in acid production[80]. Despite a continuous production of acids, the body manages to maintain normal pH through the use of various buffer systems.

When the body is presented with an acid load

there are four main buffering systems which come into play[371]. There is an immediate extracellular buffering by HCO_3^- (bicarbonate). Within a period of minutes to hours there is an increase in respiration that decreases CO_2 levels. Within 2 to 4 hours the intracellular buffers (primarily proteins and organic phosphates) and bone provide further buffering. Finally, the kidney combines hydrogen ions (H^+) with ammonia (NH3) to make ammonium (NH^{+4}) which is excreted in the urine. These buffering mechanisms keep pH within normal limits to a remarkable degree, despite significant variations in net acid excretion as reflected in 24 hour urine collections. Kurtz et al.[251] demonstrated that plasma levels of H^+, CO_2, and HCO3- remained constant despite urine net acid values that ranged from 14 *mEq/24 hr* to 154 *mEq/24 hr*. Most of such studies devoted to pH modulation only follow patients for short periods of time or involve acute loading tests, and thus, do not reflect real-life values over time.

As mentioned earlier, dietary factors can influence pH modulation. It is known that diet may contribute or detract from the fixed acid load that is generated by intermediary metabolism[80]. Carroll[72] states that endogenous acid production depends on the diet. Many researchers have known for years that meats and grains are a source of potential acids, whereas fruits and vegetables are a source of potential bases[80, 238, 297, 340]. Meats and grains contain nonmetabolizable anions (i.e., Cl^-, HPO^{2-}_4) accompanied by metabolizable cations (i.e., cationic amino acids), the absorption of which results in loss of bicarbonate. On the other hand, vegetables and fruits contain nonmetabolizable cations (i.e., Na^+, K^+, Ca^{++}, Mg^{++}) accompanied by metabolizable anions (i.e., citrate), the absorption of which results in the production of bicarbonate[72].

Although it is not well described in the literature, it appears that a diet deficient in vegetables and fruits may reduce the body's buffering capacity. Such an outcome might manifest as subtle shifts toward an acidic pH, which may enhance the nociceptive and inflammatory potential in local tissues.

INADEQUATE POTASSIUM INTAKE

General information

A total of 98% of body potassium, or 140 mEq/l, is found in the intracellular fluid and 80% of this is found in muscles. Only 2% of body potassium, or 4 mEq/l, is found in the extracellular fluid[483].

A general biochemistry text tells us that a deficiency in potassium usually occurs secondary to illness, injury or diuretic therapy and can cause muscular weakness, paralysis, and mental confusion. In contrast, symptoms of potassium toxicity include cardiac arrest and small bowel ulcers[295].

A general physiology book provides us with more detailed information about potassium function. Potassium depletion decreases insulin secretion. Potassium depleted patients, such as those with primary hyperaldosteronism, develop diabetic glucose tolerance curves. These curves are restored to normal with potassium repletion[161-p.282]. Forbes recently reported that potassium had been used at least as early as 1946 to help treat diabetic patients[621].

Potassium also influences acid-base balance. Potassium depletion appears to produce an intracellular acidosis as H^+ is secreted into the urine. As H^+ is removed from the body, HCO_3^- resorption increases which causes extracellular alkalosis[161-p.613].

Potassium has also demonstrated a dilator capacity and probably plays a role in the dilation that occurs in muscles[161-p.493]. A lack of vasodilation may result in ischemia and hypoxia. As described in Chapter 1, tissue hypoxia is pro-inflammatory. Thus, an inadequate intake of potassium may promote the pro-inflammatory state because potassium is needed to promote vasoperfusion and prevent hypoxia.

Potassium and vasoperfusion

Most physiology texts mention that potassium has a vasodilator effect on the microvasculature of muscles[31a, 161, 177-p.317]. Guyton lists several factors which cause vasodilation in local blood vessels: a lack of oxygen, excess carbon dioxide, hydrogen ions, adenosine, lactic acid, increased potassium ions and decreased body temperature[177-p.317]. Exactly which vessels respond to these metabolites is not clear. It appears that arterioles, metarterioles, capillaries and venules may all vasodilate (or vasorelax) in the presence of these metabolites[31a-p.483, 161-p.493-96, 177-p.317]. In addition, arteries, arterioles, metarterioles and veins all have sympathetic innervation. Reduced sympathetic activity can cause vasorelaxation, while increased sympathetic activity can cause vasoconstriction[177-p.331, 161-p.495]. Ganong suggests that only capillaries and venules are devoid of sympathetic vasoconstrictor innervation[161-p.495].

To what degree is potassium important in the vasodilation of muscle microcirculation? Both the Ganong and Berne texts would suggest that potassium is of neutral importance. As mentioned earlier, Ganong states that potassium has demonstrated a dilator capacity and probably plays a role in the dilation that occurs in muscles[161, p.493].

Here is how Berne's text on physiology describes potassium's dilator function. Consider the following quote:

> "Potassium release occurs with the onset of skeletal muscle contraction or an increase in cardiac activity and could be responsible for the initial decrease in vascular resistance observed with exercise or increased cardiac work. However, K+ release is not sustained, despite continued arteriolar dilation throughout the period of enhanced muscle activity. Therefore some other agent must serve as mediator of the vasodilation associated with greater metabolic activity of the tissue."[31a-p.483]

Berne[31a-p.484] suggests that adenosine may be the molecule responsible for vasodilation in exercising muscle, and that some of the prostaglandins may also function as vasodilators in certain vascular beds.

Speciality texts devoted specifically to potassium indicate that potassium is much more important than standard physiology texts would lead us to believe. The vasodilatory effect of potassium has been well studied during exercise. According to Knochel[241], at rest, normal blood flow averages only about 1 ml/100 grams of muscle weight per minute. During intense physical work, muscle blood flow may approach 40 ml/100 gm/minute. Factors other than potassium can influence blood flow during exercise such as adenine nucleotides, vasodilatory peptides, hypoxia, and a drop in pH; however, it is known that flow rate varies directly with the quantity of potassium released from contracting muscles. Experiments have demonstrated that potassium release from muscles is the key to vasodilation.

> "It can be shown clearly in the endogenously perfused isolated gracilis muscle preparation of the dog that under conditions of potassium deficiency, muscle cell contraction is not associated with release of potassium ions, and, in addition, muscle blood flow does not increase...the lack of adequate blood flow to deliver energy substrates or provide removal of heat and metabolites can lead to ischemic damage...if potassium is infused directly into the arterial supply of a working, potassium deficient muscle, blood flow is restored toward normal."[241]

The ischemic damage referred to in the previous paragraph can result in muscle cell necrosis, also called rhabdomyolysis[241]. Dorland's Medical Dictionary defines rhabdomyolysis as the disintegration or dissolution of muscle[118-p.1354]. Rhabdomyolysis is not common in humans. The majority of cases seem to occur in patients who have become potassium deficient due to diuretic use.

As rhabdomyolysis is not a common problem, it is likely that frank potassium deficiency is not commonly seen in the general population. Unfortunately, the potassium literature concentrates mostly on either overt deficiencies or toxicities. Thus, we are left to hypothesize how an inadequate intake may influence the average individual who is not extremely ill.

Information related to muscle physiology can help us better understand how potassium inadequacy may detrimentally effect the average patient. "Studies in a number of animal species and humans have shown that, when a muscle cell is depolarized immediately before contraction begins, potassium is released into the interstitial fluid, bathing muscle arterioles"[240]. Potassium release causes vasodilation and the increased muscle blood flow is required for substrate delivery, metabolic waste removal, and for muscle cooling[240]. We should consider these important functions in light of the fact that the temperature of exercising muscles can reach 106° F when a normal human works on a treadmill at 50% of maximum oxygen utilization[240].

Clearly, we should consider the problem of insufficient potassium intake when patients begin exercise or rehabilitation programs. Potassium insufficiencies may reduce vasodilation and result in some degree of ischemia and hypoxic injury. Recent evidence supports this contention. As mentioned in Chapter 1, muscle contraction normally activates KATP channels which allows for the release of potassium and a subsequent metabolic inhibition of sympathetic vasoconstriction[828].

Potassium, hypoxia and reduced ATP synthesis

On a biochemical level, hypoxia equates with reduced ATP production. This is because aerobic pathways (Krebs cycle and electron transport) are the producers of ATP. Glucose enters the cell and then anaerobic glycolysis converts glucose into pyruvate. In the presence of oxygen, pyruvate is converted into acetyl-CoA which enters the Krebs cycle. This information is relevant to our discussion of potassium because potassium deficiency can 1) impair glucose utilization, 2) impair insulin release in response to hyperglycemia, and 3) reduce glycogen stores in skeletal muscle[240]. Consider the following quote:

"Of clinical importance, potassium deficiency could induce simple glucose intolerance in otherwise normal individuals or, more importantly, result in gross

exacerbations of glucose intolerance in patients with preexistent diabetes mellitus"[240].

Inefficient glucose utilization may also play a role in the pathogenesis of musculoskeletal conditions such as fibromyalgia[1, 219]. Research has shown that tender points in muscles of fibromyalgia patients can have a 17% reduction in ATP production and a 19% reduction in phosphocreatine (PC)[28]. It has also been demonstrated that there are changes in blood flow within the muscles of fibromyalgia patients. One study showed that there is a maldistribution of capillary blood in tender points, and another study demonstrated that blood flow during exercise is reduced in fibromyalgia patients. Whether the reduction in ATP or PC was due to glucose dysregulation or reduced blood supply is not known[219]. Perhaps both play a role, and perhaps insufficient potassium intake was one of several contributing factors.

The idea that potassium inadequacy can influence the pathogenesis of muscular pain is not new. Travell states that a potassium deficiency can aggravate trigger points[449-p. 142]; however, she does not provide a mechanism. She does mention, however, that potassium deficiency disturbs the function of smooth muscle and cardiac muscle. We should remember that blood vessels contain smooth muscle cells which relax in the presence of potassium ions. Perhaps then, potassium deficiency may magnify or promote the development of trigger points by reducing vasorelaxation which may promote hypoxia. This proposal is consistent with Travell's contention that trigger points are specific regions in muscles that are characterized by increased metabolism and decreased circulation[449-p.36]. With this in mind, we should remember Dr. Travell's words when she wrote that nutritional factors "*must* be considered in most patients if lasting relief of pain is to be achieved," and that potassium is one of several "nutrients of special concern in patients with myofascial pain syndromes[449-p.114]."

Patients who have become hypokalemic due to potassium deficiency complain of malaise, muscular weakness and a poorly definable myalgia (the author did not clarify what constitutes potassium deficiency)[241]. Most patients entering a doctor's office complain of aches, pain and fatigue. This is not to suggest that these complaints are solely due to potassium deficiency; however, perhaps inadequate intake of potassium plays a role in the generation of these symptoms.

Potassium deficiency in humans

Travell suggests that potassium deficiency can develop when people consume a diet that is high in fat, refined sugar and sodium. The likelihood of becoming deficient increases if a patient takes laxatives and/or potassium wasting diuretics, and when a patient has diarrhea[449-p.142].

Potassium intake varies greatly among people around the world. The people of Scotland consume an average of 46 mEq (1,789 mg) per day and Tibetans consume approximately 20 mEq (778 mg) per day. In the United States, urban whites consume approximately 65 mEq (2527 mg) per day, while southeastern blacks average about 25-30 mEq (975-1166 mg) per day[448]. The mean intake for 15- to 20-year olds is approximately 87 mEq (3,400 mg)[481-p.256]. These values pale when compared to what hunter-gatherers are thought to have consumed. There are still a handful of humans living as hunter-gatherers, and a dietary analysis revealed that they consume between 200-285 mEq (7,778-11,083 mg) of potassium per day[448].

Based on the statistics listed in the paragraph above, it is clear that we consume approximately 75% less potassium than our hunter-gatherer ancestors who consumed low-sodium and high-potassium foods including wild game, roots, fruits, tubers, nuts, grains, and seeds[448]. It is thought that a high potassium diet is natural for man. Our modern low potassium diet is thought to be unnatural and may promote physiologic abnormalities[448]. These concerns were made clear at least as early as 1976[725]. Meneely and Batterbee explain that, "by the time man-like creatures came into being two millions years ago, many physiological mechanisms were firmly encoded in the genes"[725]. They discuss the abnormally high sodium intake of modern man and indicate that "there has hardly been enough time for the genetic material to alter in a favorable adaptation."

It must be understood that modern food consumption surveys demonstrate that our intake of vegetables and fruits is remote from recommended levels[36]. As vegetables and fruits are known to be good sources of potassium[295] the likelihood that many Americans may suffer from potassium inadequacies of varying degrees is quite large. It should also be noted that different sources of vegetables can have very different levels of potassium and sodium. In 1976, Meneely and Batterbee provided us with a table of data which demonstrates another way modern man has promoted potassium deficiency[725]. In a 100g edible portion of fresh peas there is a 380mg/0.9mg ratio of potassium to sodium. The same portion from frozen peas provides a 160/100 ratio and canned peas possess a 180/230 ratio of potassium to sodium. So, when we speak of increasing fruit and vegetable consumption, we are referring to fresh produce, *not* frozen or canned.

It is important to be aware of the fact that the Recommended Dietary Allowance (RDA) for potassium does not reflect the importance of consuming more potassium-rich foods. We are told that 40-50 mEq (1,600-2,000 mg) per day is the minimum requirement and the actual RDA for adults is 90 mEq (3,500 mg) per day[481-p.256]. In a review of the literature by Tobian[448] he indicates that the people of China and Japan have an average intake of about 45 mEq (1,750 mg) of potassium per day, a value that is accepted as the minimum daily requirement by the RDA. It is known that the stroke rate in China and Japan is very much higher than that in certain western countries [and the people of Tibet (20 mEq per day) have a higher stroke rate than the Chinese and Japanese]. One study reviewed the eating habits of two adjoining farming districts in Japan.

> "Farmers living in the Aamori district eat 8 to 10 apples per day, whereas those in the Akita prefecture do not and eat more rice instead. The consumption of this many apples would provide a greater potassium intake and possibly a lower sodium intake as well, and it is clear that the people of the apple eating district have a significantly lower stroke rate than those in the district where rice is consumed."[448]

Clearly, it is probably a wise choice to follow the eating habits of our hunter-gatherer ancestors who consumed large quantities of potassium-rich foods. Vegetarian diets somewhat resemble this historical eating pattern and it has been suggested that an optimal level of potassium consumption may be the reason for a reduced incidence of hypertension among vegetarians[741]. Based on this information, we should seriously consider the possibility that the RDAs for potassium may actually be hazardous to our health.

Cerebrovascular disease, heart disease, and cancer

Animal experiments and population studies have demonstrated that dietary deficiencies are thought to increase one's risk of developing hypertension and stroke[448]. At least as early as 1976, researchers were mobilizing to promote the consumption of a high potassium diet to reduce hypertension. "The evidence indicates that a systematic effort to reduce dietary sodium chloride intake and increase dietary potassium intake would result in the amelioration of much suffering among those who are prone and would increase both duration and quality of life for many millions of people"[725]. Unfortunately, progress was slow and people did little to change. As of 1989 there were at least seven studies that showed a decrease in blood pressure when supplemental potassium was added to the diet[448]. More recently, several papers have asserted that a so-called high potassium diet can help reduce blood pressure[439, 549, 826].

Regarding strokes, cardiovascular disease, and cancer, the following quote comes from an article published in the *New England Journal of Medicine*.

"Our findings support that hypothesis that a high incidence of potassium from food sources protects against stroke-associated death in a human population. A 10-mmol increase in daily potassium intake (approximately one serving of fresh fruit or vegetables) was associated with a 40 percent reduction in risk. These findings need confirmation and are, on their own, inadequate to support the broad recommendation of a high-potassium diet. However, there is no evidence that increasing the customary intake of potassium-rich foods — fruits and vegetables — by one or two servings a day is harmful in the general population in Western societies. Evidence suggests that whatever the mechanisms, these foods might be beneficial not only for the prevention of cardiovascular disease, but also possibly for the prevention of cancer."[230]

From one perspective, this quote is good because it suggests that Americans should consume more fruits and vegetables; however, it is ridiculous the way they subtly imply that these *foods are drugs which are possibly harmful if consumed in large amounts.* When have we ever heard of anyone becoming dreadfully ill or dying because of excessive vegetable and fruit intake?

The manner in which appropriate potassium intake can reduce the development of hypertension and stroke is not precisely understood. Suter has recently reviewed the literature and suggested that increased potassium consumption may involve several mechanisms. These include effects on natriuresis, baroreflex sensitivity, direct vasodilatory functions, catecholaminergic functions, improved glucose tolerance, and modulation of the renein-angiotensin-aldosterone system[826]. Young et al. explain that optimal levels of dietary potassium may protect against cardiovascular diseases by: 1) inhibiting free radical formation from vascular endothelial cells and macrophages; 2) inhibiting proliferation of vascular smooth muscle cells; 3) inhibiting platelet aggregation and arterial thrombosis; and 4) reducing renal vascular resistance and increasing glomerular filtration[861].

Research has also demonstrated that appropriate potassium intake may influence cardiovascular disease in a way that is not related to hypertension. Vascular endothelial cells release a substance called endothelium-derived relaxing factor (EDRF). Research has demonstrated that when EDRF is released from endothelial cells, it serves to inhibit platelet adhesion to endothelial cells and also inhibits platelet aggregation. Severe hypertension in spontaneously hypertensive stroke-prone rats (SHRsp) on a high NaCl diet causes injury to endothelial cells, causing them to release much lower quantities of endothelium-derived relaxing factor (EDRF). However, when SHRsp on a high NaCl diet were given supplements of potassium citrate, it was found that the endothelial cell's capacity for releasing EDRF was completely preserved even though blood pressure remained the same[448].

As mentioned above, optimal potassium ingestion may also prevent the development of cancer. Jansson[666, 667, 668, 669, 670, 671] has researched this subject for the past 20 years and recently explained that agents which are known to be carcinogenic act to decrease cellular concentration of potassium and increase sodium levels[671].

"In aging potassium leaves the cells, sodium enters them, and the rates of cancer increase. Patients with hyperkalemic diseases (Parkinson's and Addison's disease) have reduced cancer rates, and patients with hypokalemic diseases (alcoholism, obesity, stress) have increased cancer rates."[671]

In summary, cardiovascular disease, cerebrovascular disease and cancer constitute the leading causes of death in America and evidence suggests that insufficient potassium intake may play a pathogenic role. Insufficient potassium intake may also play an etiologic role in the development of diabetes and skeletal myopathology. Unfortunately, the approach that many will take is that *we need to treat people with high potassium diets*, as if high potassium diets are drugs. This is a ridiculous notion. We are naturally [or innately] predisposed to consume a diet rich in alkaline buffers, potassium, and antioxidants, and now we consume one that is deficient. We should simply re-learn how to eat properly.

INADEQUATE MAGNESIUM INTAKE

Elin states that, "Mg deficiency effects a *pro-inflammatory* condition with an excessive production of oxygen-derived free radicals"[129a]. Magnesium is also a key nutrient in glycolysis and the aerobic pathways which generate ATP[1, 466-p.428, 482]. Thus, it is possible that deficiencies may reduce ATP synthesis, enhance lactic acid production, and

promote tissue hypoxia, i.e., a pro-inflammatory state. Magnesium deficiency can also enhance platelet aggregation[407], which was already described in Chapter 3 as a pro-inflammatory event. Supplementation with magnesium seems to reduce the symptoms of fibromyalgia[1], increase cellular energy production[121a], and help relieve migraine headaches[612, 720, 765].

General information

"Approximately half the total Mg pool in the body is present intracellularly in soft tissues and the other half is present in bone. Less than 1% of the total body Mg is present in blood ...magnesium is the second most abundant intracellular cation and is a cofactor in more than 300 enzymatic reactions involving energy metabolism and protein and nucleic acid synthesis."[129a]

Some of these reactions involve regulation of cellular energy metabolism, complexation with phospholipids in membranes, second messenger for hormonal responses, activation of hormone receptors and many, many more[51-p.112-16]. Because magnesium is involved in so many aspects of cell function, it is likely that magnesium inadequacy plays a role in many disease processes. Indeed, Elin indicates that several diseases have been linked to a disorder in magnesium metabolism, such as chronic fatigue syndrome, diabetes mellitus, PMS, and cardiovascular disorders [acute myocardial infarction, atherosclerosis, hypertension, and arrhythmias][129a]. Accordingly, Wester and Dyckner state that symptoms of magnesium deficiency principally occur from the nervous system, skeletal muscles, digestive tract and cardiovascular system. Symptoms from the central nervous system often begin with depression as well as an inefficient memory and a lack of concentration[850], which are common presentations in the clinical setting. Rude, who describes magnesium deficiency as a cause of heterogenous disease in humans, has recently provided a list of conditions that may manifest in response to magnesium deficiency such as hypocalcemia, osteoporosis, seizures, vertigo, ataxia, depression, psychosis, cardiac arrhythmias, myocardial ischemia/infarction, hypertension, and atherosclerosis[782]. Surprisingly, the 1989 RDA book makes no mention of any relationship between magnesium deficiency and disease[481-p.187-92].

Magnesium deficiency in humans?

The best sources of magnesium are vegetables, fish, whole grains and nuts, and none are major constituents of the average American diet[406]. Green vegetables are probably the best source, as fish and meat contain protein and phosphate which interfere with magnesium absorption[850]. Several dietary factors are poor sources of magnesium and many increase magnesium need such as fat, sugar, salt, vitamin D, organic phosphate, protein and supplemental calcium, and all are high in the average American diet[406].

Magnesium excretion can be increased by various medications, diabetes mellitus, renal tubular disorders, hypercalcemia, hyperthyroidism, aldosteronism, excessive lactation, stress, and alcoholism[609]. Regarding alcohol, studies with normal subjects has demonstrated that alcohol consumption increases magnesium excretion[721]. This suggests that social drinkers with marginal magnesium intake may be at risk for developing magnesium deficiency. Additionally, it has been known for years that several diseases can reduce magnesium absorption such as ulcerative colitis, regional enteritis and gluten enteropathy[609]. It is now known that subclinical celiac disease is common[546], which may alter magnesium absorption in patients who presumed to be healthy.

Morgan simply states that a low intake of magnesium is pandemic[320]. Linder echoes this statement by indicating that many individuals consume much less magnesium than the RDA[275-p.194]. To determine if the statements of Morgan and Linder were accurate, we at NutrAnalysis performed a dietary analysis on a random sample of 44 patients and found that 64% were below the RDA for magnesium. Even the RDA book agrees; it states that the mean intake of magnesium by males and females falls short of the RDA[481-p.190-91]. More recently, Rude reported that the Food and Nutrition Board of the Institute of Medicine has increased the RDA from 280 mg/day to 320 mg/

day for women and for men the RDA has been raised from 350 mg/day to 420 mg/day[782]. These recommendations are substantially higher than estimated intakes for women and men which average 228 mg and 323 mg respectively[782]. Abraham and Grewel explain the that RDA of magnesium for Russian women ranges from 500 to 1250 mg, depending on the physiologic conditions[534]. These authors state that "the US RDA of magnesium, based on short-term balance studies, probably is the minimum daily intake of magnesium that the human body can adjust to but at the cost of increased susceptibility to stress and, very probably, postmenopausal osteoporosis"[534].

Seelig has reviewed the relationship between magnesium deficiency and stress[407]. As it turns out, mental stressors can promote magnesium deficiency and magnesium deficiency can enhance the stress response. The increased levels of catecholamines and glucocorticoids that are released during the stress response are known to reduce intestinal magnesium absorption. In addition, magnesium deficiency can cause an excessive release of stress hormones which will further lower tissue levels of magnesium. This relationship may be particularly relevant for patients with Type A personalities who maintain an ongoing level of self-sustained stress and also tend to have exaggerated responses to external stressors[407].

Cardiovascular disease and cancer

Numerous papers have discussed the relationship between magnesium deficiency and cardiovascular disease, including atherogenesis, myocardial infarction, and arrhythmias[537, 646, 658, 698, 743, 781, 804, 812, 862]. Low magnesium/calcium ratios promote an excessive release or formation of vasoconstrictive and platelet aggregating factors such as thromboxane A2. This is of particular concern for those who have increased levels of saturated fat in their diet. Magnesium deficiency can also worsen saturated fat-induced hypercoagulation and atherogenesis[407]. In 1976, Scott stated that, "as magnesium deficiency has been implicated by experimental and epidemiological evidence in the aetiology of ischemic heart disease, magnesium may in the future assume even greater importance in clinical medicine"[792]. Over 20 years later, still very few laymen and health care practitioners appreciate the prevalence or significance of magnesium deficiency.

Regarding cancer, in 1988, Elin wrote that the link between magnesium metabolism and cancer may be a fruitful areas for future studies[609]. At that time, animal studies demonstrated that deficiencies in magnesium could promote certain types of cancer, such as malignancies of the thymus. Other studies described how magnesium deficiency could alter hepatic leukopoietic maturation factors, humoral and cellular immunity, and the fidelity of DNA, and thus perhaps promote cancer. While there may be a relationship between magnesium deficiency and cancer promotion, very little research has been done in this area.

The benefits of magnesium supplementation

Studies involving the use of magnesium supplements have revealed important information. Dreosti reviewed the literature and reported that magnesium supplementation is associated with improved strength and well-being[121a]. In another study, competitive male rowers were supplemented with 500 mg of magnesium or a placebo. Results from oxygen uptake markers indicated that only the supplemented group demonstrated a more effective use of oxygen for energy production[121a]. In a similar study, moderately trained men received either 387 mg of magnesium or a placebo. Strenuous exercise on a cycloergometer demonstrated that only the supplemental group had significant reductions in heart rate, volume of oxygen consumed and volume of carbon dioxide produced[121a], which again suggests improved aerobic function. It is thought that the improvements in athletic performance from magnesium supplementation occur due to a correction of a marginal magnesium deficiency, and *not* because supplementation created a performance-enhancing, supranormal magnesium status.

The most profound results of magnesium supplementation have been reported in studies

devoted to osteoporosis. This may come as a surprise to some because calcium is always the focus nutrient for osteoporosis, to the point where women are told to consume at least 1000 mg of calcium each day [many reach this by supplementation]. Considering that the mean intake of magnesium by adult women is 207 mg/day [which is 80 mg below the RDA[481-p.187-92]], this creates a Ca:Mg ratio of greater than 4:1, rather than the recommended 2:1 ratio[121a]. Such a ratio may reduce the efficiency of magnesium absorption[121a] and therefore, exacerbate the deficiency produced by inadequate intake. Consider the outcome of magnesium supplementation on osteoporotic women.

"In a group of postmenopausal women in Israel suffering from osteoporosis who received 250-750 mg/day for 24 months, either trabecular bone increased (up to 8%) or bone loss was arrested (in 87%); in some cases both an increase in bone density and arrested bone loss occurred. Untreated controls, on the other hand, lost bone density at an average of 1% a year."[121a]

"In a group of postmenopausal osteoporotic patients in Czechoslovakia who received magnesium at levels ranging from 1500 to 3000 mg of magnesium lactate per day for 2 years, nearly 65% were classified as totally free of pain with no further deformity of vertebrae, with the condition in the remainder either arrested or slightly improved."[121a]

Although the RDA presents statistics which clearly indicate that the average American's intake of magnesium is inadequate, it does not mention that such inadequacies can promote magnesium depletion. Also, there is no mention of the potential harmful consequences of marginal intake, or the potential benefits of supplementation.

Suggestions for supplementation

The RDA states that, "there is no evidence that large oral intakes of magnesium are harmful to people with normal renal function"[481-p.192]. They do not specify what they mean by "large amounts;"

however, they state that early symptoms hypermagnesemia include nausea, vomiting, and hypotension[481-p.192], which clearly implies that one should be careful not to take too much magnesium. With this information in mind, we should recall that certain osteoporotic women in Czechoslovakia took 3000 mg of magnesium per day for up to 2 years, which allowed 65% of subjects to become pain-free. Also recall that supplementation with 387 mg of magnesium significantly improved the aerobic capacity of subjects tested on cycloergometers. Finally, recall that the RDA of magnesium for Russian women ranges from 500 to 1250 mg[534]. Based on a review of the literature, one would have to agree with Bucci who suggests that supplementation with 400-1000 mg/day in divided doses is quite reasonable[51-p.112-16].

This brings us to the topic of specific supplements. What is the best form of magnesium supplement to take? There is a long list to choose from; however, there are two general types of magnesium supplements, i.e., inorganic and organic salts. Inorganic magnesium salts include magnesium oxide, sulfate, chloride, and carbonate, while organic chelates include magnesium ascorbate, aspartate, citrate, fumarate, gluconate, lactate, malate, and orotate[51-p.112-16]. One study compared absorption from citrate and oxide, and found that there was substantially greater absorption from magnesium citrate as compared to magnesium oxide[707]. Magnesium citrate was more soluble and bioavailable than magnesium oxide[707]. Another study determined that magnesium-L-aspartate-HCL showed significantly greater absorption than magnesium oxide[733]. These studies suggest that the organic salts of magnesium offer better absorption than the inorganic variety. Shils indicates that the poor solubility and absorption of magnesium oxide and hydroxide is the basis for their use as osmotic laxatives[805].

A word on citrates and ascorbates. Most practitioners are aware that high doses of ascorbic acid can induce diarrhea by altering osmotic balance in the gut. The same seems to be true of citrates. In my experience, patients seem to tolerate magnesium fumarate and malate better than citrates and ascorbates.

FREE RADICALS

A free radical is defined as a very reactive and unstable molecule because it has an unpaired electron in its outer orbital[147]. By design, nature builds atoms and molecules such that they have paired electrons. When a free radical is formed, it very readily gives up or accepts an electron to stabilize its unpaired electron. This exchange of electrons is very damaging to cellular structures.

Free radicals are thought to damage lipids, proteins, membranes and DNA[14, 37, 92-p.10, 109, 110, 248]. In addition, it is becoming increasingly apparent that free radicals may initiate and/or amplify inflammation by upregulating several different genes involved in the inflammatory process, such as those that encode for pro-inflammatory cytokines and adhesion molecules[586]. Free radical activity is thought to be involved in the pathogenesis of a host of degenerative diseases including cancer, cataracts, aging, altered immunity, diabetes, liver disease, multiple sclerosis, heart disease, macular degeneration, Parkinson's disease, Alzheimer's disease, AIDS, and arthritis[103, 116, 121, 162, 191, 215a, 280, 287, 309, 394, 432, 460, 473, 538, 560, 586, 604, 628, 647, 648, 649, 653, 717, 732, 761, 816, 824, 836].

To many people, the term "antioxidant" is synonymous with a nutritional supplement rather than a family of nutrients found in fruits and vegetables. Scientific research often focuses around individual supplemental nutrients. In this regard, it should be understood that the use of specific supplements in the treatment of various diseases typically does not prove to be particularly effective. For example, Flagg et al. reported that the preliminary results of research trials do not support a protective effect of antioxidant supplementation against cancer[616]. Similarly, van der Vijver et al. state that general population measures involving antioxidant supplementation to prevent cardiovascular disease is not supported by the literature and is not yet justifiable[836]. Some studies show that supplementation with vitamin E, C, and beta-carotene may be of help; however, we usually hear and read about how the evidence is unconvincing and equivocal at best. It is important to put these results in the proper context.

The typical modern diet is known to be disease-promoting from several perspectives, i.e., too much of the wrongs fats, not enough of the good fats, insufficient fiber, too much alcohol, and inadequate amounts of fruits and vegetables. Smoking and lack of exercise are additional lifestyle choices that are very common. When study subjects have diets and lifestyles of such poor quality, it would be highly unlikely that a single supplement will have any positive effect; there are simply too many confounding factors. Moreover, it should be understood that this type of study is not about nutrition and lifestyle management. Instead, this type of study views vitamins as if they are drugs to be given as the sole measure to treat a given condition. When sufficient efficacy is not demonstrated in such a study, the specific antioxidant is often pronounced to be ineffective in preventing or treating a specific disease. The public and many nutrition-oriented doctors who utilize nutritional supplements would do well to accept these results for what they represent, and realize that this variety of study will *never* demonstrate the effectiveness of nutrition in the prevention and treatment of disease.

In contrast with the single antioxidant studies discussed in the previous paragraph, epidemiologic studies have demonstrated that, "one of the most consistent findings in dietary research is that those who consume higher amounts of fruits and vegetables have lower rates of heart disease and stroke as well as cancer"[628]. For example, "for most cancer sites, persons with low fruit and vegetable intake (at least the lower one-fourth of the population) experience about twice the risk of cancer compared with those with high intake, even after control for potentially confounding factors"[560]. These epidemiologic studies very often suggest that the *antioxidant component* in the fruits and vegetables was responsible for the protection against disease. This conclusion seemingly contradicts the conclusions from "single antioxidant research" which suggested that *antioxidants may not be of much benefit* in the treatment or prevention of disease.

These conflicting conclusions illustrate the problems associated with trying to study individual nutrients in the treatment of disease. No food contains just "one" nutrient. Furthermore, all

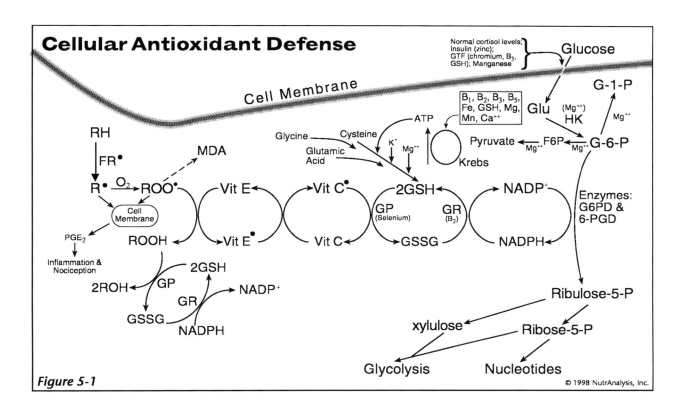

Cellular Antioxidant Defense

Figure 5-1

© 1998 NutrAnalysis, Inc.

foods, particularly fruits and vegetables, contain nutrients that cannot be found in a vitamin bottle which may have disease-fighting properties. Additionally, "single vitamin research" does not take body metabolism into account and subsequently consider that numerous nutrients work in concert with one another to generate a disease-inhibiting effect. These issues will be discussed more in the following paragraphs.

Cellular antioxidant defense

As mentioned above, it is somewhat pointless to view antioxidant defense from the perspective of individual nutrients. This is because numerous nutrients participate in the ongoing process of cellular antioxidant defense (see *Figure 5-1*). The information in this image was derived from several sources[57, 82, 108, 134, 155, 182, 232, 270, 275-p.249, 332, 343, 382, 482, 498]. Sen refers to this defense system as an antioxidant chain reaction. Sen provides a similar image and includes lipoic acid in the chain reaction, such that lipoic acid may play a role in reducing oxidized vitamin E and glutathione[802].

It is well known that polyunsaturated fatty acids (RH) in cell membranes are susceptible to free radical (FR·) attack, the result being the production of a fatty acid or lipid radical (R·). If R· is exposed to oxygen, it will be converted into a lipid peroxyl radical (ROO·). One way in which such free radicals can promote inflammation, nociception, pain, and various diseases is by the liberating arachidonic acid from cell membranes which promotes the production of PGE-2.

Vitamin E is capable of reducing R· back to RH, and ROO· into a lipid hydroperoxide (ROOH). If ROO· is not reduced, then it can be converted into malondialdehyde (MDA). MDA is a nasty molecule, known as a bifunctional aldehyde, which can efficiently and irreversibly cross-link biological macromolecules such as proteins, phospholipids and nucleic acids[270-p.37-38]. MDA is considered to be cytotoxic, mutagenic and tumorigenic. It is also thought to be involved in the formation of aging pigments[498-p.79]. It is known that MDA is a major metabolite of arachidonic acid[498-p.68].

Notice that both R· and ROO· can also interact with cell membranes. Free radicals are thought to stimulate membrane phospholipase A-2 which causes arachidonic acid release, and the subsequent formation of prostaglandin E-2[108]. Once again, recall that PGE-2 plays a role in the sensitization of nociceptors and acts to drive the inflammatory process, both of which play a role in the pathogenesis of joint complex dysfunction.

When vitamin E reduces ROO· to ROOH, it then becomes oxidized (Vit E·). In essence, Vit E now becomes a free radical (Vit E·). Vitamin C is known to convert Vit E· back into its reduced state (Vit E), after which, Vit C becomes a free radical (Vit C·). Similarly, reduced glutathione (GSH) converts Vit C· back into its reduced state (Vit C), after which, GSH becomes oxidized (GSSG). The enzyme glutathione peroxidase (GP) (selenium-dependent) is required for this conversion. GSSG is then converted back into GSH through the action of riboflavin-dependent glutathione reductase (GR) which utilizes NADPH.

Notice how the body makes GSH and NADPH. GSH production requires ATP synthesis which occurs during the oxidation of glucose via glycolysis, the Krebs cycle, and the electron transport chain. Several nutrients are required for ATP synthesis including vitamins B1, B2, B3, B5, K, Mg, Ca, and GSH itself (see Chapter 8). Amino acids which serve as substrates for GSH production include cysteine, glycine and glutamic acid. The enzymes involved in GSH synthesis utilize magnesium and potassium.

NADPH is synthesized by the hexose monophosphate shunt (HMS). The enzymes which convert $NADP^+$ into NADPH include glucose-6-phosphate dehydrogenase (G6PD) and 6-phosphogluconate dehydrogenase. Recall that the "N" in NADPH stands for niacin, also known as vitamin B-3.

We should keep in mind that both glycolysis and the HMS require the presence of glucose. Glucose entry into cells requires appropriate insulin sensitivity and the glucose tolerance factor (GTF). Zinc deficiency may impair insulin function[232] and several nutrients constitute the GTF moiety including chromium, niacin and GSH[275]. Both experimentally and clinically, manganese deficiency has been shown to impair glucose utilization; the exact mechanism of which is unknown[134, 332]. Also, recall that potassium deficiency can impair glucose utilization[240].

We should also be aware that hypercortisolemia can impair glucose utilization. Glucocorticoids are known to counteract the effects of insulin at numerous steps in glucose homeostasis, such that gluconeogenesis appears to be the net effect. Cortisol may also decrease the quantity of insulin receptors and reduce receptor affinity[57]. Cortisol will be discussed in more detail in Chapter 6.

In summary, numerous nutritional and metabolic factors influence free radical production. Clearly, the recommendation to take antioxidants to prevent free radical formation should be considered in light of the factors illustrated in *Figure 5-1*. Additionally, research efforts should take these biochemical pathways into consideration and avoid trying to test individual nutrients in the treatment of complex disease processes.

Phytochemicals

Vegetables and fruits are known to contain an abundance of antioxidant nutrients, including the vitamins and minerals listed in *Figure 5-1*. One common mineral that was not mentioned in *Figure 5-1* is potassium. While potassium is not a classic antioxidant, i.e., it does not provide reducing equivalents to oxidized molecules like vitamin C, E, and reduced glutathione, it does influence free radical activity. Research has led to the conclusion that "physiological increases in potassium concentration inhibit the rate of superoxide anion formation by cell lines derived from endothelium and from monocytes/macrophages and reactive oxygen species formation by human white blood cells"[718]. It is quite possible that this antioxidant benefit is derived from potassium's role as regulator of vasomotor tone.

In addition to important antioxidant vitamins and minerals, vegetables and fruits also contain a bewildering amount of important phytochemicals. Unfortunately, the average American's dietary intake of these foods is *remote* from recommended levels[36].

Craig refers to phytochemicals as the "guardians of our health"[590]. Vegetables, fruits, whole grains, and nuts contain an abundance of phenolic compounds, terpenoids, and carotenoids, which have been associated with protection against and/or treatment of many chronic diseases including heart disease, cancer, diabetes, hypertension, and many other diseases[590]. With respect to cancer, the types of fruits or vegetables which appear to offer the most protection include raw vegetables in general, followed by allium vegetables (garlic and onions), carrots, green vegetables, cruciferous vegetables (broccoli, Brussels sprouts, cabbage, cauliflower), and tomatoes[816]. Ginger, garlic, soybeans, cilantro, and parsley are thought to possess some of the highest anticancer activity[590]. The phytonutrients thought to be involved in cancer prevention include dithiolthiones, isothiocyanates, indole-3-carbinol, allium compounds, isoflavones, saponins, phytosterols, D-limonene, glucarates, lignins, carotenoids, lycopene, ellagic acid, and flavonoids[590, 816]. Most of the same foods and phytochemicals are thought to protect against heart disease, premenstrual syndrome, macular degeneration and other degenerative diseases. For example, earlier in this chapter a study was described in which rheumatoid arthritis patients were switched to a vegetable-based diet and subsequently had dramatic and long lasting reductions in pain and inflammation[237]. It is likely that phytochemicals were partly responsible for this beneficial response. In particular, flavonoids may have played a significant anti-arthritic role as they are known to act as antioxidants, reduce platelet aggregation, and have anti-inflammatory action[576, 590, 597, 706, 711, 714, 774].

Citrus fruits should be of special interest to most people as ascorbic acid is one of the most commonly used vitamin supplements. A quick review of the phytochemicals found in citrus will demonstrate why supplements cannot take the place of food. There are more than 170 phytochemicals in citrus fruits including some 60 different flavonoids, 40 limonoids, and 20 carotenoids[590]. No vitamin C supplement will ever by able to offer the same nutritional benefit as eating fresh citrus. The fact that people have become so enamored with vitamin C is surprising, for research in the late 1930's and early 1940s suggested that the flavonoid component of citrus fruits and certain vegetables offered health-promoting and disease-preventing benefits[739]. Back then, flavonoids were referred to as vitamin P. It appears that hesperidin and rutin were among the first flavonoids to receive attention[739].

Herbs and spices are substances which receive little attention as health promoting and disease preventing substances. Rosemary, sage, oregano, thyme, ginger, onion, and garlic possess many antioxidants, terpenoids, and phenols[590]. Liberal use of these substances instead of table salt is highly recommended. Numerous studies have been devoted to garlic and it appears that garlic consumption offers a significant anti-inflammatory and cytoprotective effect[535, 536, 562, 742]. Bordia et al. suggest that garlic and onions should be consumed raw rather than cooked to achieve a beneficial effect[562]. It appears that small amounts of garlic and onions should be consumed on a consistent basis to derive ongoing benefits. With respect to ginger, powdered ginger has been shown to provide significant anti-inflammatory effects[431].

In recent years, lycopene has received an increasing amount of attention. Lycopene is one of some 600 different members of the carotenoid family[573]. Beta carotene is the most well known carotenoid. Unlike beta carotene, lycopene and most other carotenoids do not have provitamin A activity. It is likely that lycopene functions as an antioxidant and may be of benefit in preventing cancer, heart disease, and other free radical generated diseases[579, 626, 629]. Tomatoes are the major source of lycopene in the diet, and the highest concentrations of lycopene are found in tomato paste and sauces. The uptake of lycopene was found to be greatest when sauces and paste are heated[626]. In addition to lycopene, tomatoes also contain vitamin E, trace elements, flavonoids, phytosterols, and several water soluble vitamins[552].

Examples of phenolic compounds include vanillin, sesamol, caffeic acid, ferulic acid, quercetin, epicatechin, epigallocatechin, ellagic acid, and curcumin[595]. These are found in berries, grapes, cloves, wine and tea. In recent years, wine has been a focus of attention due to the so-called "french paradox." Red wine drinkers in France were shown to have a reduced incidence of cardiovascular disease. At first, some thought that alcohol was responsible for this effect, but now it is generally agreed that the high concentration of phenolic compounds provided protection against heart disease[590, 656]. It should be understood that red wine and grape juice, but not white wine, contain significant levels of phenolic flavonoids and red anthocyanin pigments[590]. A recent study suggests that green tea may provide more phenols than grape juice or wine[840]. Phenols found in tea include gallic acid, catechin, epicatechin, epicatechin gallate, epigallocatechin, and epigallocatechin gallate[840].

While most view olive oil as a source of monounsaturated fatty acids, it is also known that olive oil contains an abundance of phytochemicals, and the highest concentration is found in extra virgin olive oil[842]. For example, extra virgin olive oil contains tocopherols, alkanols, sterols, terpenes flavonoids, anthocyanins, and phenols such as hydroxytyrosil, tyrosil, vanillic acid and caffeic acid[842]. Wiseman et al. suggest that perhaps only extra virgin olive oil contains appreciable amounts of phenols[852]. There are thought to be numerous biologic effects of olive oil phenolics including inhibition of LDL oxidation, inhibition of platelet aggregation, reduced TXB2 and LTB4 production by activated leukocytes, enhanced nitric oxide generation by lipopolysaccharide-challenged murine macro-phages, and reduction of free radicals[759, 841, 842]. The radical scavenging properties of olive oil's polyphenols proved to be equally or more effective than vitamins C, E, and BHT (butylated hydroxytoluene)[842]. Olive oil is also known to be rich in squalene and Newmark[738] has recently proposed that it may play a major role in the cancer risk-reducing effect of olive oil.

This section on phytochemicals focussed on those found in vegetables, tomato sauce, herbs and spices, fruits, wine, tea, and olive oil, most of which constitute the mainstay of the traditional Mediterranean diet[645]. The Mediterranean diet is also naturally low in saturated fat and sugar, and high in omega-3 fatty acids[599, 601, 811]. A recent randomized trial suggests that patients following a cardioprotective Mediterranean diet have a prolonged survival rate and may also be protected against cancer[600].

In contrast, the standard American diet is high

in saturated fat, high in sugar (average intake is over 100 pounds/year per person), high in light beer, high in omega-6 fatty acids, high in *trans* fatty acids, low in extra virgin olive oil, extremely low in omega-3 fatty acids, and extremely low in vegetables and fruit. Block went as far as to say that our consumption of vegetables and fruit is *remote* from recommended levels[36]. Indeed, Craig recently explained that the average American eats only about 1 1/2 servings of vegetables per day and less than 1 serving of fruit per day[590]. A recent survey demonstrated that only 1 in 11 Americans meet the guidelines of at least 3 servings of vegetables per day and 2 servings of fruit. In fact, 1 in every 9 people surveyed said they ate no fruit or vegetable on the day of the survey. Finally 2 of 3 Americans surveyed stated that only 2 or fewer servings of vegetables and fruit were sufficient for good health[590].

Based on this information, it should not be a surprise to anyone that the American population is stricken with chronic pain, inflammation, obesity, chronic fatigue, and numerous degenerative diseases. To "remedy" (sic) this situation, the new food guide pyramid, in part, recommends that we consume a variety of refined grain products, various desserts, vegetable oils, margarine, and choose our remaining fat calories from whatever sources we want (see Chapter 7). There is no mention of olive oil, omega-3 fatty acids or phytochemicals.

The free radical-musculoskeletal connection

Of interest to chiropractors is the fact that free radicals promote the release of arachidonic acid from cell membranes with the subsequent production of prostaglandin E-2 and leukotriene B-4[96, 108, 248], both of which, as mentioned earlier, have the ability to sensitize nociceptors and drive the inflammatory process.

There is also evidence that free radical activity can directly promote spinal dysfunction. At the time of surgery, lipofuscin has been found in the nucleus pulposus and the inner and middle layers of the anulus fibrosis, regions associated with strong histologic degeneration. Lipofuscin was found in the discs of individuals older than 20 years of age. Lipofuscin is produced by the oxidation of lipids

or lipoprotein and is commonly referred to as the aging pigment[860].

In the past researchers have hypothesized that antioxidant abnormalities may be involved in the pathogenesis of fibromyalgia, as antioxidant supplementation has been effective in treating this condition. However, studies have demonstrated that lipid peroxidation levels are normal in fibromyalgia patients. In a recent study, researchers set out to determine if protein peroxidation is present in fibromyalgia patients. The results showed evidence of increased protein peroxidation, associated with thiol abnormalities and decreased levels of nitric oxide[610].

It is now common for chiropractors to include exercise in the office treatment plan and/or recommend that patients begin exercising at the home or gym. Practitioners need to be aware of the growing literature devoted to free radicals, antioxidants, and exercise. A recent review article discussed this issue in detail[802]. Animal studies have shown that antioxidant deficiencies increase free radical damage in exercising muscles. For example, vitamin E deficiency is known to enhance tissue lipid peroxidation, increase susceptibility of skeletal muscle to damage, increase fragility lysosomal membranes, compromise respiratory control ratio in skeletal muscle, increase sarcoplasmic and endoplasmic reticulum lesions, increase erythrocyte hemolysis, decrease oxidative phosphorylation in liver, and decrease exercise performance[802]. Human studies have shown that supplementation with antioxidant vitamins has favorable effects on lipid peroxidation after exercise, such that antioxidants and antioxidant enzymes can protect against exercise-induced muscle damage[898]. Dekkers et al. indicate that sufficient evidence warrants the use of antioxidant supplements for those who engage in regular heavy exercise[898]. Packer explains that, "there is little evidence that antioxidant supplementation can improve performance, but a large body of work suggest that bolstering antioxidant defences may ameliorate exercise-induced damage, suggesting that the benefits of antioxidant intervention may be for the long term rather than the short term"[744]. The prudent use of antioxidant supplements can provide insurance against a suboptimal diet and/

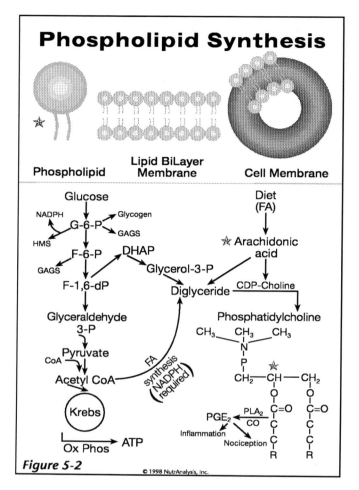

Phospholipid Synthesis

Phospholipid | Lipid BiLayer Membrane | Cell Membrane

Figure 5-2

© 1998 NutrAnalysis, Inc.

or the elevated demands of exercise training[679]. These considerations may be particularly applicable to patients with diabetes, pre-diabetes, and the aging population.

Research has demonstrated that diabetics and aging cells have a weakened antioxidant defense system. Atalay et al. explain that insulin depended diabetic patients have impaired antioxidant defences that may predispose these patients to increased resting and exercise-induced oxidative stress[747]. In addition, complications of diabetes may be generated, in part, by reduced antioxidant status and increased lipid peroxidation. Newly diagnosed NIDDM patients were suspected of having altered antioxidant status[545]. Improving glycemic regulation (see Chapter 6) and supplementing with antioxidants may be advisable for such patients.

Research has demonstrated that aging is associated with a decline in muscle mass, a reduction in functional capacity, and a decrease in cellular antioxidant defense, which makes the elderly more susceptible to oxidative stress and muscle injury. Exercise is recommended to reduce physical deconditioning, and dietary changes and antioxidant supplements should be included to help fight free radical pathology and to slow the age-dependent decline of functional capacity[727].

FATTY ACID IMBALANCES

Phospholipid synthesis

All cell membranes in the human body contain phospholipids. Cells have the inherent ability to produce their own phospholipids through various biochemical pathways. *Figure 5-2* demonstrates how glucose is taken through the glycolytic pathway and is converted into ATP. Notice that pathway and is converted into ATP. Notice that the six carbon fructose-1,6-diphosphate (F-1,6-diP) molecule is converted into glyceraldehyde-3-phosphate (G-3-P) and dihydroxyacetone phosphate (DHAP), both of which are three carbon molecules. G-3-P is ultimately converted into acetyl CoA and DHAP is converted into glycerol-3-phosphate.

Observe how a diglyceride is formed from the interaction of glycerol-3-phosphate, acetyl CoA and an essential fatty acid from the diet, in this case arachidonic acid. The diglyceride is then acted upon by CDP-choline to form phosphatidylcholine, which is a phospholipid found in cell membranes.

Depending upon the nature of the essential fatty acid, a phospholipid can be pro-inflammatory or anti-inflammatory. The phospholipid will be pro-inflammatory if arachidonic acid is incorporated. This is because arachidonic acid is converted into pro-inflammatory prostaglandin E-2 (PGE-2), prostacyclin (PGI-2), prostaglandin F-2 (PGF-2), leukotriene B-4 (LTB-4), and thromboxane A-2 (TXA-2). As mentioned earlier in this book, both PGE-2 and LTB-4 can sensitize nociceptors and drive the inflammatory process.

Arachidonic acid is found preformed in animal products, especially meat. In addition, linoleic acid can be converted into arachidonic acid. Linoleic acid is found in seeds, grains, nuts, and certain vegetables. Linoleic acid is also a precursor of dihomogamalinolenic acid (DGLA). DGLA is a precursor of PGE-1 and TXA-1, both of which are anti-inflammatory. Both arachidonic acid and linoleic acid are referred to as omega-6 (n-6 for short) fatty acids.

Cold water fish such as salmon, sardine, and mackerel contain preformed eicosapentaenoic acid (EPA) and docosahexaenoic acid (DHA). Green leafy vegetables and certain nuts and seeds contain α-linolenic acid which is a precursor to EPA. EPA, DHA and α-linolenic acid are referred to as omega-3 (n-3 for short) fatty acids, which are precursors for PGI-3, TXA-3, PGE-3 and LTB-5, all of which are anti-inflammatory.

This information regarding dietary sources of essential fatty acids and their inflammatory potential is well known[64, 127, 209, 248, 275-p.76, 318, 350, 414, 419, 485].

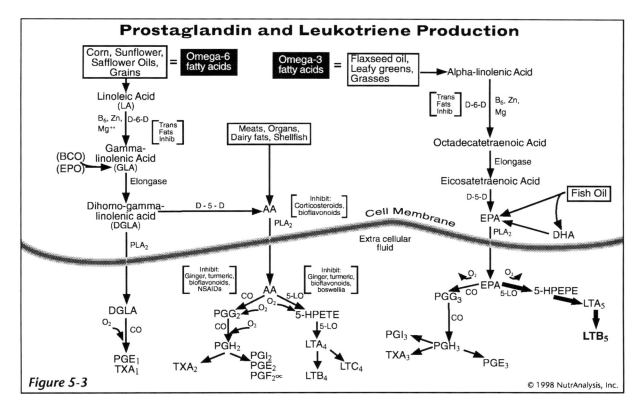

Prostaglandin and Leukotriene Production

Figure 5-3

© 1998 NutrAnalysis, Inc.

Prostaglandin production

Figure 5-3 illustrates the metabolic machinery involved in eicosanoid synthesis. Note that PLA-2 is an enzyme that is located near the cell membrane. PLA-2 stands for phospholipase A-2, which is the enzyme that cleaves the unsaturated fatty acid from position-2 of cell membrane phospholipids for conversion into an eicosanoid[318]. Depending on dietary habits, this unsaturated fatty acid can be DGLA, EPA or arachidonic acid.

Linoleic acid is found in seeds, grains, nuts, and most plants[417]. Through processes known as desaturation and elongation, linoleic acid is converted into dihomogammalinolenic acid (DGLA). If acted upon by cyclooxygenase, DGLA is converted into the anti-inflammatory PGE-1. If acted upon by delta-5-desaturase (D-5-D), DGLA will be converted into arachidonic acid which is then converted into pro-inflammatory eicosanoids such as PGE-2, PGI-2, LTB-4, TXA-2, and PGF-2α. It should be remembered that arachidonic acid also comes preformed in the various products that we get from grain-fed animals[417].

Linolenic acid is found in flaxseed oil and green vegetables[417, 811]. Via desaturation and elongation, linolenic acid is converted into eicosapentaenoic acid (EPA). EPA comes preformed in fish and fish oil supplements. As mentioned above, EPA is the precursor of the anti-inflammatory PGE-3, PGI-3, LTB-5, and TXA-3. While conversion of EPA to DHA occurs, it seems that this conversion is slow[284], while the conversion from DHA to EPA occurs rapidly[737-p.94-95]. For this reason, many feel that it is best to eat fish or take fish oil supplements in order to get adequate amounts of DHA.

Fatty acid consumption patterns

It should be understood that there are three main essential fatty acids which can ultimately become part of cell membrane phospholipids. These include linoleic acid, linolenic acid and arachidonic acid. In addition to these classic essential fatty acids, one might add eicosapentaenoic acid (EPA) and docosahexaenoic acid (DHA) to the list. Normal life is not possible unless essential fatty acids are consumed in sufficient quantities, i.e., approximately 3-4% of caloric intake[97].

Naturally, our food choices determine the concentration of specific fatty acids in our diets, which, in turn, determines the types of eicosanoids we will produce. Unfortunately, it appears that the average American diet shifts the fatty acid balance

Table 5-1
Plasma choline phosphoglycerides (12 vegans & 12 controls)
mg/g total fatty methyl esters

	VEGETARIANS	MEAT EATERS
Linoleic acid	333	260
DGLA	32	34
arachidonic acid	106	91
EPA	2	13
DHA	14	40

Table 5-2
Erythrocyte lipid fatty acids (18 vegans & 18 controls)
mg/g total fatty methyl esters and dimethyl esters

	VEGETARIANS	MEAT EATERS
Linoleic acid	113	87
DGLA	13	12
arachidonic acid	126	125
EPA	1	8
DHA	19	58

---

towards excessive production, storage and utilization of arachidonic acid; the end result being the generation of pro-inflammatory eicosanoids.

"Several sources of information suggest that man evolved on a diet with a ratio of n-6 to n-3 fatty acids of approximately 1:1, whereas today, this ratio is approximately 10:1 to 20-25:1, indicating that Western diets are deficient in n-3 fatty acids compared with the diet on which humans evolved and their genetic patterns were established"[417].

Clearly, the n-6:n-3 ratios in our diets may help to create a pro-inflammatory state. Budowski and Crawford recommend that we consume less than a 5:1 ratio of n-6 to n-3[64]. Eaton et al. also suggests that man historically consumed a 1:1 ratio[608]. In Linder's text, she cites researchers who recommend a 4:10 ratio of n-6 to n-3 intake[275-p. 56], which significantly favors n-3 fatty acids. More recently, Simopoulos stated that an n-6:n-3 ratio above 4:1 would promote changes in gene activity that would promote cancer and heart disease[811-p.25].

Vegetarian diets -- fatty acid profile

As mentioned earlier in this chapter, a clinical trial was recently performed to see how patients with rheumatoid arthritis would respond to a vegetarian diet. Kjeldsen-Kragh et al. concluded that, "a switch to a vegetarian diet causes an extensive change of the profile of the fatty acids of the serum phospholipids. These changes may favor the production of prostaglandins and leukotrienes with less inflammatory activity."[237] It should be understood that Kjeldsen-Kragh et al. were not precise about the n-6:n-3 ratio of the subjects' meals, and thus, we do not have precise information regarding fatty acid profiles.

I have been able to locate only one paper devoted to the subject of fatty acid balance in vegetarians versus meat eaters. Researchers analyzed plasma choline phosphoglycerides and erythrocyte fatty acids and found that both vegetarians and meat eaters incorporated linoleic acid, DGLA, arachidonic acid, EPA and DHA into the respective phospholipids[384]. The vegetarians used in this study had not eaten meat for at least 1 year. The results can be found in *Table 5-1* and *Table 5-2*.

These results indicate that vegetarians have significantly more linoleic acid than meat eaters. These values also demonstrate that vegetarians are quite capable of converting linoleic acid into arachidonic acid; which means that D-6-D, elongase, and D-5-D are functional. This is an important point because many say that these enzymes do not work well, particularly D-6-D.

Of importance to note is the fact that vegetarians actually have higher concentrations of arachidonic acid, equal amounts of DGLA, and less EPA and DHA than their meat eating counterparts. From these values alone, it appears that vegetarians may be more pro-inflammatory than meat eaters. However, a sound vegetarian diet will also supply significant amounts magnesium, potassium and phytochemicals, all of which offer anti-inflammatory and health-promoting benefits.

The vegetarian lifestyle may also offer additional health benefits. Generally speaking, vegetarians tend to be active and they usually do not smoke, drink alcohol or consume fat and sugar-laden desserts. Meat eaters tend toward these particularly unfavorable, disease-promoting lifestyle and eating patterns. Baring arguments about pesticides and hormones, I believe the main difference between vegetarians and meat eaters is the addition of these disease-promoting habits by meat eaters.

There are, however, drawbacks associated with vegetarianism that should be mentioned. Some of my sickest patients were vegetarians. It is very difficult to consume sufficient amounts of vegetables, fruits and grains so that all macro and micronutrient requirements will be met. Vegetarians also tend to be hypoglycemic compared to their meat eating counterparts and many continuously crave sweets. My experience suggests that most, if not all vegetarians, should at least add modest amounts of eggs, egg whites, yogurt and cheese to their diets. This contention is supported by the work of Kjeldsen-Kragh et al.[237]. Recall that most participants in their study needed to switch to a lactovegetarian diet to insure nutritional adequacy.

Trans fatty acids

Fatty acids with the *trans* configuration are also thought to be pro-inflammatory. Certain members of the food industry might argue that such a claim is not well founded[18], and responsible biochemists indicate that the *trans* fatty acid controversy is not resolved[275]. Therefore, a brief discussion of trans fats is warranted. It should also be noted that new editions of premier nutrition texts do not discuss *trans* fats[126].

Most of the unsaturated fatty acids found in vegetable and animal fats contain *cis* isomers. Generally speaking, trans isomers are not found in nature; man has introduced these fats to the food chain. *Trans* fatty acids are formed during the hydrogenation of vegetable oils, a process that transforms the oil into a semisolid state that more closely resembles saturated animal fat. Margarine is an example of a hydrogenated oil and nutrition contents listed on packaged foods usually indicate the presence of hydrogenated or partially hydrogenated oils. Holman indicates that the concentration of *trans* isomers reaches 17% in commercial vegetable oils, 47% in margarine, and 58% in vegetable shortenings[203].

Although the precise degree to which *trans* fatty acids may participate in the pathogenesis of certain diseases, such as heart disease, has not been determined, it has been known for many years that *trans* isomers are capable of altering normal fatty acid metabolism. In 1956 it was suggested that *trans* fatty acids could cause essential fatty acid deficiency[202]. At that time, laboratory experiments with rats demonstrated that *trans* fatty acids inhibited normal growth, caused skin problems and reduced spermatogenesis[202].

In recent years, more definitive evidence about *trans* fatty acids has surfaced in the literature. Katan, Zock and Mensink state[681]:

> "*Trans* fatty acids raise plasma low-density lipoprotein (LDL) cholesterol levels in volunteers when exchanged for *cis* unsaturated fatty acids in the diet. In addition, *trans* fatty acids may lower high-density lipoprotein (HDL) cholesterol levels and raise triglyceride and lipoprotein(a) levels in plasma. *Trans* and *cis* unsaturated fatty acids are thus not equivalent, and diets aimed at reducing the risk of coronary heart disease should be low in both *trans* and saturated fatty acids."

Khosla and Hayes state that, "*trans* fatty acids appear to raise LDL-C like saturated fatty acids, but unlike saturated fatty acids they tend to lower HCL-C, thus adversely affecting CHD risk"[686]. Another recent article explained that, "our findings suggest that replacing saturated and *trans* unsaturated fats with unhydrogenated monounsaturated and polyunsaturated fats is more effective in preventing coronary heart disease in women than reducing overall fat intake"[659]. Researchers at the University of North Carolina at Chapel Hill recently determined that women with high levels of *trans* fatty acids had a 40% increased risk of breast cancer[690]. In 1995, Trichopoulou et al. stated that olive oil consumption may reduce the risk of breast cancer, while margarine intake increases the risk of developing breast cancer[834]. Sampugna and Teter have recently urged the food industry to include the trans fatty acid content on food labels[789].

Current estimations suggest that approximately 5.5% of the fat consumed by Americans consists of *trans* fatty acids[275-p.78]. Others suggest that *trans* fats make up about 2 percent of our caloric intake[359]. *Trans* fats are able to incorporate into the tissues of humans and may compose up to 14% of certain lipids[203].

It is thought that *trans* fats compete with linoleic and linolenic acids to be acted upon by delta-5-desaturase (D-5-D) and delta-6-desaturase (D-6-D) and subsequently reduce the conversion of linoleic acid to DGLA and arachidonic acid[275-p.78]. Other authors have found that feeding rats an omega-3 trans fatty acid made by heating linseed, would result in increased arachidonic acid incorporation into cell membranes and reduce n-3 incorporation. These researchers found that an n-3 trans fatty acid did not significantly affect D-6-D but tended to increase the activity of D-5-D[38]. Whichever the case may be, it is still likely that arachidonic acid will be incorporated into cell membranes, as it comes preformed in meat which is a dietary emphasis, especially in America[275].

Diseases promoted by fatty acid imbalances

A diet that is highly concentrated with n-6 fatty acids and elevated n-6:n-3 fatty acid ratios is known to promote the production of disease-promoting, pro-inflammatory *eicosanoids* (see *Figure 5-3*), *growth factors*, i.e., platelet-derived growth factor (PDGE), and *cytokines*, i.e., TNF and IL-1[572, 573, 614, 636, 728, 729, 810]. The list of diseases that are promoted by n-6:n-3 imbalances is seemingly endless: cancer, heart disease, arthritis, chronic pain, diabetes, schizophrenia, psychiatric illnesses, chronic gastrointestinal diseases, lupus, respiratory diseases, gingivitis[417, 556, 574, 575, 592, 614, 688, 728, 753, 754, 784, 785, 817] Additionally, n-6 fatty acids also promote hyperinsulinemia and insulin resistance (see Chapter 6). Clearly, the great majority of chronic diseases which strike down modern man are driven, in part, by an excessive intake of n-6 fatty acids and a deficient intake of n-3 fatty acids.

The musculoskeletal system does not escape from the ravages of n-6 overload. Rheumatoid arthritis is one of the most inflammatory of all musculoskeletal diseases and it is driven by the pro-inflammatory mediators derived from n-6 fatty acids. Accordingly, research has conclusively demonstrated that n-3 fatty acid supplementation can provide RA patients with significant relief, even to the point of discontinuing NSAID therapy[693].

Even more basic pathologies of the skeletal system seem to be enhanced by n-6 excess. For example, both herniated discs and inflammatory synovial fluid from degenerative joints contain phospholipase A-2[378]. Saal indicates that human lumbar disc phospholipase A-2 is 20- to 100,000-fold more active than any other phospholipase yet to be described[378], and that this enzyme is particularly pro-inflammatory[154].

As spinal injury is very common, it would be prudent to insure that cell membrane phospholipids are endowed with sufficient amounts of EPA. Sierkerka suggests that nutritional therapy should accompany any chosen treatment regime to accelerate the healing of a damaged disc, the most integral aspect of acute therapy being the dietary addition of foods containing n-3 and n-6 fatty acids and the avoidance of those that contain arachidonic acid[414]. Naturally, it would be best to focus on n-3 fatty acids and not the n-6 family.

Monounsaturated fatty acids

Recall that Jeppesen et al. recommend that half of total fat intake should come from monounsaturated fatty acids[673]. In essence, these researchers suggest that we replace a high saturated fat diet with foods rich in monounsaturated fat (n-9 fatty acids), i.e., we should use olive oil instead of butter, lard, margarine and vegetable oils. Some of the antioxidant benefits of olive oil were discussed earlier in the section on free radicals. While the data is not definitive, studies do suggest that the monounsaturated fat component of olive oil and other substances may help protect against heart disease, cancer, and diabetes[615, 682, 709, 834, 855, 625]. These findings are consistent with the belief that the high-monounsaturated fat, low saturated fat content of the Mediterranean diet plays a role in the prevention of chronic disease.

A recent review article describes how a diet high in oleic acid, i.e., the main dietary monounsaturated fatty acid, reduces LDL oxidation, compared to diets rich in n-6 fatty acids[823]. In another study, a high-carbohydrate, very-low-fat diet (10% of total calories from fat) was compared to a low fat diet (26% of total calories) supplemented with olive oil and olive-oil base margarine. While both diets resulted in significant reductions in LDL cholesterol and total cholesterol compared to the baseline diet, only the olive oil-enriched low fat diet prevented significant reductions in HDL cholesterol[731]. Another study demonstrated that olive oil may favorably enhance tissue levels of coenzyme Q-10[716], which is known to be a cardioprotective substance. A recent study compared the putative protective effects of virgin olive oil versus sunflower oil against free radical damage in rats[715]. Olive oil-fed sedentary and exercising rats had less free radical damage than those fed n-6 fatty acid-rich sunflower oil. The researchers also suggest that virgin olive oil offers more antioxidant protection than alpha-tocopherol.

Many may recall that some of the original work on dietary fats and atherosclerosis involved rabbits. In one study, researchers fed rabbits three different cholesterol-free diets, supplemented by either North American peanut oil, South American peanut oil, or olive oil for 8 months[694]. The rabbits fed olive oil had higher levels of serum and hepatic lipids compared to the peanut oil-fed rabbits; however, the olive oil group exhibited significantly lower levels of aortic atherosclerosis.

It should be understood that monounsaturated fatty acids are not acted upon by the desaturase and elongase enzymes, so they do not play a direct role in eicosanoid synthesis; however, they do play a role in controlling eicosanoid-driven inflammation. For example, in both animal and human studies, it was shown that diets rich in olive oil promoted the incorporation of n-3 fatty acids into membrane phospholipids[735, 786]. A recent article also describes how the oleic acid component of olive oil may reduce unwanted immune-driven inflammatory processes involving the adhesion molecule ICAM-1, which may help prevent/treat inflammatory conditions such as rheumatoid arthritis and atherosclerosis[859].

SUMMARY

Vegetables and fruits contain an abundance of important nutrients. Accordingly, a diet that is deficient in vegetables and fruits, i.e., the average American diet, will necessarily be deficient in many key nutrients. In this chapter we focussed on potassium, magnesium, antioxidants, phytochemicals, and various fatty acids. Researchers have studied each nutrient and determined that *excesses* of saturated fats and omega-6 fatty acids, and *deficiencies* in potassium, magnesium, antioxidants, phytochemicals, omega-3 fatty acids and omega-9 fatty acids can have general pro-inflammatory consequences and in certain cases, even promote specific diseases such as heart disease, cancer and diabetes.

Epidemiologic studies demonstrate that diets rich in vegetables and fruits prevent disease; however, research into specific nutrients for the treatment of specific diseases are rarely conclusive. This outcome should be expected. The deficiencies associated with the standard American diet cannot be overcome by supplementing with 500 mg of vitamin C or 5000 IU of beta carotene. Such supplementation studies will also be "equivocal" at best. Unfortunately, doctors too often focus on recommending supplements and spend too little time modifying dietary habits. The information in this chapter should have made it clear that dietary modification is the most important nutritional intervention. Chapter 6 focuses on an additional dietary factor that needs to be carefully considered, i.e., glycemic regulation.

Chapter 6

GLYCEMIC DYSREGULATION AND ITS PRO-INFLAMMATORY POTENTIAL

HIGH CARBOHYDRATE DIETS

In recent years, a significant amount of public attention has been directed at the subject of carbohydrate consumption and glycemic regulation. Our discussion will begin with the work of Barry Sears because he has had a lot to do with this focus. He has recently published papers[404, 800] and a new text entitled *The Zone* [799], which have extolled the negative properties of high-carbohydrate diets that are rich in breads and pasta.

The standard recommendations for the distribution of total calories typically consist of 55-70% from carbohydrate, 10-15% protein, and 20-30% from fat. Sears flatly derides these ratios in favor a 40:30:30 balance of intake. In short, Sears claims that high carbohydrate diets increase insulin output and reduce the output of glucagon. As a consequence this will stimulate delta-5-desaturase (*see Figure 6-1*) and increase the conversion of DGLA into arachidonic acid, a precursor of pro-inflammatory eicosanoids. In addition, Sears contends that hyperinsulin responses will also promote diabetes, heart disease, cancer, obesity and a host of other chronic diseases[404, 799, 800].

Needless to say, Sears' recommendations are viewed as radical by many. In particular, Coleman[580, 581, 582, 583] has written several articles which strongly disagree with Sears. She states that, "the metabolic pathways that supposedly connect

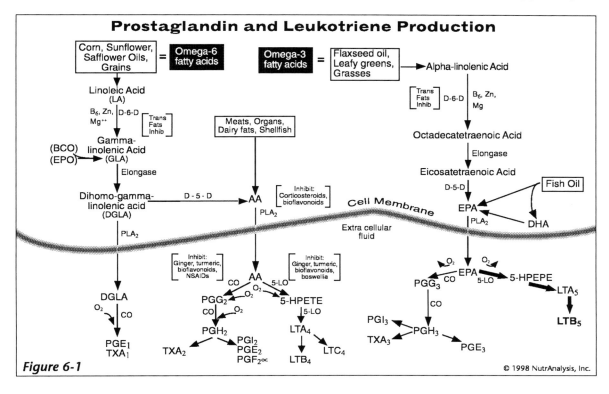

Figure 6-1

© 1998 NutrAnalysis, Inc.

diet, insulin-glucagon, and eicosanoids do not exist in standard nutrition or biochemistry texts"[582]. Coleman cites two references to support her claims; one is a standard dietitian text[503] and the other is a basic biochemistry text[294]. She also looks askance at the idea that dietary protein will increase glucagon levels, and states that high carbohydrate diets do not increase insulin levels; high carbohydrate diets do not promote fat deposition due to increased insulin output; and the insulin-glucagon axis does not control the production of eicosanoids[583].

In fact, none of what Coleman says is accurate. Numerous texts and articles refute her contentions (each issue will be discussed under a separate heading). Understand that because Coleman is wrong, it does not mean that Sears is correct in all of his assertions or recommendations. In fact, I personally do not think that the 40:30:30 ratio is the optimal balance for all people. For example, well-respected researchers at Stanford University suggest that a 45:15:40 balance may be the best for all[673]. Additionally, Sears appears to inappropriately downplay the importance of vitamins and minerals in favor of overall macronutrient balance.

Dietary regulation of insulin and glucose

In brief, the endocrine pancreas contains islet cells which are involved in blood sugar control. Insulin is found in beta-cells, while glucagon is found in alpha-cells[444]. Insulin is one of the body's anabolic hormones, while the counter regulatory hormones are characterized as catabolic. Insulin can also oppose the catabolic activity of the counter regulatory hormones, thus acting in an anticatabolic fashion[113]. Insulin *increases* glycogen, protein, and fatty acid synthesis[113], and *inhibits* lipolysis in adipose tissue[294].

Insulin and glucagon have antagonistic activities, and epinephrine and cortisol often work in concert with glucagon. Glucagon, epinephrine, and cortisol are referred to as counter regulatory hormones, i.e., they counter regulate the actions of insulin. Various factors can influence the release of these different hormones resulting in imbalances

that can lead to metabolic problems and diseases.

Modern Nutrition in Health and Disease is viewed as one of medicine's authoritative texts on nutrition. The last two editions explain that, "carbohydrate metabolism is finely regulated by interactions between insulin, the hormone promoting fuel storage, and the counter regulatory hormones, such as glucagon, epinephrine, cortisol, and growth hormone"[57, 113]. Additionally, "the ingestion of carbohydrate produces a prompt increase in plasma insulin and a decrease in glucagon concentrations"[57, 113]. When a diet contains a high proportion of refined carbohydrates, which have high glycemic indices, the body's insulin response will be enhanced[223]. On the contrary, "when a carbohydrate-free protein meal is ingested, insulin concentrations increase slightly and promote protein synthesis in skeletal muscle, with a parallel rise in glucagon, which prevents hypoglycemia"[57]. It should be mentioned that the second to last edition of this text was published in 1988[57], so this information has been available for many years.

An endocrinology text published in 1987 stated that, "if pure carbohydrate is taken, insulin (and somatostatin) is secreted selectively, and the combination of glucose and insulin inhibits glucagon secretion"[444]. The response to a protein meal is different. All three islet hormones, i.e., insulin, somatostatin, and glucagon, are secreted[444], which indicates that protein is required in the diet to elicit a glucagon response.

In addition to the information found in these standard texts, research trials have demonstrated that the carbohydrate to protein ratio of a meal can dramatically influence the release of both regulatory and counter regulatory hormones. Westphal, Gannon, and Nutthal examined the metabolic responses associated with different ratios of carbohydrate to protein[479]. They found that their results were in agreement with other published studies, i.e., protein ingesting stimulates glucagon production while the ingestion of glucose suppresses glucose secretion. "In addition, our data confirm the observation that the circulating glucagon concentration depends on the ratio of protein to carbohydrate in the meal"[479]. In this study, human subjects consumed breakfasts consisting of 50 grams of glucose and various amounts of beef protein (0 g, 10 g, 30 g, 50g), and also with 50 grams of beef alone. It appears that a beneficial insulin/glucagon ratio of secretion followed the consumption of a 50:30 ratio (or 1.7/1) of glucose to beef[479]. Naturally, it is difficult to apply these findings to the typical meal because no one eats pure glucose. Fortunately, other studies have examined metabolic responses to meals.

Studies have also been performed in which subjects ate standard meals prior to being evaluated for glucose, insulin and other markers related to blood sugar control. For example, back in 1983, Coulston et al.[589] subjected 11 healthy volunteers to diets containing two different levels of carbohydrate for an ingestion period of 10 days on each diet. One diet contained 60% carbohydrate, 19% protein, and 21% fat, while the other diet contained a 40:19:41 balance. Nearly identical foods were used in each diet; only the amounts varied, which allowed for the differences in the high- and low-carbohydrate diets. The purpose of the study was to determine how the two diets would affect plasma glucose, insulin, cholesterol, triglyceride, and high density lipoprotein (HDL)-cholesterol concentrations. Fasting blood samples were taken on days 8, 9, and 10 of each diet period. Plasma glucose, insulin and triglyceride concentrations were also determined before and three hours after the noon meal in days 8 and 10. While no differences were seen in fasting plasma glucose, insulin, and cholesterol, the subjects on the high-carbohydrate diets had significantly elevated fasting triglyceride levels and significantly decreased levels of HDL-cholesterol. In addition, post-meal levels of insulin and triglycerides were also significantly higher with the 60% carbohydrate diet.

The results of a similar study were published in a 1994 issue of the *Journal of the American Medical Association*[624]. The subjects in this four-center randomized crossover trial were all non-insulin dependent diabetic patients. The high carbohydrate diet contained a 55:15:30 balance of carbohydrates, protein, and fats. The other diet, which contained a 40:15:45 balance, was referred to as the high-monounsaturated fat diet. The results indicated that the high-carbohydrate diets caused a persistent deterioration of glycemic control and accentuation of hyperinsulinemia, as well as increased triglyceride and VLDL-cholesterol levels.

In a more recent paper, Jeppesen et al. reported the results of a study that compared the metabolic responses to a high and low carbohydrate diet in healthy postmenopausal woman[673]. The two diets were isoenergetic. The first diet consisted of 60% of calories from carbohydrate, 15% protein and 25% fat, resulting in a 4:1 ratio by weight of carbohydrate to protein. The second diet consisted of 40% of calories from carbohydrate, 15% protein and 45% fat, resulting in a 2.7:1 ratio by weight of carbohydrate to protein. The results demonstrated that the 60% carbohydrate diet caused a reduction in HDL-cholesterol concentrations and an increase in plasma levels of insulin, glucose, triacylglycerol, and very-low-density-lipoproteins, all of which are thought to increase the risk of ischemic heart disease in postmenopausal women. These researchers question the utility of high carbohydrate diets and concluded that, "an isoenergetic diet containing (as a % of total energy) 15% protein, 45% carbohydrate, 10% saturated fat, 10% polyunsaturated fat, and 20% monounsaturated fat might be the best (and simplest) for all"[673]; that is a 3:1 ratio by weight of carbohydrate to protein.

Reaven recently reviewed the literature and outlined how insulin resistance is promoted by high-carbohydrate, low-fat diets[769]. These findings are consistent with other researches who suggest that a high-monounsaturated fat diet should be used instead of a high-carbohydrate diet in the treatment of diabetes[623, 625]. In general, it seems that protein intake should stay the same, and calories should be shifted from carbohydrates to monounsaturated fat, while total caloric intake should remain the same.

Thus far, it should be evident that the balance of carbohydrate, protein and fat can significantly influence glucose regulation. However, the story of glycemic control does not end here. In addition, the glycemic index of each food and meal can influence blood glucose and insulin responses.

The glycemic index is defined as, "the blood

glucose response to a 50 gram available carbohydrate portion of a food expressed as a percentage of the response to the same amount of carbohydrate from a standard food, which has been either glucose or white bread"[223]. In practical terms, this means that each food's glycemic response has been compared to that of a reference food. White bread is the typical reference food and it has a glycemic index (GI) of 100. Comparatively speaking, glucose has a GI of 138, while a grapefruit has a GI of 36[543, 622]. Recent articles have published the GI for extensive lists of foods[622, 853]. Wolever et al. first list the ratio of carbohydrate:protein:fat in each food and then list the glycemic index[853].

In general, the GI increases as a carbohydrate is refined, such that the GI for refined carbohydrates is high and comparatively low for complex carbohydrates. The higher the glycemic index, the higher the glucose response, and the higher the insulin response. Jenkins et al. list the benefits of consuming foods with a low GI[223]:

1. Insulin secretion is reduced.

2. Overall blood glucose control improves in insulin-dependent and noninsulin-dependent diabetes mellitus (NIDDM) subjects.

3. There is a reduction of abnormal blood glucose, insulin, and amino acid levels in patients with cirrhosis.

4. Blood lipids are reduced in hyper triglyceridemic patients.

5. Urinary urea excretion is reduced, presumably by increasing nitrogen trapping by colonic bacteria.

6. Low GI foods may enhance satiety.

7. Low GI foods may increase athletic performance.

The benefits of consuming low GI foods is obvious. Most studies have found the GI concept to be accurate and useful in the management of diabetes and hyperlipidemia[622]. Additionally, in men without NIDDM or cardiovascular disease, diets with a high glycemic load and low cereal fiber

were shown to promote the development of NIDDM. The researchers conclude that these findings, "suggest that grains should be consumed in a minimally refined form to reduce the incidence of NIDDM"[787]. The same conclusions were reached when these researchers performed a similar study in women[787].

Despite this information, dietitians do not typically utilize the glycemic index[503-p.443, 583, 854]. For example, in Coleman's recent article on carbohydrates for sports and exercise, she implies that GI is of no utility[583]. Wolever states that "it is time for the ADA to take an objective look at the data rather than evading the issue"[854].

In summary, it should be clear that Coleman's assertions about insulin and glucagon regulation are short-sighted and inaccurate. Similar errors can be found in her assertion that insulin plays no role in fat gain and obesity.

Do high carbohydrate diets increase fat deposition by promoting insulin secretion?

In the previous paragraphs, it was been established that high-carbohydrate diets enhance insulin release. This is particularly the case for refined carbohydrates and for high glycemic index carbohydrates. Many other dietary factors promote hyperinsulinemia and insulin resistance, some of which included deficiencies of specific vitamins, minerals and fatty acids, and an excessive intake of certain fatty acids. These additional factors will be discussed in the section below entitled *Insulin resistance syndrome*.

In short, insulin resistance and its related hyperinsulinemia is thought to precede and promote the development of numerous disease including obesity, NIDDM, hypertension and coronary artery disease[638, 809]. Regarding obesity, as far back as 1971, research suggested that dietary factors, in this case a high-carbohydrate diet, could promote a state of hyperinsulinemia which could in turn promote obesity[635].

In 1998, McGarry stated that, "it is widely held that although obesity and type 2 diabetes are polygenic in origin, the primary defect causing both conditions is insulin resistance, which in turn gives rise to a constellation of other abnormalities including hyperinsulinemia, dyslipidemia, glucose intolerance, and (in the genetically predisposed) frank hyperglycemia"[723]. McGarry then goes on to propose that a different order of events may take place. It is proposed that hyperinsulinemia begets insulin resistance, and that hyperinsulinemia is caused by a signaling defect within the pancreas and/CNS. He then goes on to describe how hyperinsulinemia and insulin resistance may promote obesity. For example, it is suggested that hyperinsulinemia promotes an excessive production of hepatic VLDLs by stimulating fatty acid biosynthesis and reesterification of circulating fatty acids which are then taken up by adipose tissue[723].

By examining some of the metabolic machinery involved in lipogenesis and its modulation, we can begin to appreciate how high-carbohydrate, low-fat diets, especially when they are rich in refined carbohydrates, can promote fat gain and obesity. A recent review of the literature explains how high-carbohydrate, low-fat diets induce the genetic expression of lipogenic enzymes in both the liver and adipose tissue[833]. In general, glucagon inhibits the activity of lipogenic enzymes, while insulin induces the lipogenesis of dietary carbohydrates. Acetyl-coenzyme A carboxylase (ACC) is an enzyme that is central to the process of lipogenesis and it is known that glucose stimulates ACC, and that insulin strongly potentiates this effect[833].

Unlike carbohydrates, dietary fat inhibits lipogenesis. More specifically, dietary polyunsaturated fatty acids (PUFA) repress the activity of lipogenic enzymes, such as ACC. The authors do not indicate which PUFA is most responsible for this inhibition[833]. However, Simopoulos has recently reviewed the literature and states that the suppression of fatty acid synthase is greater with DHA, EPA, and arachidonic acid than with linoleic or linolenic acids[810]. DHA appears to be the most potent inhibitor of lipogenic enzymes. In addition, DHA appears to be the most potent inducer of acyl-CoA oxidase, which is the enzyme involved in beta-oxidation[810], i.e., fat oxidation or fat burning.

Although n-6 fatty acids can reduce lipogenesis and enhance beta-oxidation, it should be understood that n-6 fatty acids have numerous pro-inflammatory effects (see Chapter 5). Additionally, it is thought that high n-6 linoleic acid consumption, which is reflected as a high n-6:n-3 ratio, will aggravate hyperinsulinemia and insulin resistance[758, 809, 821, 823, 857]. In other words, n-6 fatty acids promote hyperinsulinemia, and as stated above, insulin stimulates lipogenic enzymes. In addition, a high percentage of saturated fats in the diet appears to promote hyperinsulinemia. "If saturated fatty acids as a percentage of total energy were to decrease from 14% to 8%, there would be an 18% decrease in fasting insulin, and a 25% decrease in postprandial insulin"[747].

In 1981, Ruderman et al.[783] wrote an interesting article that describes the "metabolically obese" normal weight individual. They indicated that obesity is typically associated with NIDDM, hypertension, and hypertriglyceridemia. However, there are people with these disorders who are not obese. It is proposed that these individuals might be characterized by hyperinsulinism and possibly by increased fat cell size. Ruderman et al. suggest that high-carbohydrate diets characterized by increased levels of refined carbohydrates and physical inactivity can promote hyperinsulinemia.

In summary, there is ample evidence to suggest that high-carbohydrate diets and the wrong fats will promote hyperinsulinemia, insulin resistance, and numerous metabolic disorders, including obesity. This is not say that insulin, in and of itself, is a "bad" hormone. Quite to the contrary, insulin is necessary to sustain life; however, when insulin control and sensitivity is compromised due to poor lifestyle choices, a variety of diseases can develop.

The final issue raised by Coleman had to do with modulation of eicosanoids. She contends that insulin and glucagon do not control eicosanoid synthesis.

Does the diet and insulin-glucagon connection control eicosanoid synthesis?

Sears was the first to go to the general public with the concept that insulin and glucagon could control eicosanoid synthesis[799]. It should be understood that this is not a concept that Sears concocted out of thin air. However, as far as I can tell, he uses only one article by Brenner to support this contention[565]. In 1974, Brenner published an article that outlined how certain nutritional and hormonal factors would influence the desaturation of unsaturated fatty acids during their conversion into eicosanoids[55]. He found that when glucose was given to fasting rats, it provoked insulin secretion which subsequently promoted an increase in delta-6-desaturase (D-6-D) activity. It was determined that delta-5-desaturase (D-5-D) responded in a similar fashion. So, for at least 25 years it has been know that insulin could stimulate D-6-D and D-5-D activity. Look at *Figure 6-1* so you know where these enzymes function in eicosanoid synthesis.

Then, in 1981, Brenner published a similar article in a journal entitled *Progress in Lipid Research*[565]. Brenner introduces the discussion by indicating that he and other researchers have shown that desaturase activity is modified by these nutritional and hormonal factors. Brenner provides diagrams of D-6-D and D-5-D to show how they are induced or depressed. For example, he illustrates how D-6-D is induced by insulin and depressed by glucagon, epinephrine, glucocorticoids, and thyroxine.

Brenner illustrates the hormonal control of D-5-D in a different fashion. For example, he indicates that D-5-D is activated by *reduced* levels of glucagon, epinephrine, and glucocorticoids. This leads one to infer that increased insulin levels would stimulate D-5-D, although he never states it openly. However, our inference is supported by his statement that, as far as they can tell, the various hormones produce similar effects on both enzymes.

Since the time Brenner published his work, several other similar articles have been published which echoed the results of Brenner. For example, like Brenner, Dutta-Roy[606] provides a figure that illustrates how insulin stimulates D-6-D and D-5-D. He goes on to explain that, "since the delta 6 and delta 5 desaturation steps of EFA metabolism are regulated by insulin, the relative availability of polyunsaturated fatty acids for membrane incorporation is itself controlled by the hormone"[606]. Bezard et al. state that, "with regard to hormones, insulin and thyroxine are necessary to D-6-D and D-5-D activities, whereas other hormones (glucagon, epinephrine, ACTH, glucocorticoids) inhibit desaturation"[557]. Borkman et al. write about insulin's stimulatory affect on desaturase activity as if it is well-known[563]. Peterson explains that it is well-known that administering insulin will stimulate desaturase activity in IDDM, but it is not known if hyperinsulinemia associated with NIDDM will also stimulate desaturase[758].

Based on this evidence, it is reasonable to suggest that hyperinsulinemia may promote arachidonic acid production when sufficient amounts of linoleic acid are present. As indicated in Chapter 5, arachidonic acid is the precursor for a host of pro-inflammatory eicosanoids.

INSULIN RESISTANCE SYNDROME

Reaven coined the term syndrome X in 1988 to describe the cluster of abnormalities occurring in nondiabetic persons that increase the risk of coronary heart disease[767, 769]. The common feature of the syndrome was insulin resistance, which is why syndrome X is also called the insulin resistance syndrome. The metabolic changes which occur in Syndrome X include glucose intolerance, hyperinsulinemia, increased VLDLs, decreased HDLs, and hypertension[767]. In 1995, Reaven published an extensive review article in which Syndrome X was characterized by insulin resistance, hyperinsulinemia and has the following manifestations: hypertriglyceridemia, small dense LDLs, decreased HDLs, postprandial lipemia, increased plasminogen activator inhibitor, increased uric acid levels, and hypertension[768].

Groop et al. refer to syndrome X and the insulin resistance syndrome as the prediabetic state[638]. In a review of the literature, Preuss lists the diseases that may be promoted by insulin resistance with hyperinsulinemia and/or hyperglycemia: NIDDM, obesity, hypertension, lipid abnormalities, and atherosclerosis[763 p. 397]. Hyperinsulinemia may also be involved in the pathogenesis of cancer[763 p. 393, 820, 821, 857].

What causes hyperinsulinemia and insulin resistance? No one knows for sure, but dietary and lifestyle factors seem to play a key role. Preuss states that,

> "ingestion of sugars, fats, and sodium have been linked to decreased insulin sensitivity, while caloric restriction, exercise, ingestion of chromium, vanadium, soluble fibers, magnesium, and certain antioxidants are associated with greater insulin sensitivity. Thus, manipulation of diet by influencing the glucose/insulin system may favorably affect life-span and reduce the incidence of chronic disorders associated with aging." [763-p. 397]

The high-carbohydrate and fatty acid connections to hyperinsulinemia were discussed earlier in this chapter. In addition, deficiencies in certain nutrients may also promote hyperinsulinemia including magnesium [745, 779] and chromium [541, 772, 542]. Diets high in simple sugars are known to increase urinary chromium losses [691]. A deficiency in biotin [863, 864] and potassium [240] may impair glucose utilization, and vitamin E supplementation improves insulin action [571].

It is commonly believed that insulin resistance is a condition that develops in adulthood. This notion is patently incorrect. Several papers have discussed the prevalence of insulin resistance in adolescents [554, 684, 764, 866]. First it should be appreciated that a degree of hyperinsulinemia may be a normal developmental consequence. Insulin is characterized as an anabolic hormone and it is known to have a growth hormone-like effect which may explain why increased insulin appears to be related to the pubertal growth spurt [544]. However, it is also known that features of syndrome X appear in overweight adolescents in particular [544].

In another study [764], the authors explain that obesity indices were strongly associated with insulin levels in children (6-12 years), adolescents (15-18) and young adults (21-24 years). However, high insulin levels associated with high triglycerides, elevated systolic blood pressure, and lowered HDL-cholesterol were significantly clustered independent of obesity. These results support the concept that a specific syndrome with multiple metabolic disorders exists already in the young [764]. Other authors have commented that

signs of syndrome X cluster in even supposedly healthy children and adolescents [684].

Perhaps the same dietary imbalances involved in promoting syndrome X in adults also apply to children. Research has demonstrated that mental stress may also be related to the development of insulin resistance [684, 730]. This is probably because both epinephrine and cortisol can cause insulin resistance [684]. In addition, certain people may be genetically predisposed to develop insulin resistance. For example, children of NIDDM patients show signs of syndrome X, indicating that genetics can play a significant predisposing role [757].

PRO-INFLAMMATORY ASPECTS OF THE INSULIN RESISTANCE SYNDROME MAY IMPACT UPON THE MUSCULOSKELETAL SYSTEM

A recent trial involving healthy human subjects, demonstrated that hyperinsulinemia and elevated levels of proinsulin "were associated with higher levels of fibrinogen and plasminogen activator inhibitor (PAI) activity and lower tissue plasminogen activator activity, implicating a prothrombotic and hypofibrinolytic condition" [611]. In addition to playing a role in cardiovascular disease [611], reduced fibrinolysis is thought to promote inflammation and pain in several musculoskeletal conditions including osteoarthritis [164,347], rheumatoid arthritis [347, 193], and chronic back pain [90, 178, 213, 221, 222, 352]. Several additional lifestyle factors may add to a hypofibrinolytic state including smoking [178, 221, 153], high levels of triglycerides [178] and cholesterol [153], and reduced fiber intake [153, 254].

Proteoglycan synthesis may also be impaired by insulin resistance. A recent paper explains that diabetic patients have proteoglycans with lower buoyant density and substantially undersulfated glycosaminoglycans, which might lead to an increased susceptibility to disc prolapse [776]. Proteoglycans are complex sugar molecules that are formed by the cell's glycolytic pathways. Glucose-6-phosphate and fructose-6-phosphate are the precursor molecules for glycosaminoglycans and proteoglycans. Thus, it would seem natural that alterations in glucose metabolism could negatively impact upon proteoglycan synthesis.

CORTISOL CONNECTION

As mentioned earlier in this chapter, mental stress can lead to an increase in epinephrine and cortisol output from the adrenal gland. Epinephrine is produced in the adrenal medulla which constitutes about 10% to 20% of the gland, while cortisol is produced by the adrenal cortex which makes up the other 80% to 90% of the gland.

The adrenal medulla is basically an enlarged and specialized sympathetic ganglion. However, the neurons of the medulla do not contain axons and instead release their catecholamines directly into the blood; thus, acting like an endocrine gland and not a ganglion. Cholinergic preganglionic fibers from the greater splanchnic nerve enter the medulla and depolarize catecholamine-containing chromaffin cells via the release a acetylcholine[31]. Stressful events drive this pathway such that the organism responds with the so-called "fight or flight" response. This component of the stress response can be activated to different degrees by various stressors such as mental stressors, traumatic injury and hypoglycemia. Via different mechanisms, each stressor will ultimately stimulate the hypothalamus which then coordinates the stress response.

Regarding hypoglycemia, not everyone develops symptoms and not all people who develop symptoms suffer from the same ones. Severe symptoms typically involve sweating, weakness, hunger, tachycardia, and anxiety. Such symptoms are thought to be due to hyperepinephrinemia and sympathetic nervous system activity, which respond to rapid falls in blood glucose[444]. Some patients develop these symptoms when meals are skipped and after high glycemic foods are consumed. When blood glucose falls more slowly, it is thought that cerebral symptoms may predominate such as headache, blurred vision, diplopia, confusion, incoherent speech, and sometimes coma and convulsions[444]. Sometimes a combination of symptoms appear. In my experience, hunger, mild anxiety, headache and loss of mental concentration are common. Eating a balanced meal or snack often eliminates the symptoms within a few minutes to 30 minutes.

The adrenal cortex is made up of three zones. The outermost zone is the zona glomerulosa, which mainly secretes mineralocorticoids such as aldosterone. The middle zone is the zona fasiculata, which mainly secretes glucocorticoids such as cortisol. The inner zone is the zona reticularis which mainly secretes androgens such as dehydroepiandrosterone (DHEA)[31].

Cortisol is normally released in a circadian rhythm via autonomic control involving the paraventricular nucleus of the hypothalamus which releases corticotropin-releasing hormone (CRH) into the pituitary portal system. In response to CRH, the anterior pituitary gland releases adrenocorticotropic hormone which stimulates the zona fasiculata. Stressful situations override the normal diurnal pattern of cortisol release to help meet the behavioral needs of the organism. Common stressors include pain, nociception, fear, apprehension, anxiety and hypoglycemia[31, 48]. Burt explains that the hippocampus, a component of the limbic system, is responsible for overriding the normal controls by directly stimulating the parvosecretory cells of the paraventricular nucleus[570]. Over time, it is possible that hypoglycemia, cumulative mental stressors, and pain could disrupt proper cortisol regulation and promote an ongoing state of hypercortisolemia (see below).

Whereas cortisol release in normal amounts is physiologically beneficial, a continuous excess of cortisol will produce a continuous drain on body protein stores, most notable in muscle, bone, connective tissue, and skin[31]. An excess of endogenous cortisol reduces REM sleep; reduces cell mediated immunity by inhibiting the production of interleukin-1, interleukin-2, and gamma interferon; increases glomerular filtration rate; decreases the proliferation of osteoblasts; reduces collagen synthesis, and reduces glucose utilization[31]. Muscle protein synthesis is also reduced. In particular, the ratio of slow oxidative type I muscle fibers to fast glycolytic type II-B muscle fibers is decreased. Cortisol also promotes fat deposition around the mid section of the body[31].

Hypercortisolemia is also thought to inhibit secretory IgA (sIgA) output from the gut[113a]. Normally, gut immunocytes produce and secrete sIgA. Secretory IgA has been referred to as the "blocking antibody", as one of its major functions is to prevent antigen absorption. Numerous authors agree that sIgA can prevent the absorption of food antigens[85, 132, 326]. In this regard, the absorption of food antigens have been shown to be associated with the release of prostaglandins and the subsequent development of joint pain[65].

Germane to this chapter is the fact that stress[730] and hypoglycemia[31, 596] promote cortisol release which can promote insulin resistance[730]. Glucocorticoids are known to counteract the effects of insulin at numerous steps in glucose homeostasis, such that gluconeogenesis appears to be the net effect. Cortisol may decrease the production of glucose transporters. Cortisol decreases insulin binding to its receptor by reducing the quantity of insulin receptors and by reducing receptor affinity[57]. The outcome is hyperglycemia which will be amplified in the presence of increased levels of glucagon, epinephrine or growth hormone[57].

Pregnenolone is the precursor for all steroid hormones, i.e., cortisol, progesterone, estrogen, testosterone, aldosterone, and dehydro-epiandrosterone (DHEA). During severe illness and chronic stress, the body preferential produces cortisol at the expense of the other hormones. For example, over time, cortisol levels will rise and DHEA levels will fall[748]. This may serve to amplify insulin insensitivity as DHEA is known to promote insulin sensitivity. Researchers suggest that DHEA therapy may be beneficial in the treatment of some forms of insulin resistance[569]. DHEA is also typically viewed as an anti-glucocorticoid as it counteracts the negative effects of excess cortisol output. Naturally, this protective effect is lost during chronic stress when DHEA synthesis is reduced in favor of the cortisol pathway.

Not surprisingly, many believe that stabilizing insulin, glucagon, cortisol, and DHEA output can have a dramatic effect on health and longevity. Aging and chronic diseases are thought to be driven by imbalances in these hormones. A Russian researcher named Dilman has studied and

researched this area since the early 1950's. He is widely published in American medical journals and recently co-authored a text with an American physician named Ward Dean[115]. Dilman coined the term "hyperadaptosis" to describe a stress-induced diseased state.

> "Hyperadaptosis is a disease characterized in its latent state by excessive and prolonged elevation of glucocorticoid levels in response to stressors, and in the overt state by elevation of basal glucocorticoid levels in the absence of apparent stressors. Conditions which are characterized by increased basal cortisol levels include ischemic heart disease, various cancers, hypertension and depression."[115]

Obesity, pre-diabetes, and latent type II diabetes are also thought to be promoted by hyperadaptosis. Low DHEA levels are thought to have similar pathologic effects[115].

The degree to which hyperadaptosis exists in our population is surprisingly high. Diagnos-Techs, A clinical and Research Laboratory which performs salivary cortisol and DHEA testing, indicates that a significant number of patients suffer with adrenal malfunction[215]. For this test, saliva samples are taken four times per day to assess the circadian release of cortisol in a real-life fashion. Results from over 30,000 salivary cortisol tests indicate that approximately 45% to 55% of the population have adrenal hyperfunction which is reflected by demonstrable cortisol elevations. Another 15% have flattened curves which is representative of patients that have passed through the hyperfunction phase and on toward adrenal fatigue. The remaining patients have either normal values or have circadian rhythms with specific pathological aberrancies. Many researchers suggest that saliva is the optimal body fluid for testing free cortisol[561, 639, 676, 697, 839, 845].

EXERCISE ENHANCES INSULIN SENSITIVITY

Several studies suggest that exercise promotes insulin sensitivity and thereby reduces insulin resistance. Broughton and Taylor explain that exercise training can increase insulin sensitivity up to 40%[568]. Cononie et al. state that hyper-insulinemia associated with aging can be blunted significantly by regular exercise and is not dependent on changes in body composition[587]. Other studies have reported similar findings[832, 777].

THE FACTS ON FATS

The information presented in this chapter has demonstrated that insulin and cortisol promote fat gain and obesity. This relationship is not typically considered by the various weight management programs. Fat is the main focus, and it is promoted that fat in the diet will make one fat. This assertion needs to be amended in several ways. For example a recent article explained that, "at this stage there is no conclusive evidence from epidemiologic studies that under isoenergetic conditions dietary fat intake promotes the development of obesity more so than other macronutrients"[801].

Willet has recently reviewed the literature and presents convincing evidence that high fat diets do not directly or consistently cause increased fat gain and obesity[851]. In the past 25 years, the prevalence of obesity has dramatically increased in the United States; a period of time in which fat consumption as a total percent of calories has declined. Among European men, there is no observed association between fat intake and body mass index (BMI), even though fat intake ranges from 25%-47% of energy. In European women, there is actually an inverse relationship, such that women with low fat diets (35% of total calories) had the highest BMI. There are few long-term trials on low-fat diets and weight loss, and those that exist do not demonstrate the effectiveness of a low-fat diet in fat reduction. Willet concludes that, "diets high in fat are not the primary cause of excess body fat in our society, nor are reductions in dietary fat a solution." Instead, exercise seems to be the most viable physiological alternative. However, research does suggest that certain fatty acids play different roles in fat metabolism. For example, in animal studies, n-3 fatty acids are apparently protective against weight gain, whereas the n-6 fatty acids, linoleic acid, lead to weight

gain[809]. Earlier in this chapter we also discussed how DHA is a potent inhibitor of lipogenesis and an equally potent activator of beta-oxidation.

Monounsaturated fats also seem to be beneficial for fat loss. Using NIDDM patients as subjects, one study compared a high-carbohydrate, low-fat diet, i.e., 23% of energy, versus a 35% fat diet that was high in monounsaturated fat[844]. Each group lost fat despite a marked difference in fat consumption, which demonstrates that total caloric intake is more important that fat intake. However, the distribution of fat loss was very different between the two groups. The high monounsaturated fat group lost fat evenly between the upper and lower half of the body, while the high-carbohydrate, low-fat group only lost fat in the lower body[844]. Other studies have reported that low-carbohydrate, high monounsaturated fat diets provide better glycemic regulation and allow for fat loss[625, 631].

High levels of saturated fat in the diet seems to be the main concern. Recall that Jeppeson et al. recommend that saturated fats do not exceed 10% of total calories[673]. Saturated fatty acids raise plasma cholesterol levels and reduce LDL receptor activity[613]. As mentioned earlier in this chapter, saturated fatty acids also promote hyperinsulinemia[747]. Animal studies (mice) have shown that beef fat, which is high in saturated fatty acids, leads to an increase in body fat gain, while a diet rich in monounsaturated fat does not. Furthermore, when these mice exercise, the ones on a monounsaturated fat diet lose more fat than those on saturated beef fat[553]. A recent study suggests that a high intake of saturated fat and a low intake of n-3 fatty acids are associated with an increased risk of dementia[677]. Clearly, reductions in saturated fatty acid intake is highly advisable. Unfortunately, the battle cry against fats typically refers to all fats and not just saturated fats and n-6 fatty acids.

Taking a broad approach to fat restriction can have disastrous consequences. For example, Wells et al.[849] recently reported that reducing dietary fat content from 41% to 25% energy may have adverse effects on mood. Ratings of anger-hostility significantly increased when female subjects were place on the low-fat diet. Several studies have also discussed the relationship between a low n-3 fatty acid diet and depression[754, 784, 657].

No discussion about fats could approach completeness without devoting some time to the much-maligned egg. Pelletier et al. determined the effect of egg consumption on gastric emptying and on glycemic and hormonal responses. Four different diets were assessed on 12 healthy male subjects ranging from age 18-29 years. Diet C, the standard breakfast, consisted of 80 g white bread with 25 g of butter, 10 g of sugar and 250 ml of black coffee, and no eggs. The percent of calories was distributed as approximately 45% from carbohydrate, 6% protein, and 49% fat (45:6:49). Diet E, for whole egg, consisted of the standard breakfast plus *2 eggs* resulting in a 33:13:54 distribution of caloric intake. Diet Y, for yolk, consisted of the standard breakfast plus *2 egg yolks* resulting in a 35:9:56 distribution. Diet W, for egg white, consisted of the standard breakfast plus *2 egg whites* resulting in a 42:12:46 distribution.

The rise in blood sugar was significantly greater after Diets C or W than after Diets E or Y ingestion. Diets E and Y also significantly delayed gastric emptying compared to Diets C or W. Additionally, Diet Y significantly reduced insulin peaks. "The results indicated that egg ingestion, especially yolk ingestion, may be of interest in regulating metabolic variables of glucose metabolism"[755]. In other words, fat content of the diet can have a beneficial affect on glycemic regulation.

With respect to egg yolks, these beneficial results contradict the extremely negative characterization that eggs have received. In fact, studies suggest that egg consumption may not have the negative consequences that are so often promoted. Recent research indicates that eating up to 14 eggs per week had no untoward effects on lipoprotein metabolism in 70 healthy young African men who are part of a population group at high risk for coronary heart disease[843]. These findings echo the work of Flynn et al.[617] who, back in 1979, studied the effects of egg consumption on 116 male volunteers between the ages of 32 and 62 years. These men consumed 2 whole eggs daily in their customary diets for 3 months. There were no significant changes in mean serum cholesterol levels

and there was no association of dietary cholesterol intake with either serum cholesterol or triglyceride[617]. The authors conclude by stating,

> "our data further support the suggestion that indiscriminate exclusion of eggs may be a useless preventive measure to maintain low serum cholesterol in all normal healthy men."

It should be remembered that many different dietary factors influence lipoprotein metabolism, and not just cholesterol levels in the diet. As discussed earlier in this chapter, lipoprotein metabolism is greatly influenced by glycemic regulation and the composition of specific fatty acids in the diet. Additional dietary factors can positively influence lipoprotein metabolism including garlic, dietary fiber, and psyllium husk as a fiber source[535, 539, 593, 672]. Additionally, it is now possible to buy eggs that are rich in n-3 fatty acids[811].

SUMMARY

This chapter provided an overview of the topic of glycemic dysregulation. Clearly, numerous dietary, nutritional and lifestyle factors are involved. During patient care, practitioners should urge patients to 1) reduce the intake of refined carbohydrates, 2) reduce total carbohydrate consumption to less than 50% of total calories, 3) maintain a 3:1 to 2:1 ratio of carbohydrate to protein, 4) focus on fruits and vegetables as the main carbohydrate sources and consume minimal amounts of grain products, 5) pursue a 1:1 ratio of n-6:n-3 fatty acids, 6) consume extra virgin olive oil to increase monounsaturated fatty acid and phytochemical intake, 7) consume garlic, onions, and ginger to reduce inflammation and platelet aggregation, 8) insure adequate fiber intake, 9) insure adequate intake of all vitamins and minerals, particularly magnesium, chromium, and biotin, and 10) exercise regularly.

Of interest to note is that these recommendations are very similar to those used to treat patients with cancer, heart disease, rheumatoid arthritis, and many other degenerative conditions. The exact same recommendations are made to those who wish to pursue health and stay free of degenerative disease.

For more details about insulin resistance see a new sports medicine text by Maffetone[713]. In addition to providing a thorough scientific and clinical discussion, Maffetone also focuses on important considerations related to exercise and physical training.

Chapter 7

THE FOOD GUIDE PYRAMID
SAFE OR PRO-INFLAMMATORY?

INTRODUCTION

The information presented in this chapter will demonstrate that following the USDA's food guide pyramid is unsafe and pro-inflammatory, particularly as it relates to fatty acid imbalances. This concern was actually voiced in the December, 1994 issue of the *American Journal of Clinical Nutrition*. Siguel and Lerman[807] wrote an open letter to the editor stating that, "as usually interpreted by most people, the pyramid may encourage an essential fatty acid (EFA)—deficient diet and lead to an increased incidence of atherosclerotic disease, among other health-related problems." These authors contend that, "EFA insufficiency is associated with significant disease states and may underlie many of the chronic diseases prevalent in Western societies."

In response to this letter, Kennedy, Shaw, and Davis defended the pyramid and stated that ample amounts of EFAs are available when one follows the pyramid guidelines[685]. In fact, we are told that the food pyramid will ensure EFA consumption that exceeds the currently estimated requirements. Incidentally, Shaw and Davis were two of the authors of the USDA publication that promotes the food guide pyramid, which you can download from the USDA web site (http://www.nalusda.gov/fnic/Fpyr/pyramid.html).

I recently searched this USDA publication for essential fatty acids, linoleic acid, linolenic acid, etc., and nothing came up. In other words, this book that is supposed to be a resource for nutrition educators does not discuss EFAs in connection

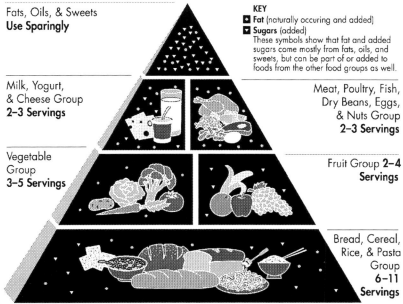

Figure 7-1   SOURCE: U.S. Department of Agriculture/U.S. Department of Health and Human Services

with the food pyramid. Siguel and Lerman seem to be aware of this fact, for in their response to Kennedy et al. letter they thoroughly dismantle the arguments of the USDA writers and subsequently discredit the USDA[808].

THE PROBLEM WITH THE FOOD PYRAMID

The main problems are quite obvious. One has to do with their recommendations for fat intake as alluded to in the above section, and the second problem has to do with their approach to carbohydrate intake.

Fats

Regarding fats, the general impression one gets from the food pyramid is that fats are bad and should be avoided. Fats and oils are located at the top of the food pyramid and are supposed to be used sparingly (see *Figure 7-1*). This recommendation is consistent with the standard battle cry against fats, i.e., that fats cause heart disease and cancer. This concern has been passed on to the food industry which produces numerous varieties of fat-free foods for a public that has been conditioned to consume copious amounts of these foods.

The latest edition of the RDA states that we should consume no more than 30% of our calories from fat and less than 1/3 of those calories should come from saturated fats, and no more than 1/3 of those calories from linoleic acid, i.e., an n-6 fatty acid. Nothing precise is mentioned about which type of fats should comprise the remaining 1/3 of fat calories[481].

The food guide pyramid is much more liberal in its recommendations for fat content in the diet. "Rather than prescribe specific low fat foods (such as nonfat milk), the guide permits consumers to decide which foods they prefer as sources of fat and added sugars, while keeping their total fat intake to no more than 30% of calories"[803]. This naturally suggests that consumers understand the differences and sources of the various fatty acids and their health or disease-promoting qualities. However, it is a mystery as to where this knowledge

should come from, particularly when we consider that the RDA book and the food guide pyramid do not discuss this subject in sufficient detail. Moreover, neither publication discusses the significant health-promoting benefits of monounsaturated fats and omega-3 fatty acids, or makes recommendations regarding levels of intake.

In particular, there is no mention of n-6:n-3 ratios and their importance, despite the existence of volumes of research on this subject. For example, there were some 576 papers published between January 1985 and May 1989 on the subject of fish oil consumption by humans [no animal studies were included in this database search][417]. In the five year period before Simopoulos published this paper, a total of more than 1500 studies had been reported[417]. Of course, there were many animal and human studies performed before 1985. Unfortunately, none of this research is discussed in the RDA book or the food pyramid publication. Additionally, Simopoulos stated that the current data, i.e., circa 1990, supported the need to make recommendations for the general public regarding n-3 fatty acids. As of 1990, the Canadian nutrition recommendations already included information on n-6 and n-3 fatty acids. This has yet to occur in the United States and has been ignored by the USDA, the ADA, and those who publish the RDAs. USDA writers even down play the importance of this issue when questioned[685].

Quick fatty acid review

The topic of fatty acid consumption patterns was already discussed in Chapter 4. It was made clear that our current ratio of n-6:n-3 intake ranges from 10:1 to 25:1. Numerous chronic diseases as well as chronic inflammation are promoted by such ratios (see Chapter 5).

Recall that Budowski and Crawford published a paper in 1985, recommending that n-6:n-3 ratios should be less than 5:1[64]. Linder[275-p.56] cited a 1988 article by Neuringer et al. which recommends a 4:10 ratio of n-6:n-3 fatty acid intake. In 1991, Simopoulos indicated that we are genetically predisposed to consume a ratio of 1:1[417]. In 1996, Eaton et al. explain that our hunter-gatherer ancestors consumed a 1:1 ratio[608]. In 1998, Simopoulos published *The Omega Plan*, which reviewed all the important omega-3 literature to date. She indicates that the n-6:n-3 ratio must be less than 4:1 to prevent changes in genetic expression that promote cancer and heart disease[811].

Carbohydrates

The food guide pyramid urges people to consume massive amounts of grain products and minimal fats. Clearly this suggests that bread, cereal, rice, and pasta should be the main foods consumed by humans. As far as I can tell, there is no evidence to support this arbitrary notion and much evidence suggests that only minimal to moderate amounts of grains should be consumed.

Research suggests that man has historically consumed a diet that contained minimal grain products[608]. "For Paleolithic humans, vegetables and fruit provided the bulk of dietary carbohydrate, cereal grains were used only in extraordinary circumstances and there was no refined flour or sugar at all"[608]. Additionally, the n-6:n-3 fatty acid ratio was about 1:1[608]. The addition of grain foods into the human diet brought with it an extraordinary increase in n-6 consumption, for grains contain only n-6 fatty acids[811].

Consumption of grain products as the mainstay of the diet brings with it additional concerns that need to be addressed. Chapter 6 already discussed how high-carbohydrate diets and diets high in omega-6 fatty acids have been shown to promote hyperinsulinemia and insulin resistance. An increase in grain consumption also means that there will be an associated increased ingestion of gliadin and phytic acid.

Gliadin is the toxic agent found in gluten[858]. Gluten is found in wheat, rye, oats, barley, graham, wheat germ, malt or malt flavoring, kasha, bulgur, buckwheat, millet, amaranth, quinoa, spelt and teff[544]. There are several subfractions of gliadin, all of which appear harmful to the intestinal mucosa[858].

The general perspective on gluten/gliadin is that it is only harmful to those with gluten enteropathy, i.e., celiac disease, and their offspring who may be genetically predisposed. Recent evidence suggests that gluten sensitivity is far more widespread than previously thought. In one study, gliadin antibodies were measured in 200 randomly selected adults[546]. Those with the highest antibody levels (48 subjects) were compared to negative controls. A significantly higher proportion of gliadin-positive individuals reported unexplained attacks of diarrhea and an increased prevalence of chronic fatigue. Compared to negative controls, the positive group also showed significantly decreased transferrin saturation, mean corpuscular volume and mean corpuscular hemoglobin. Additionally, headaches were more common in the gliadin-positive group[546].

While the incidence of elevated gliadin antibodies is about 3% in healthy subjects, researchers discovered that 11 of 92 patients (12%) with osteoporosis had elevated gliadin antibodies. Additionally, intestinal biopsy verified Celiac disease in this group at levels tenfold higher than in the healthy population[708].

A more recent study indicates that the incidence of elevated gliadin antibodies may be as high as 5.7% in the healthy population in Northern Ireland[724]. The incidence was shown to increase with advancing age. These authors state that, "gluten sensitivity is thought to be significantly under-diagnosed in the population." The same authors found that a variety of non-gastrointestinal symptoms may be related to gluten sensitivity[847].

Diagnos-Techs, a private clinical laboratory, has reported that between 14-18% of the population may have increased gliadin antibodies. This lab has developed a simple non-invasive saliva test to determine gliadin sensitivity[602].

Phytic acid is found mainly in grains and may influence the availability of iron and calcium[275-p.325]. Most nutrition texts mention phytates and their influence on mineral absorption, including iron, calcium, zinc and other elements. The extent to which phytic acid may promote deficiency states is unknown.

The information in this section demonstrates that there is no historical evidence to suggest that modern man should be consuming huge amounts of grains as recommended in the food pyramid. Furthermore, contemporary research indicates that many additional problems are associated with diets that are rich in breads, pastas and other grain products. None of these issues are discussed in the RDA book or the Food Guide Pyramid publication.

COMPOSITION OF DIETS BASED ON THE FOOD PYRAMID

The USDA provides three different 5-day diets based on caloric intake levels, i.e., 1600 kcal, 2200 kcal, and 2800 kcal[803]. Naturally, food selection was based upon the food guide pyramid. We

analyzed these sample diets and generated reports on caloric distribution, fats and fatty acids, and vitamins and minerals.

Table 7-1A contains the USDA diet that provides 1600 kcal per day, and the results from our analysis are presented in *Figures 7-1A thru C*. *Table 7-2A* contains the USDA diet that provides 2200 kcal per day, and the results from our analysis are presented in *Figures 7-2A thru C*. *Table 7-3A* contains the USDA diet that provides 2800 kcal per day, and the results from our analysis are presented in *Figures 7-3A thru C*.

Food Pyramid 1,600 Calorie Diet (Female 52)

FIVE DAYS' MENUS AT 1,600 CALORIES

Day 1	Day 2	Day 3	Day 4	Day 5
BREAKFAST				
Orange juice ....3/4 c	Grapefruit juice ....3/4 c	Grapefruit 1/2	Fresh sliced strawberries ....1/2 c	Cantaloupe............1/4 melon
Oatmeal.....................1/2 c	*Breakfast pita .....1 sandwich	Ready-to-eat cereal flakes ....1 oz	Whole-grain cereal flakes ....1 oz	*Whole-wheat pancakes.....2
White toast ....1 slice	Skim milk.......................1 c	Toasted english muffin with raisins 1/2	Toasted plain bagel........1/2	*Blueberry sauce..........1/4 c
Margarine....................1 tsp		Jelly.............................1 tsp	Cream cheese..........1/2 tbsp	Skim milk.........................1 c
Jelly.............................1 tsp		Skim milk...................1/2 c	2% fat milk ....1 c	
Skim milk.....................1/2 c				
LUNCH				
*Split pea soup................1 c	*Turkey pasta salad ....1-1/4 c	*Taco salad greens..........................1 c	Broiled chicken fillet sandwich 1	*Chili-stuffed baked potato...1
*Quick tuna and sprouts sandwich 1	Tomato wedges on lettuce leaf..........1 serving	chili ....3/4 c	Mayonnaise ....1 pkt	*Spinach-orange salad .....1 c
Mixed green salad ....1 c	Hard roll 1	Sherbet.......................1/2 c	*Confetti coleslaw ....1/2 c	Wheat crackers 6
Reduced-calorie italian dressing ....1 tbsp	Margarine....................1 tsp		2% fat milk ....1 c	
*Chocolate mint pie.........................1 serving	Skim milk.......................1 c			
DINNER				
*Savory sirloin............. 3 oz	*Creole fish fillets...........3 oz	*Pork & vegetable stirfry mixture............................1 c	*Lentil stroganoff mixture ....1-1/2 c	*Apricot-glazed chicken..3 oz
*Corn and zucchini combo.......... 1/2 c	Small new potatoes with skin 2	rice ....3/4 c	noodles ....3/4 c	*Rice-pasta pilaf......... 3/4 c
Tomato and lettuce salad ....1 serv.	Cooked green peas......1/2 c with margarine ....1 tsp	Cooked broccoli...........1/2 c	Cooked whole green beans................1/2 c	Tossed salad ....1 c
Reduced-calorie french dressing ....1 tbsp	*Whole-wheat cornmeal muffin 1	White roll........................1	Tomato and cucumber salad.........1 serv.	Reduced-calorie italian dressing ....1 tbsp
Whole-wheat roll 1	Margarine....................1 tsp	Minted pineapple chunks.......................1/2 c	Reduced-calorie vinaigrette dressing ......1 tbsp	Hard roll 1
Margarine.....................1 tsp	*Peach crisp ....1/2 c		Honeydew...........1/8 melon	Vanilla ice milk.............1/2 c
*Yogurt-strawberry parfait.........................1 c				
SNACKS				
Graham crackers ....3 squares	Bagel ....1 medium	Wheat crackers 6	Roast beef sandwich........1/2	Fig bar 1
Skim milk.......................1 c	Margarine....................1 tsp	Skim milk.......................1 c		Skim milk....................3/4 c
	Jelly............................1 tsp			

Source: *Using the Food Pyramid: A Resource for Nutrition Educators*, U.S. Department of Agriculture Food, Nutrition, and Consumer Service Center For Nutrition Policy and Promotion p.91

* Recipes included in Appendix 2.

Table 7-1A

Food Pyramid 2,200 Calorie Diet (Female 30)

FIVE DAYS' MENUS AT 2,200 CALORIES

Day 1	Day 2	Day 3	Day 4	Day 5
BREAKFAST				
Orange juice ....3/4 c	Grapefruit juice ....3/4 c	Grapefruit 1/2	Fresh sliced strawberries ....1/2 c	Cantaloup.............1/4 melon
Oatmeal......................1/2 c	*Breakfast pita .....1 sandwich	Banana..................1 medium	Whole-grain cereal flakes ....1 oz	*Turkey patty...........1-1/2 oz
White toast................2 slices	2% fat milk ....1 c	Ready-to-eat cereal flakes ....1 oz	Toasted plain bagel ....1 medium	*Whole-wheat pancakes......2
Margarine....................2 tsp		Toasted english muffin with raisins........................1	Cream cheese.............1 tbsp	*Blueberry sauce..........1/4 c
Jelly............................1 tsp		Margarine....................2 tsp	2% fat milk ....1 c	Margarine....................1 tsp
2% fat milk ....1/2 c		Skim milk....................1/2 c		Skim milk........................1 c
LUNCH				
*Split pea soup...............1 c	*Turkey pasta salad ...1-1/4 c	*Taco salad greens............................1 c	Broiled chicken fillet sandwich 1	*Chili-stuffed baked potato.............................1
*Quick tuna and sprouts sandwich 1	Tomato wedges on lettuce leaf..........1 serving	chili .... 3/4 c	Mayonnaise ....1 pkt	Lowfat, low-sodium cheddar cheese ....3 tbsp
Mixed green salad ....1 c	Hard rolls...........................2	Gingersnaps.......................2	*Confetti coleslaw ....1/2 c	*Spinach-orange salad .....1 c
Reduced-calorie italian dressing ....1 tbsp	Margarine................... 2 tsp		Fresh orange 1	Wheat crackers 6
*Chocolate mint pie.........................1 serving	Oatmeal cookies................4		2% fat milk ....1 c	Skim milk........................1 c
	2% fat milk ....1 c			
DINNER				
*Savory sirloin...............3 oz	*Creole fish fillets...........4 oz	*Pork and vegetable stirfry mixture ....1 c	*Lentil stroganoff mixture ....1-1/2 c	*Apricot-glazed chicken ....3 oz
*Corn and zucchini combo........................3/4 c	Small new potatoes with skin 2	rice ....3/4 c	noodles ....3/4 c	*Rice-pasta pilaf...........3/4 c
Tomato and lettuce salad ....1 serv	Cooked green peas ......1/2 c with margarine ....1 tsp	Cooked broccoli...........1/2 c	Cooked whole green beans.................1/2 c with margarine ....1 tsp	Tossed salad ....1 c
French dressing............1 tbsp	*Whole-wheat cornmeal muffins 2	White rolls 2	Tomato and cucumber salad ....1 serv.	Reduced-calorie italian dressing ....1 tbsp
Whole-wheat rolls 2	Margarine....................2 tsp	Margarine....................2 tsp	Reduced-calorie vinaigrette dressing ....1 tbsp	Hard rolls...........................2
Margarine....................1 tsp	*Peach crisp.................1/2 c	Minted pineapple chunks.........................1/2 c	Pumpernickel roll.................1	Margarine....................2 tsp
*Yogurt-strawberry parfait.............................1 c			Margarine....................1 tsp	Vanilla ice milk.............1/2 c
			Honeydew ....1/8 melon	
SNACKS				
Graham crackers ....6 squares	Bagel ....1 medium	Wheat crackers 6	No-salt-added vegetable juice.............3/4 c	Soft pretzel ....1 large
2% fat milk ....1 c	Margarine....................2 tsp	Cheddar cheese ......1-1/2 oz	Roast beef sandwich 1	Fresh apple 1/2
Peanut butter ....2 tbsp	Fresh pear.........................1	Turkey sandwich 1/2	2% fat milk ....1 c	
Fresh peach........................1		No-salt-added tomato juice.................3/4 c		
Carrot sticks ....7–8 medium				

Recipes included in Appendix 2.

Source: *Using the Food Pyramid: A Resource for Nutrition Educators*, U.S. Department of Agriculture Food, Nutrition, and Consumer Service Center For Nutrition Policy and Promotion p.92

Table 7-2A

Food Pyramid 2,800 Calorie Diet (Male 23)

FIVE DAYS' MENUS AT 2,800 CALORIES				
Day 1	**Day 2**	**Day 3**	**Day 4**	**Day 5**
BREAKFAST				
Orange juice ....3/4 c	Grapefruit juice ....3/4 c	Grapefruit 1/2	Fresh sliced strawberries ....1/2 c	Cantaloup............1/4 melon
Oatmeal......................1/2 c	*Breakfast pita .....1 sandwich	Banana.................1 medium	Hard cooked egg...............1	*Turkey patty...........1-1/2 oz
White toast................2 slices	Bran muffin ....1 large	Ready-to-eat cereal flakes ....1 oz	Whole-grain cereal flakes ....1 oz	*Whole-wheat pancakes......3
Margarine.....................2 tsp	Margarine....................1 tsp	Toasted english muffin with raisins........................1	Toasted plain bagel ....1 medium	*Blueberry sauce ....6 tbsp
Jelly.............................2 tsp	2% fat milk ....1 c	Margarine....................2 tsp	Cream cheese............2 tbsp	Margarine.....................2 tsp
2% fat milk ....1/2 c		Skim milk.........................1 c	2% fat milk ....1 c	2% fat milk ....1 c
LUNCH				
*Split pea soup...............1 c	*Turkey pasta salad ...1-1/4 c	*Taco salad greens.............................1 c	Broiled chicken fillet sandwich 1	*Chili-stuffed baked potato...1
*Quick tuna and sprouts sandwich 1	Tomato wedges on lettuce leaf..........1 serving	chili ....3/4 c	Mayonnaise ....1 pkt	Lowfat, low-sodium cheddar cheese ....3 tbsp
Mixed green salad ....1 c	Hard rolls...........................2	Sherbet......................1/2 c	*Confetti coleslaw ....1/2 c	*Spinach-orange salad .....1 c
Italian dressing ....1 tbsp	Margarine....................2 tsp	Gingersnaps.........................3	Fresh orange 1	Fresh grapes.....................12
*Chocolate mint pie ....1 serving	Tangerine 1	Skim milk.........................1 c	*Lemon pound cake.....1 slice	Wheat crackers 6
2% fat milk ....1 c	Oatmeal cookies................6		2% fat milk ....1 c	Fig bars 2
	2% fat milk ....1 c			2% fat milk ....1 c
DINNER				
*Savory sirloin...............4 oz	*Creole fish fillets...........4 oz	*Pork and vegetable stirfry mixture...........................1 c	*Lentil Stroganoff mixture ....1-1/2 c	Honeydew ....1/4 melon
*Corn and zucchini combo ....1 c	Small new potatoes with skin 2	rice ....3/4 c	noodles ....3/4 c	*Apricot-glazed chicken..3 oz
Tomato and lettuce salad ....1 serv.	Cooked green peas ......3/4 c with margarine ....1 tsp	Cooked broccoli..............1 c	Cooked whole green beans ....1 c with margarine ....1 tsp	*Rice-pasta pilaf..........3/4 c
Reduced-calorie french dressing......................1 tbsp	*Whole-wheat cornmeal muffins 2	White rolls 2	Tomato and cucumber salad ....1 serv.	Steamed zucchini ....1/2 c
Whole-wheat rolls 2	Margarine....................2 tsp	Margarine....................2 tsp	Reduced-calorie vinaigrette dressing ......1 tbsp	Tossed salad ....1 c
Margarine.....................1 tsp	*Peach crisp ....1/2 c	Minted pineapple chunks........................1/2 c	Pumpernickel rolls 2	Italian dressing ....1 tbsp
*Yogurt-strawberry parfait................................1 c			Margarine.....................2 tsp	Hard rolls............................2
				Margarine.....................2 tsp
				Vanilla ice milk.............1/2 c
SNACKS				
Graham crackers ....6 squares	Bagel ....1 medium	Wheat crackers 6	No-salt-added vegetable juice.............3/4 c	Fresh apple 1/2
Peanut butter-banana sandwich 1	Margarine....................2 tsp	Orange juice ....3/4 c	Roast beef sandwich 1	Soft pretzel 1large
Fresh peach.........................1	Jelly.............................2 tsp	Cheddar cheese ......1-1/2 oz	2% fat milk ....1 c	Lemonade........................1 c
Nonfat fruit-flavored yogurt ....8 oz	Fresh pear...........................1	Turkey sandwich 1	Lemonade........................1 c	2% fat milk ....1 c
Carrot sticks ....7–8 medium	Lowfat fruit-flavored yogurt ....1/2 c	Raw vegetables ....6 pieces		
	Unsalted roasted peanuts ....2-1/2 tbsp (1/2 oz)	Spinach dip................2 tbsp		

* Recipes included in Appendix 2.

Table 7-3A

Source: *Using the Food Pyramid: A Resource for Nutrition Educators*, U.S. Department of Agriculture Food, Nutrition, and Consumer Service Center For Nutrition Policy and Promotion p.93

Caloric balance

Figures 7-1A thru 7-3A illustrate the percent of total calories from carbohydrates, protein and fat, and the ratio of carbohydrate to protein. Regarding total caloric intake, recall that Jeppesen et al. recently suggested that a 45:15:40 percent balance was desirable. In each of the three food pyramid diets, carbohydrates represent more than 50% of calories. Additionally, a closer look at the sources of dietary carbohydrate reveals that a significant percentage of calories came from grain products and desserts, many of which have a high glycemic index, i.e., bagels, white bread/rolls, soft pretzels, and chocolate mint pie. These carbohydrates also represent sources of empty calories. It is hard to imagine that the USDA can actually promote the consumption of these foods as components of a healthy diet.

Food Pyramid
1,600 Calorie Diet (Female 52)

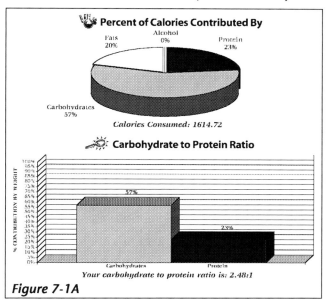

Figure 7-1A

Food Pyramid
2,200 Calorie Diet (Female 30)

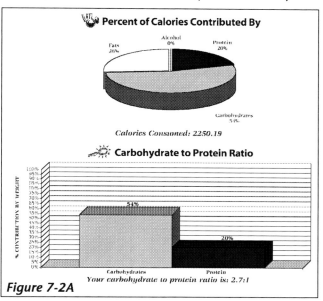

Figure 7-2A

Food Pyramid
2,800 Calorie Diet (Male 23)

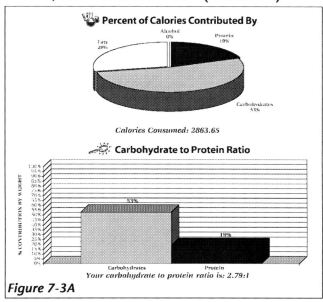

Figure 7-3A

While protein intake is reasonable, notice that fat intake ranges from 20-28% of total calories. This is significantly lower then the recommended 40 percent. The problems with low fat diets were discussed in Chapter 6.

Fats and fatty acids

Figures 7-1B thru 7-3B illustrate percentages of total fats and a breakdown of individual fatty acids. The overall balance of fats is reasonable;

Food Pyramid
1,600 Calorie Diet (Female 52)

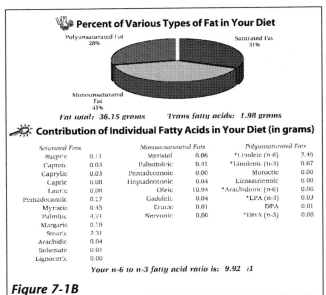

Figure 7-1B

Food Pyramid
2,200 Calorie Diet (Female 30)

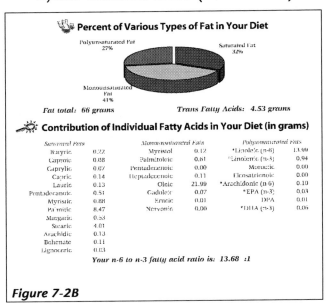

Figure 7-2B

Food Pyramid
2,800 Calorie Diet (Male 23)

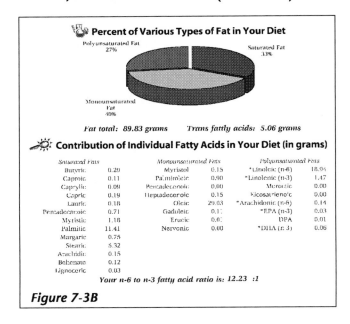

Figure 7-3B

however, carefully examine the ratio of n-6:n-3 fatty acids. Each diet provides at least a 10:1 ratio which, as stated above, is pro-inflammatory and known to promote cancer, heart disease, diabetes and many other diseases.

Comparison to RDA nutrients

Figure 7-1C thru 7-3C illustrates vitamin and mineral levels found in food pyramid diets. As you can see, many nutrients are low or borderline when compared to the RDA.

It should be mentioned that food packages compare their nutrient density to the 1968 RDA and not the 1989 version. Additionally, in recent years, new recommendations have come forth from the Food and Nutrition Board at the Institute of Medicine-National Academy of Sciences. The information in Appendix C outlines the RDAs from 1968 and 1989, the recommendations from two different nutrition

texts, and the new dietary reference intakes (DRI) from 1997-98.

If you go to Appendix C and look at folic acid recommendations, you will see an interesting trend. In 1968 we were told that 400 mcg was the RDA. This number changed over the years and eventually ended up being ~200 mcg in 1989. Then in 1997-98 the new DRI level for folic acid increased back up to 400 mcg, which is exactly what it was some 30 years ago. A similar trend can be seen with calcium. Will this be the same with other nutrients? It is difficult to say at this point, but the DRI for magnesium is higher than the 1989 RDA.

Regarding nutrient levels, it is important to remember that the RDAs are well below toxicity levels for all nutrients. This means that there is a significant margin between

Food Pyramid 1,600 Calorie Diet (Female 52)

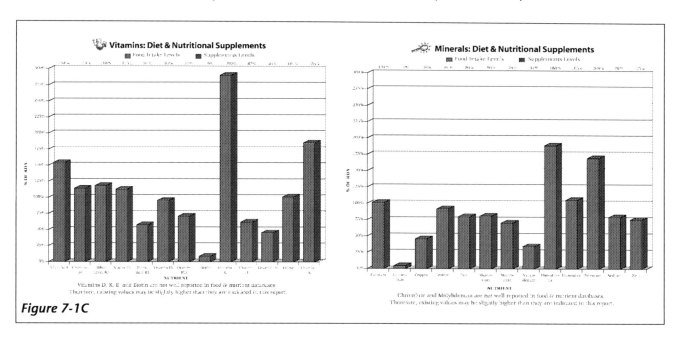

Figure 7-1C

adequate intake and toxicity. Thus, it would always be wise to err on the high side rather than the low. In our reports we compare dietary levels to the 1968 RDAs, or one of the other recommendations if it is higher than the 1968 recommended level.

If you look at *Figure 7-1C thru 7-3C* you will see that the nutrient levels provided by the food guide pyramid barely meet 100% of recommended levels and many nutrients fall short. Clearly, we should have serious concerns about the food pyramid.

Food Pyramid 2,200 Calorie Diet (Female 30)

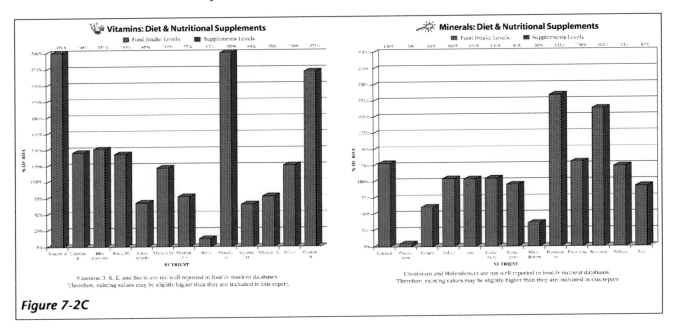

Figure 7-2C

Food Pyramid 2,800 Calorie Diet (Male 23)

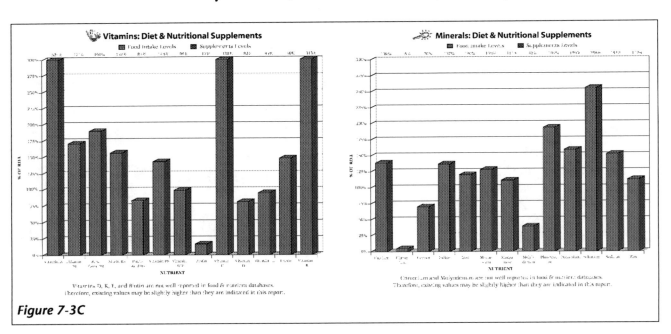

Figure 7-3C

Trans fatty acids

The potential dangers related to *trans* fatty acids were discussed Chapter 5. *Trans* fatty acids are also discussed in this chapter because the food pyramid recommends that we 1) spread margarine on our high glycemic grain products, and 2) use margarine in the preparation of various food pyramid recipes. In addition, some of breads, cereals and crackers recommended by the food pyramid also contain *trans* fatty acids.

At the present time, *trans* fatty acids are only reported in about half of the foods found in most databases. Regarding margarine, levels for *trans* fatty acids varies among the many different products. In our database, trans fatty acids comprise anywhere from 2.7g to 36g of the total weight of 100 g samples of margarine. We used a medium level sample, i.e., 12.05g, as the margarine in the food pyramid diet plans. Trans fatty acid levels are listed in *Figures 7-1B* thru *7-3B*.

COMPOSITION OF A NATURAL DIET CONTAINING NO MARGARINE, GRAIN PRODUCTS, OR PACKAGED FOODS

We created a 7-day diet that is high in fruits, vegetables, fish, and olive oil. *Table 7-4* contains the natural diet and *Figures 7-4A* thru *7-4C* illustrate the results of our analysis.

Caloric balance

As illustrated in *Figure 7-4A*, the caloric intake was 2,200 kcal with a distribution of about 40:20:40 among carbohydrates, proteins and fats. Compare this diet to the 2,800 kcal diet from the food guide pyramid.

The majority of carbohydrate calories came from fruits and vegetables as there were no grain products in this diet, and thus it is a gliadin-free diet and contains significantly less phytates compared with the food pyramid diet. Potatoes in the natural diet represented the carbohydrate food that most closely resembled the grain products found in the food pyramid diet.

Fats and fatty acids

Figure 7-4B illustrates fat intake. First, notice that the natural diet contains only 0.76 grams of trans fatty acids versus 5.06 grams from the food pyramid. The balance of fats is approximately what is recommended by Jeppesen et al.[673], and has less saturated fatty acids than the food pyramid diet. The balance of polyunsaturated fatty acids represents a significant departure from the food pyramid. Whereas the n6:n3 fatty acid ratio in the food pyramid diet is 11.73:1, the natural diet provides an almost perfect 1.56:1

Natural Diet (Male 23)

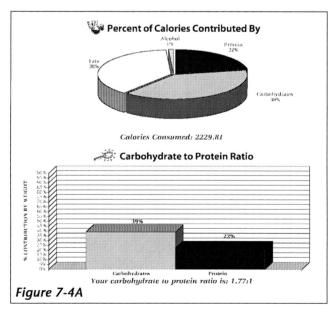

Figure 7-4A

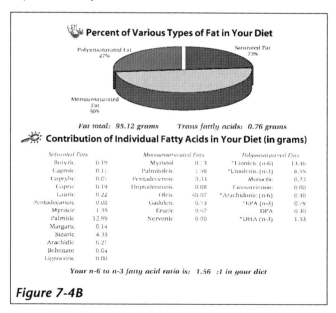

Figure 7-4B

NATURAL DIET

BREAKFAST

DAY 1
- Plain lowfat yogurt ..... 1 c
- Fresh blueberries ..... 1 c
- Fresh pineapple ..... 1 c
- Banana ..... 1 med
- Raw sunflower seeds ..... 1 oz
- Green tea ..... 8 oz

DAY 2
- Omelet ..... 3 eggs
- Onions/sauteed ..... 1/4 c
- Carrots/sauteed ..... 1/4 c
- Red peppers/sauteed ..... 1/4 c
- Mushrooms/sauteed ..... 1/4 c
- Green tea ..... 8 oz
- Olive oil ..... 1 Tbsp

DAY 3
- Plain lowfat yogurt ..... 1 c
- Fresh strawberries ..... 1 c
- Fresh pineapple ..... 1 c
- Raw sunflower seeds ..... 1 oz
- Green tea ..... 8 oz

DAY 4
- Cottage cheese/2% fat ..... 1 c
- Fresh strawberries ..... 1 c
- Fresh blueberries ..... 1 c
- Kiwifruit ..... 1 med
- Green tea ..... 8 oz

DAY 5
- Plain lowfat yogurt ..... 1 c
- Fresh strawberries ..... 1 c
- Fresh grapes ..... 1 c
- Kiwifruit ..... 1 med
- Green tea ..... 8 oz

DAY 6
- Omelet ..... 3 eggs
- Onion/sauteed ..... 1/4 c
- Carrots/sauteed ..... 1/4 c
- Red peppers/sauteed ..... 1/4 c
- Mushrooms/sauteed ..... 1/4 c
- Green tea ..... 8 oz
- Olive oil ..... 1 Tbsp

DAY 7
- Cottage cheese/2% fat ..... 1 c
- Fresh strawberries ..... 1 c
- Fresh raspberries ..... 1 c
- Banana ..... 1 med
- Green tea ..... 8 oz

LUNCH*

DAY 1
- Lentil Soup ..... 1 1/2 c
- Salad w/:
- Romaine lettuce ..... 3 c
- Red peppers ..... 1/2 c
- Broccoli ..... 1/2 c
- Onions ..... 1/2 c
- Olive oil ..... 1 Tbsp
- Flaxseed oil ..... 1 Tbsp
- Vinegar ..... 1 Tbsp

DAY 2
- Tuna/can/in water ..... 6 oz
- Celery ..... 1/4 c
- Onions ..... 1/4 c
- Red peppers ..... 1/4 c
- Mayonnaise ..... 2 Tbsp
- Salad w/:
- Raw spinach ..... 3 c
- Flaxseed oil ..... 1 Tbsp
- Mushrooms ..... 1/2 c
- Olive oil ..... 1 Tbsp
- Vinegar ..... 1 Tbsp

DAY 3
- Salad w/:
- Raw spinach ..... 3 c
- Garbanzo Beans ..... 1 c
- Watercress ..... 1/2 c
- Red peppers ..... 1/2 c
- Onions ..... 1/2 c
- Flaxseed oil ..... 1 Tbsp
- Olive oil ..... 1 Tbsp

DAY 4
- Chili & Beans ..... 1 c
- Onions/sauteed ..... 1/2 c
- Olive oil ..... 1 Tsp
- Salad w/:
- Romaine lettuce ..... 2 c
- Red peppers ..... 1/2 c
- Broccoli ..... 1/2 c
- Carrots ..... 1/2 c
- Flaxseed oil ..... 1 Tbsp
- Olive oil ..... 1 Tbsp
- Tomato ..... 1/2 med
- Lemon juice ..... 1 Tsp

DAY 5
- Broiled herring ..... 6 oz
- Salad w/:
- Raw spinach ..... 2 c
- Arugula ..... 1 c
- Romaine lettuce ..... 1 c
- Red peppers ..... 1 c
- Broccoli ..... 1/2 c
- Carrots ..... 1/2 c
- Flaxseed oil ..... 1 Tbsp
- Olive oil ..... 1 Tbsp
- Vinegar ..... 1 Tbsp

DAY 6
- Hamburger patty ..... 4 oz
- Dill pickle ..... 2 med
- Ketchup ..... 1 Tbsp
- Salad w/:
- Romaine lettuce ..... 3 c
- Mushrooms ..... 1/2 c
- Onions ..... 1/2 c
- Tomato ..... 1/2 med
- Olive oil ..... 1 Tbsp
- Flaxseed oil ..... 1 Tbsp
- Vinegar ..... 1 Tbsp

DAY 7
- Grilled salmon ..... 6 oz
- Onions/sauteed ..... 1/2 c
- Olive oil ..... 1 Tbsp
- Salad w/:
- Raw spinach ..... 2 c
- Arugula ..... 1 c
- Broccoli ..... 1/2 c
- Red peppers ..... 1/2 c
- Flaxseed oil ..... 1 Tsp
- Olive oil ..... 1 Tbsp
- Vinegar ..... 1 Tbsp

DINNER*

DAY 1
- Grilled Salmon ..... 6 oz
- Sweet Potato ..... 1 med
- Butter ..... 1 pat
- Kale/sauteed ..... 2 c
- Garlic/sauteed ..... 1 clove
- Mushrooms/sauteed ..... 1/2 c
- Onions/sauteed ..... 1/2 c
- Olive oil ..... 1 Tbsp
- Red wine ..... 4 oz

DAY 2
- Beef Stir Fry w/:
- Ground Beef ..... 6 oz
- Onions ..... 1/2 c
- Mushrooms ..... 1/2 c
- Red Peppers ..... 1/2 c
- Carrots ..... 1/2 c
- Olive oil ..... 1 Tbsp
- Salad w/:
- Garlic/sauteed ..... 1 clove
- Olive oil ..... 1 Tsp

DAY 3
- Sausage and Peppers w/:
- Turkey sausage ..... 6 oz
- Onions ..... 1 c
- Red Peppers ..... 1 c
- Mushrooms ..... 1/2 c
- Butter ..... 1 pat
- Salad w/:
- Raw spinach ..... 2 c
- Onions ..... 1/2 c
- Olive oil ..... 1 Tbsp
- Flaxseed oil ..... 1 Tbsp
- Vinegar ..... 1 Tbsp

DAY 4
- Grilled Halibut ..... 6 oz
- Broccoli/steamed ..... 1 c
- Kale/steamed ..... 1 c
- Baked potato ..... 1 med
- Butter ..... 1 pat
- Salad w/:
- Raw spinach ..... 2 c
- Onions ..... 1/2 c
- Olive oil ..... 1 Tbsp
- Flaxseed oil ..... 1 Tbsp
- Vinegar ..... 1 Tbsp

DAY 5
- Grilled sea trout ..... 6 oz
- Broccoli/steamed ..... 1 c
- Spinach/steamed ..... 1 c
- Salad w/:
- Romaine lettuce ..... 2 c
- Olive oil ..... 1 Tbsp
- Vinegar ..... 1 Tbsp
- Flaxseed oil ..... 1 Tsp

DAY 6
- Chicken breast/grilled ..... 6 oz
- Onions/sauteed ..... 1/2 c
- Mushrooms/sauteed ..... 1/2 c
- Garlic/sauteed ..... 1 clove
- Olive oil ..... 1 Tbsp
- Salad w/:
- Romaine lettuce ..... 2 c
- Mushrooms/sauteed ..... 1/4 c
- Olive oil ..... 1 Tbsp
- Vinegar ..... 1 Tbsp
- Red wine ..... 4 oz

DAY 7
- Oysters/steamed 8
- Shrimp/steamed 10
- Broccoli/steamed ..... 1 c
- Kale/sauteed ..... 1 c
- Salad w/:
- Mushrooms/sauteed ..... 1/4 c
- Olive oil ..... 1 Tbsp
- Vinegar ..... 1 Tbsp
- Red wine ..... 4 oz

SNACKS

DAY 1
- Dried figs 6
- Apple ..... 1 med
- Fresh vegetable juice ..... 12 oz
- Carrots ..... 3 long
- Celery ..... 3 long
- Beet ..... 1/2 med
- Fresh ginger root ..... 1/8 c

DAY 2
- Fresh cantaloupe ..... 1/2 med
- Apple ..... 1 med
- Banana ..... 1 med
- Fresh vegetable juice ..... 12 oz
- Carrots ..... 3 long
- Celery ..... 3 long
- Beet ..... 1/2 med
- Fresh ginger root ..... 1/8 c

DAY 3
- Fresh cantaloupe ..... 1/2 med
- Raw almonds ..... 1 oz
- Banana ..... 1 med
- Dried figs 6

DAY 4
- Fresh grapefruit ..... 1 med
- Fresh cantaloupe ..... 1/2 med
- Apple ..... 1 med
- Fresh vegetable juice ..... 12 oz
- Carrots ..... 3 long
- Celery ..... 3 long
- Beet ..... 1/2 med
- Fresh ginger root ..... 1/8 c

DAY 5
- Raw almonds ..... 1 oz
- Plain lowfat yogurt ..... 1 c
- Banana ..... 1 med
- Fresh cantaloupe ..... 1 c
- Fresh vegetable juice ..... 12 oz
- Carrots ..... 3 long
- Celery ..... 3 long
- Beet ..... 1/2 med
- Fresh ginger root ..... 1/8 c

DAY 6
- Peach ..... 1 med
- Raw almonds ..... 1 oz
- Fresh cherries 20
- Apple ..... 1 med
- Fresh vegetable juice ..... 12 oz
- Carrots ..... 3 long
- Celery ..... 3 long
- Beet ..... 1/2 med
- Fresh ginger root ..... 1/8 c

DAY 7
- Dried Figs 6
- Plain lowfat yogurt ..... 1 c
- Fresh cantaloupe ..... 1 c
- Fresh vegetable juice ..... 12 oz
- Carrots ..... 3 long
- Celery ..... 3 long
- Beet ..... 1/2 med
- Fresh ginger root ..... 1/8 c

*Season to taste with low sodium condiments

Natural Diet (Male 23)

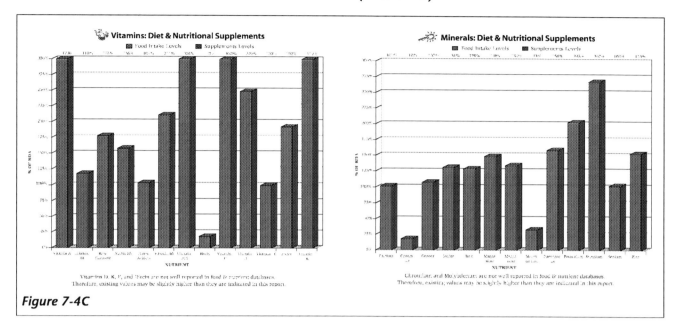

Figure 7-4C

Comparison to the RDA nutrients

Figure 7-4C illustrates that the natural diet, while being 600 kcal less than the 2,800 kcal food pyramid diet, provides significantly more vitamins and minerals. Notice that potassium intake reached the levels consumed by our hunter gatherer ancestors, ratio. Readers should be aware of the fact that the n-3 levels achieved in the natural diet were due to the use of flaxseed oil in the salad dressings. However, it is possible to stay below the desired 4:1 ratio with diet alone. For example, the natural diet without flaxseed oil provided a 3.3:1 ratio of n-6:n-3 fatty acids. In most diets, however, it does not seem possible to get sufficient amounts of n-3 fatty acids unless either flaxseed or fish oil supplements are used.

which is significantly more than what is derived from the food guide pyramid. In addition, the natural diet also provides significantly less sodium compared to the food pyramid diet. Although food databases do not determine phytochemical content in the diet, it is likely that the natural diet also contains significantly more phenols, flavonoids, terpinoids, carotenoids, etc., compared with the food pyramid diet.

SUMMARY

While no one knows if this "natural" diet represents the best diet, it is clear that the benefits far exceed those offered by the food guide pyramid. It is time the USDA and ADA improve their recommendations and overall approach to dietary practices.

Chapter 8

CHEMICAL IRRITANTS - GENERATION AND NUTRITIONAL INHIBITION

While reading or referring to the information in this chapter, keep in mind that the inflammatory process is a complex chemical phenomena, involving numerous chemical mediators. Chapter 5 demonstrated that our dietary habits can enhance the production of a variety of chemical mediators which are pro-inflammatory in nature. With such a pro-inflammatory state, it is likely that the body will release an excess of chemical mediators of inflammation when the bodily tissues are injured via micro or macrotrauma.

This chapter deals with each specific chemical mediator and nutritional supplements that can act as mediator inhibitors. It should be understood that it is foolhardy to attempt to inhibit one or more chemical mediators without first addressing the diet-induced pro-inflammatory state. The nice part about this approach to nutritional supplementation is that a doctor does not need to stock more than five to nine supplements. The seven main supplements include a multiple vitamin/mineral, magnesium, anti-oxidant (vitamin C and bioflavonoids), fish oil (i.e., EPA/DHA), an anti-inflammatory botanical, chondroitin/glucosamine, and bromelain. You may also want to supplement with vitamin E and coenzyme Q10, which would bring the total to 9 supplements. Most nutrition companies provide these supplements, and it is possible to get all of these supplements from the same company. However, I would consider using a variety of companies as certain ones specialize in the production and development of different products.

Before beginning this discussion about the biochemical irritants, it should be reemphasized that these biochemicals are not bad molecules. In fact, it appears that the various biochemicals become irritants only when they are produced in excess. Readers might also infer from what is written that the purpose of supplementation is to absolutely inhibit the production of the various biochemical irritants. Albeit, the term "nutritional inhibition" may be used; however, the purpose is really to try to normalize the production of the various inflammatory mediators. Please keep this in mind while reading the text that follows.

Readers should also keep in mind that the nutritional recommendations in this chapter are provided as an adjunct to the dietary modifications described in Chapters 5-7. Additionally, it should be understood that nutrition supplement research has been done with both animal and human subjects. Both types of studies are referenced in this chapter. Whenever possible, human studies are highlighted and used to help develop supplementation recommendations.

LACTIC ACID

Introduction

Lactic acid is probably one of the most well known biochemicals. Any layman who has ever exercised has heard of lactic acid in the context of it being responsible for pain production during exercise...this notion is probably incorrect. It is bradykinin that is thought to be most responsible for pain production during exercise. Bradykinin is also thought to be the most potent chemical mediator[433]. Of interest to note is the fact that tissue acidity is known to activate prekallikrein which is then converted into bradykinin. The accumulation of lactic acid during exercise is thought to initiate this conversion which results in pain[433, 434]. Although lactic acid itself can depolarize nociceptors[146, 408, 424, 504], it is thought to be the *least* potent of all chemical irritants in terms of nociception[491].

Another common misconception is that lactic acid causes fatigue. Some evidence exists to support the theory that lactate accumulation is involved in the fatigue associated with *anaerobic exercise*[331-p.364-66, 438, 298-p.111]. McArdle states that, "fatigue is probably mediated by increased acidity that inactivates various enzymes [phosphorylase and phosphofructokinase[438]] involved in energy transfer as well as the muscles' contractile properties"[298]. Stewart suggests that lactic acid-induced bradykinin production is the major factor that inhibits further exercise[433, 434]. The lactic acid-bradykinin connection is most likely involved when pain develops during anaerobic exercise. In contrast, the fatigue that develops during *aerobic exercise* most likely occurs due to a depletion of glycogen stores over the course of a given activity[298-p.516,331-p.370], and has nothing to do with lactic acid accumulation or bradykinin production.

Lactic acid is produced during anaerobic metabolism via glycolysis. The glycolytic pathway functions to convert intracellular glucose into pyruvate. If oxygen is *not* present, pyruvate will be converted into lactic acid. In the presence of oxygen, pyruvate and coenzyme-A join to form acetyl-CoA. Acetyl-CoA then joins with oxaloacetic acid to form citric acid, the first step in the Krebs cycle. Through a series of oxidation reactions, citric acid is ultimately converted into oxaloacetic acid which can then join with another acetyl-CoA molecule to form citric acid. The cycle will then repeat itself. During specific conversion steps, NADH and $FADH_2$ are produced which are then shuttled into the electron transport chain where the hydrogen molecules (protons) are used to make ATP.

ATP Production

As alluded to above, understanding ATP production requires a degree of familiarity with glycolysis, the Krebs cycle and the electron transport chain. To many clinicians, the thought of studying these pathways is bothersome because most of us were taught biochemistry incorrectly, such that we were led to believe that biochemical pathways are not clinically relevant in most cases.

We should, in fact, embrace biochemical pathways because our patients **are** patients because they have biochemical aberrations. The following quote will help put ATP production into a more clinical context:

> "The energy in food is not transformed directly to the cells for biologic work. Rather, this "nutrient energy" is harvested and funneled through the energy-rich compound adenosine triphosphate or ATP. The potential energy within the ATP molecule is then utilized for all the energy-requiring processes of the cell. This energy receiver-energy donor cycle, in essence, represents the two major energy-transforming activities in the cell: [1] to form and conserve ATP from the potential energy in food, and [2] to use the chemical energy for biologic work."[298-p.101]

Very simply, our bodies make ATP from food, and without ATP our bodies would die. Indeed, "oxidation of pyruvate is a central step in the energy metabolism of all cells, and major impairment of this step is not likely to be compatible with life in most instances"[174].

A closer examination of carbohydrate metabolism reveals that glycolysis, the Krebs cycle and the electron transport chain are driven by enzymes that require the presence of specific vitamins and minerals. In other words, a variety of additional nutrients must be present in our foods if ATP is to be made from the carbon molecules in that food.

Figure 8-1 provides a method to learn and understand the basics of ATP synthesis. Part 1 illustrates the basic skeleton for glycolysis (the vertical line), the Krebs cycle (the circle), and the electron transport chain (the horizontal line). Understanding glycolysis, the Krebs cycle and the electron transport chain is as simple as line-circle-line. Part 2 illustrates the line-circle-line-ATP flow, to which we add more information in a piecemeal fashion. Parts 3 & 4 in *Figure 8-1* illustrate a manner in which additional information can be added to the line-circle-line skeleton.

An interesting fact about glycolysis and the Krebs cycle is that each pathway is involved in the

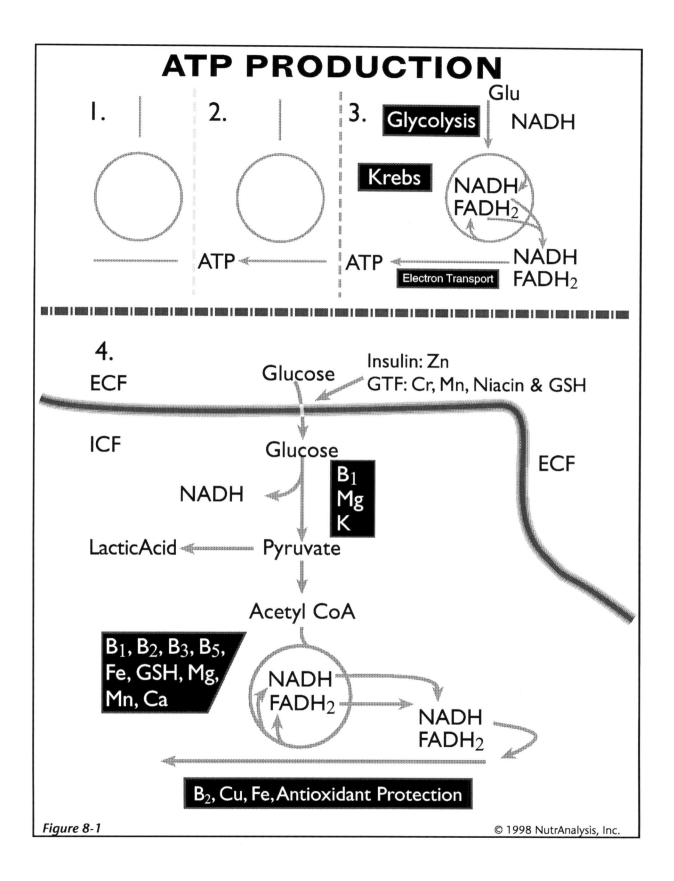

Figure 8-1

© 1998 NutrAnalysis, Inc.

synthesis of many more molecules than just ATP, including phospholipids, glycogen, glycosaminoglycans, nucleotides, coenzyme Q10, various hormones, and NADPH (one function of NADPH is antioxidant in nature). *Figure 8-2* demonstrates how these important molecules are synthesized and also lists the nutrients required to run the pathways [275, 343, 466-p.428, 482].

Factors associated with increased lactic acid production

Figure 8-2 illustrates how glucose is converted into pyruvate, which can then be converted into either acetyl-CoA or lactic acid. Most of us remember that if oxygen is not present, pyruvate will be converted into lactic acid. Additionally, if key nutrients are not present, even if there is sufficient oxygen available, the end result will be lactic acid production. For example, several authors have indicated that a deficiency in vitamin B-1 can promote lactic acid production [174, 277, 398, 484]. van der Beek et al. demonstrated that dietary deficiencies in thiamin, riboflavin, pyridoxine and vitamin C resulted in a significant decrease in aerobic power and an earlier onset of blood lactate accumulation [457].

The interesting aspect of van der Beek's study is that the healthy male volunteers consumed a diet that contained approximately 3,070 kcal/day; well in excess of the 2,000 kcal/day that many people try to consume (the actual RDA ranges from 1,900-2,200 kcal/day for women and 2,300-2,900 for men [481-p.3]). The food content of the basal diet used in this study differs little with what the average American consumes on a daily basis. This particular diet was selected because it contained a maximum of 32.5% of the Dutch RDA for the vitamins mentioned earlier. Subjects remained on this diet for 8 weeks; however, "within 3-6 weeks deterioration of the vitamin status was indicated by decreased vitamin concentrations in blood, decreased erythrocyte enzyme activities, elevation of stimulation tests of these enzymes, and lower vitamin excretion in the urine." The authors made it clear that, "no vitamin-specific clinical signs and symptoms of deficiency were observed." This suggests that numerous individuals in America may be sub-clinically deficient in several nutrients and completely unaware of the problem.

More recently, van der Beek et al. [837] performed a similar study, this time supplying a diet with no more than 55% of the RDA for thiamin, riboflavin, and pyridoxine for 11 weeks. The subjects included 24 healthy males with a mean age of about 24 years. Vitamin restriction resulted in a significant overall decrease in aerobic power, onset of blood lactate accumulation, oxygen consumption at this power output, peak power and mean power. The authors propose that B-vitamin restriction may reduce mitochondrial metabolism and thereby influence exercise performance [837]. See Aw and Jones for a review of the nutritional factors related to mitochondrial function [548].

This information demands that we update our view towards vitamin deficiencies. Many view nutrient deficiencies as being present only when overt, classical signs of deficiency are evident. For example, in the case of thiamin, many suggest that thiamin deficiencies do not exist unless the neurological signs/symptoms of beriberi are present. Consider this view while reading the following list of symptoms associated with a subclinical deficiency, and also consider how much money is probably spent on diagnostic tests and treatments that do not address the underlying subclinical deficiency state. In experimental studies designed to create a thiamin deficiency, the following symptoms appeared: paresthesia, giddiness, soreness of the muscles, backache, insomnia, anorexia, nausea and vomiting, generalized weakness, reduced capacity for muscular work, and emotional signs (irritability, moodiness, quarrelsomeness, lack of cooperation, agitation, mental depression); however, no physical signs of neuropathy developed which are classically associated with beriberi [449-p.117,484].

Please realize that the purpose of presenting this list is not to motivate doctors to begin a massive thiamin supplementation campaign; rather, this list was presented to alert doctors to the fact that just one sub-clinical deficiency can reek havoc on physiologic function. Most of our patients have multiple sub-clinical deficiencies. The reason for this is very clear.

"Many essential nutrients, especially minerals, are distributed widely in our food supply, but low in concentration. It is,

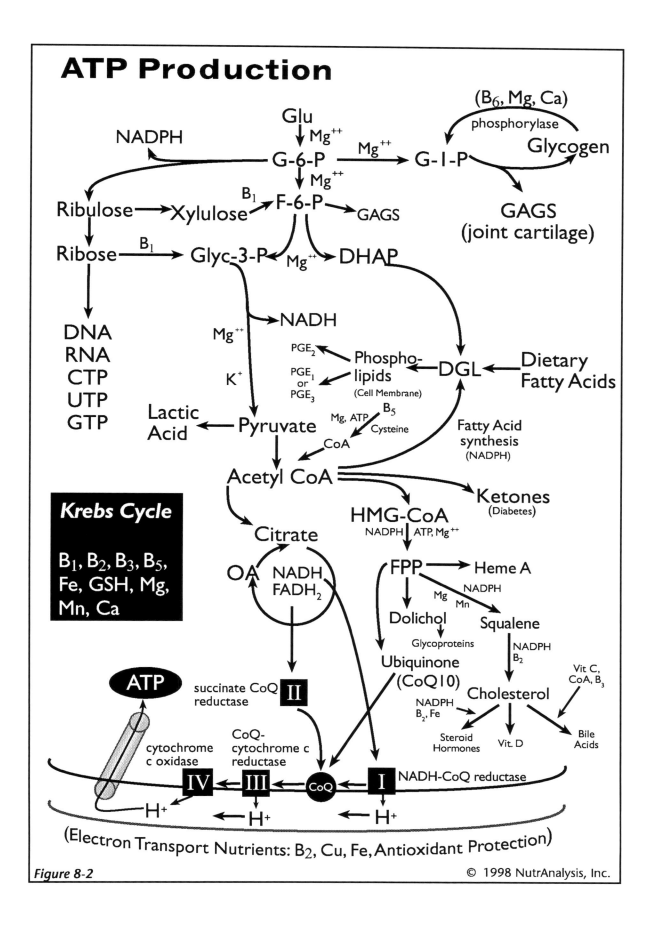

ATP Production

Figure 8-2

© 1998 NutrAnalysis, Inc.

therefore, difficult and often impossible to assure nutritional adequacy of diets that are low in energy content. Adequate essential nutrients may not be available in diets of less than 2,000 kcal for adults and adolescents."[425]

An adequate caloric intake will not cure the problem cited above. In 1971, Schroeder conducted a detailed investigation of the effects of food processing on nutrient quantity in foods; his conclusions were staggering:

"It is apparent that American diets may be marginal in respect to adequate intakes of several micronutrients essential for optimal function...Trace elements in foods usually follow build elements, and it is likely that marginal intakes existed in many school lunches (300 schools were studied)...Large losses of magnesium and most trace metals apparently resulted from the refining or partitioning of foods into two or more fractions...These data demonstrate the dietary needs for the use of whole grains and unprocessed foods of most varieties."[400]

Schroeder's concerns were echoed by Linder in 1991 when she wrote:

"the tendency in our society to refine whole grains and other carbohydrate sources, our dietary emphasis on meats, and methods of food preparation that overcook or leach the vitamins from foods are the main factors responsible for the existence of vitamin deficiencies within the United States population"[275-p.113-14].

Travell reviewed nutritional data on a randomly selected municipal hospital population[449-p.114]. She states that, "the prevalence of unrecognized hypovitaminosis is distressingly high." Out of 120 patients, 88% (105 patients) were deficient in one or more of 11 vitamins. Greater than 50% were deficient in two or more vitamins. Only 39% percent of the patients gave a history of inadequate intake.

Although magnesium was discussed earlier, it is important to state here that *magnesium is known to*

be the key mineral involved in glycolysis and the Krebs cycle[1, 466-p.428, 482]. Oral supplementation with magnesium has shown to improve symptoms associated with fibromyalgia[1] and lower lactate levels in competitive swimmers[95]. Intravenous magnesium treatment in patients with chronic fatigue syndrome improves energy and emotional status and reduces muscle cramps and myalgia[95].

A fact that is not well-known is that free radicals are formed during the activity of many normal metabolic reactions. Germane to the topic of lactate and ATP production is that free radicals are formed by the electron transport chain during the synthesis of ATP[108, 109, 110, 155]. It is thought that the decline in oxidative capacity in aging muscle may be caused by free radical production. Unfortunately, we Americans do little to prevent free radical damage. We choose to avoid those foods that would help to afford us with antioxidant protection.

"It is clear that the nutrients in fruits and vegetables, probably particularly the antioxidant micronutrients, are associated with real and substantial disease protection. And it is clear that in the United States, the population's intake of these foods is remote from the recommended levels."[37]

Perhaps free radical damage in the mitochondria may reduce ATP production. For this reason, supplementation with an anti-oxidant (preferable a vitamin C/bioflavonoid combination) would probably be a wise preventive measure.

Research has demonstrated that there is decreased ATP and increased AMP in trigger point zones[416], and muscles in fibromyalgia patients have low oxygen, low ATP and low phosphocreatine[197]. An interesting paper discusses the possibility that fibromyalgia is caused, in part, by a glycolytic impairment[740]. Compared to normal controls, red blood cells in fibromyalgia patients produce less ATP despite a significant upregulation of pyruvate kinase activity. Additionally, fibromyalgia patients have nearly twice as much pyruvate compared to normal subjects[740], suggesting a reduced entry into the Krebs cycle and a reduction in ATP synthesis. Although it has yet to be studied, muscle changes associated with joint complex dysfunction probably suffer from similar metabolic disturbances.

One way in which local ATP deficiencies influence muscle function has to do with the relationship between actin and myosin[163, 330]. Cross bridge formation between actin and myosin occurs in the presence of the calcium ions that are released by the sarcoplasmic reticulum. If ATP is unavailable, the calcium ions cannot be pumped back into the sarcoplasmic reticulum and the result is contracture of the sarcomere(s) in question, causing local muscle dysfunction that we refer to as trigger points, tender points or myopathology. We must appreciate that a variety of nutrients may play a role in reducing cellular ATP production associated with these conditions. Below is a quote from Dr. Janet Travell that emphasizes the importance of nutrition regarding the treatment of musculoskeletal problems:

> "Nutrients of special concern in patients with myofascial pain syndromes are the water-soluble vitamins B-1, B-6, B-12, folic acid, vitamin C; and certain elements, calcium, iron, and potassium...Nearly half of the patients whom we see with chronic myofascial pain require resolution of vitamin inadequacies for lasting relief...Although nutritional factors are not mentioned in many chapters of this manual, they **must** be considered in most patients if lasting relief of pain is to be achieved (emphasis is Dr. Travell's)...Vitamin inadequacy requires the body to make some degree of metabolic adjustment because the amount of the coenzyme (vitamin) is limited. The patient with a serum vitamin level at the low end of, but within, "normal" limits may show no metabolic evidence of deficiency, yet the level may be inadequate for optimal health. Myofascial trigger points are aggravated by inadequate levels of at least four B-complex vitamins, listed above."[449-p.114]

A small number of human and animal studies have demonstrated that B-vitamin supplementation may reduce nociception and pain[550, 675, 712, 791, 865]. Zimmerman suggests that B-vitamins may influence both peripheral and central antinociceptive mechanisms[865].

Nutritional supplementation:

Clearly, based on the information present above, we can conclude that the average American diet creates a metabolic predisposition to numerous problems including a greater probability of lactic acid production. Our goal with nutrition in the context of this section is to ensure the presence of nutrients that are needed for ATP synthesis. Recommendations include the consumption of large quantities of vegetables, fruits, and modest portions of animal proteins.

What about supplementation? This is a difficult question to answer. Being that so many nutrients are involved in ATP synthesis, targeting specific nutrients to supplement is a difficult task. I believe that a multiple vitamin and mineral supplement, as well as a magnesium supplement, is the best choice to ensure nutrient adequacy. It would also be wise to take an anti-oxidant supplement (i.e., C/bioflavonoids) because, as mentioned above, free radicals are formed during the synthesis of ATP. Finally, you might consider supplementing with coenzyme Q10 (CoQ10), because of the crucial role it plays in ATP synthesis. In summary, based on the information discussed in the lactic acid section, it appears that most, if not all patients would do well to take the following supplements:

1. Multiple vitamin/mineral

2. Magnesium

3. Anti-oxidant (Free-form bioflavonoids with vitamin C)

4. CoQ10

The most common question encountered is how much of a supplement should we take? This is the $64,000 question. There are people who say that we do not need supplements at all. However, based on the information presented in the lactic acid discussion, it appears clear that we should take supplements to make sure that we reach adequate levels. The following paragraphs provide more information regarding each type of supplement. For the remainder of this chapter, only the type of the supplement will be mentioned if that particular supplement is discussed below. However, when a new/different supplement is discussed for the first time (i.e., EPA and Boswellia in Prostaglandin E-2 discussion], more information will be provided.

1. *Multiple vitamin/mineral*: To start, we need to understand the definition of RDA. RDAs refers to "the level of intake of essential nutrients that, on the basis of scientific knowledge, are judge by the Food and Nutrition Board to be adequate to meet the known nutrient needs of practically all healthy persons"[481-p.1]. Based on this definition, you should be able to figure out why the RDAs are a poor guideline system.

Notice that the RDAs refer to the needs of "healthy" persons. However, the RDA book never defines a "healthy person," so we do not know what they mean by "health." The inherent fault of the RDA definition is that it presumes that there are truly "healthy" people in our population. A more accurate definition for RDA would probably be something like the *level of nutrient required to prevent the development of deficiency diseases.*

Another major fault in the RDA book is that it only focuses on general signs of deficiency. In the case of thiamin, for example, they only discuss the characteristic signs of beriberi. This is completely inappropriate. In 1943, Williams et al.[484] published a paper which described an experiment in which they induced thiamin deficiency in two subjects. As part of their introduction they discussed some of the their previous work (see Arch Int Med 1942; 39:721-38). In the 1942 paper, Williams et al. examined the outcome of reducing thiamin intake to about half of the RDA. The subjects consumed .22 mg/1000 kcal for six months. Consider the following quote from this paper:

"In this study moderate, prolonged restriction of thiamine, but not calories, was associated with states of emotional instability, reflected by irritability, moodiness, quarrelsomeness, lack of cooperation, vague fears progressing to agitation, mental depression, variable restriction of activity and numerous somatic complaints. Detectable metabolic disturbances, occurring irregularly, were of variable degrees of severity and were reflected in disturbance of function of various tissues of the body. None of these signs, symptoms or metabolic disorders were observed in the control subjects when their intakes of thiamin exceeded .5 mg/1000 calories."

Believe it or not, the 1989 RDA book references the 1942 study by Williams et al. and never mentions these bizarre symptoms associated with marginal thiamin status[481].

We need to put this information about thiamin into perspective. If we go below the RDA of .5 mg/1000 kcal (they set 1mg/day as the minimum) bizarre [non-beriberi] deficiency symptoms may appear. According to the RDA, the average adult consumed slightly less than 0.7mg/1000 kcal per day. However, Linder states that between 17-27% of Americans may have marginal thiamin deficiency[275-p.116]. In addition, it should be appreciated that several factors can influence thiamin status. For example, thiamin losses occur during food processing and storing[87a-p.254]. Sulfites and certain flavonoids (quercetin and rutin) are known to be thiamin antagonists[87a-p.254]. Additional factors may reduce thiamin status including stress, perhaps smoking, genetics, refinedcarbohydrate diets, the status of other vitamins (i.e., B-6, B-12 and folic acid), and intake of tea, coffee and alcohol[175a]. Based on all of these factors, it makes sense to take a multiple vitamin/mineral that contains thiamin. This suggestion is very reasonable, particular when we consider that there is no evidence of thiamin toxicity by oral administration[481-p.129]. Let us be safe, rather than sorry and take appropriate supplements to prevent a subclinical deficiency state.

Although this discussion focussed on thiamin, it is likely that similar cases can be made for most other nutrients (space does not permit a detailed discussion of each nutrient). Consider the information discussed earlier under the heading *Factors associated with increased lactic acid production* and also, take for example the following data on nutrient intake for women. It has been found that 78% consume less then 100% of the RDA for calcium; 95% consume less then 100% of the RDA for iron; 96% consume less then 100% of the RDA for zinc; 55% consume less then 100% of the RDA for vitamin A; 76% consume less then 100% of the RDA for vitamin E; 44% consume less then 100% of the RDA for vitamin C; 94% consume less then 100% of the RDA for vitamin B-6; and 96% consume less then 100% of the RDA for folic acid[302a]. So, it seems obvious that a multiple vitamin/mineral supplement would be a wise choice for all of us.

2. *Magnesium*: As mentioned in Chapter 5, it may be wise to supplement with magnesium (up to 1000 mg/day in divided doses). To obtain the highest degree of absorption, it is best to take magnesium [and calcium] about 20 minutes before eating a meal. For a review of magnesium and information on supplementation, see Chapter 5.

3. *Anti-oxidant*: Most multiples contain vitamin E, beta-carotene and selenium, as well as the other nutrients found in *Figure 5-1* in Chapter 5. Recall that phytochemicals such as flavonoids and phenols act as antioxidants. Bucci suggests that it is reasonable to consume 1-2 grams of flavonoids per day[51-p.207]. He also states that the upper limit for toxicity has not been found and is probably beyond practical reach. Vitamin C can also be taken with flavonoids. For a couple of reasons, I would not suggest taking more than 500-1000 mg/day in divided doses. First, vitamin C absorption is reduced as greater amounts are taken. Second, oxidation of ingested vitamin C is possible when taken in gram amounts. Third, megadoses of C can create osmotic changes in the gut and cause diarrhea.

4. *Coenzyme Q10*: Examine *Figure 8-1* and you will see that ubiquinone (CoQ or CoQ10) is synthesized in the body from acetyl-CoA. It is intimately involved in the function of the electron transport chain and is required for ATP synthesis. Bucci states that, "coenzyme Q10 is the single most important metabolic component of ATP production." Researchers explain that coenzyme Q10 is indispensable in mitochondrial energetics and required for human life to exist[620, 696].

A human double-blind and open crossover trial with CoQ10 involving patients with progressive muscular disease and associated cardiac disease revealed the benefits of CoQ10 supplementation[619]. Improved physical well-being was observed for 4/8 in the treatment group while none of the placebo patients (0/4) benefited, and 5/6 on CoQ10 in crossover maintained improved cardiac function[619]. CoQ10 supplementation is useful in cardiovascular disease and as an immunomodulating agent. As with cardiovascular and muscle disease, benefits of CoQ10 on immune function probably involve improving mitochondrial energetics in white blood cells[619]. Patients with angina pectoris received 150 mg of CoQ10 per day for 4 weeks. In this double-blind, placebo-controlled, randomized, crossover trial, patients taking Coq10 had less anginal attacks and improved exercise capacity compared to controls[678].

According to Bucci, "of interest for practical applications is the finding that normal levels of CoQ10 do not saturate the respiratory chain and, thus, energy production, thereby leading to a working hypothesis that additional CoQ10 may lead to increased cellular energy output, tissue function, organ function and clinical benefits for healing"[51-p.59]. After 8 to 12 weeks of supplementation with 60 to 100 mg of CoQ10 per day led to a doubling or tripling of serum and gingival tissue levels[51-p.59].

Coenzyme Q10 production appears to be antagonized by several medications including adriamycin (used to treat cancer)[619], betablockers[835], and HMG-CoA reductase inhibitors such as lovastatin, pravastatin, and simvastatin[618, 630, 760]. HMG-CoA reductase, which is considered to be a rate-limiting enzyme in cholesterol synthesis, can be seen in *Figure 8-1*. Many people do not realize that reducing cholesterol levels with HMG-CoA reductase inhibitors also serves to significantly reduce CoQ10 production. Researchers suggest that these medications may create a new cardiac risk by lowering CoQ10 levels[618].

POTASSIUM IONS

Potassium's relationship to the generation of the pro-inflammatory state was discussed earlier. Recall that a potassium deficiency can reduce appropriate vasorelaxation in working muscles. The end result being tissue hypoxia which is pro-inflammatory.

This section will discuss how potassium itself may act as a nociceptor irritant. Approximately 98% of the body's potassium supply is in the intracellular fluid and 80% of that is in muscles. The extracellular fluid contains only 2 percent[483]. The concentration between intracellular and extracellular compartments is maintained by the Na/K-ATPase pump (Na/K-pump), which requires ATP and magnesium to function properly[483]. Potassium continuously leaks out of cells and thus, a continuous supply of ATP and magnesium is required to maintain the appropriate concentrations.

Free radical activity can damage the Na/K-pump[110]. As free radical activity is linked to the aging process[103], this may be why Na/K-pump activity has been shown to decrease with age[418] and thus, perhaps another reason to increase antioxidant consumption.

Alterations in the phospholipid content of the cell membrane may alter the activity of the Na/K-ATPase pump:

"The intact enzyme contains a significant amount of phospholipid and cholesterol; some estimates indicate as much as one third of the total molecular mass may be lipid in nature. Procedures that remove phospholipid, such as solvent or detergent extraction or phospholipase treatment, inhibit the enzyme activity. Such partially inactivated enzyme preparations can be reactivated by the addition of phosphatidylserine or, to a lesser degree, by phosphatidylethanolamine. Phosphatidylcholine is not capable of restoring enzyme activity. Much of the cholesterol can be removed by oxidation in situ to cholestenone or by extraction, without loss of activity. The conclusion is that acidic phospholipids are the only essential lipids, but the precise nature of their protective effect is not well established."[317]

Because the Na/K-pump is specifically sensitive to the type of phospholipid incorporated in the membrane, perhaps essential fatty acid deficiency may alter the enzymes activity, as is the case with other membrane bound enzymes[9]. If this is the case, then increased consumption of trans-fatty acids, which are known to promote essential fatty acid deficiency[204], might alter the Na/K-pump activity. Research has also demonstrated that an increased cholesterol/phospholipid ration can markedly inhibit Na/K-pump activity[130].

Certain foods, when tested in vitro, inhibit Na/K-pump activity. These include tea, cocoa, and red wine[189]. The degree to which these effects occur in vivo is unknown.

The clinical relevance of the data presented in this section on potassium is not known. I am unaware of research that has looked at the Na/K-pump from the perspective of the musculoskeletal system. Conclusions about this data must be guarded. I would hypothesize that in the region of injured tissue, where there is increased potassium levels, depressed pump activity might perpetuate the exposure of potassium ions to local nociceptors.

Nutritional supplementation:

To reduce nociceptor exposure to potassium ions, the most logical recommendation would be to provide the appropriate nutrients that help to drive ATP production (see previous section). Fatty acid consumption patterns should also be considered as the ATPase enzyme depends on phospholipids as part of its matrix. Dietary factors associated with fatty acids have already been discussed in Chapter 5.

PROSTAGLANDIN E-2

Prostaglandins and leukotrienes are among the most potent and ubiquitous of the inflammatory mediators, and appear whenever animal cells are damaged, and can also be found in increased concentrations in inflammatory exudates[137-p.31-87]. Certain aspects of prostaglandin E-2 were already discussed in Chapter 5. In this section, various supplements will be described which may act as inhibitors of PGE-2 synthesis.

History

Prostaglandins were discovered in 1930; however, their specific structures were not elucidated until after 1960. In 1962, PGE-1 was

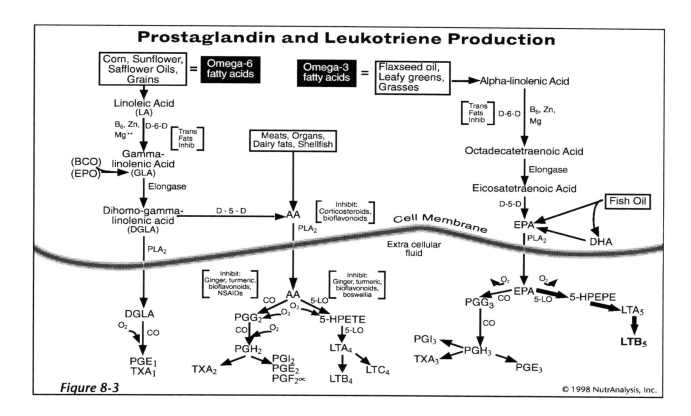

Prostaglandin and Leukotriene Production

Figure 8-3

© 1998 NutrAnalysis, Inc.

described; in 1964, PGE-2 was described; in 1975, TXA-2 was described; and in 1983, LTB-4 was described. It was not until 1971 that it was discovered that aspirin inhibited cyclooxygenase[316].

Synthesis and inhibition of prostaglandins

Please examine *Figure 8-3* and notice that phospholipase A-2 (PLA-2) and cyclooxygenase (CO) are the two key enzymes involved in PGE-2, PGI-2, and $PGF_2\alpha$ production. Recall that PLA-2 cleaves the unsaturated fatty acid off of position two of cell membrane phospholipids. This fatty acid will then be acted upon by CO, which will convert arachidonic acid into pro-inflammatory PGE-2 and $PGF_2\alpha$. DGLA will be converted into anti-inflammatory PGE-1 and EPA will be converted into anti-inflammatory PGE-3. Thus, we need to consume a diet that facilitates the incorporation of anti-inflammatory fatty acids into cell membrane phospholipids. The specific dietary recommendations were discussed in Chapter 5.

Various authors mention different mechanisms by which PLA-2 can be activated. I should mention that the specific details by which the activation occurs are not well described in the papers and texts I have read. The following factors are thought to activate PLA-2:

- Mechanical, electrical, chemical, and immunological stimuli[92-p.55]

- Free radicals[108]

- Immunological stimuli such as IgE[353] and IgG[156]

- Chemical stimuli such as bradykinin, thrombin, angiotensin II, leukotriene C-4 and D-4, and noradrenaline[370]

The following drugs and nutrients are thought to inhibit PLA-2 activity:

- Corticosteroids; some side effects include hyperglycemia, peptic ulceration, myopathy, suicidal tendencies, osteoporosis/compression fractures, and inhibition of DNA synthesis[195]

- Bioflavonoids[51-p.206, 311, 263] (also see phytonutrient section in Chapter 5)

The following drugs and nutrients are thought to inhibit cyclooxygenase activity:

- Aspirin and NSAIDs (see Chapter 4)

- Ginger[149, 218, 431], turmeric[51-p.214, 148], and bioflavonoids[51-p.206, 194]

It is worthwhile to mention ginger and turmeric is some detail. Both have been used for centuries in India. In the Ayurvedic and Tibb systems of medicine, ginger is used as an anti-rheumatic and anti-inflammatory agent. A recent study examined the effectiveness of ginger in the treatment of rheumatoid arthritis, osteoarthritis and muscular discomfort[431]. Whereas three-quarters of the arthritis patients experienced varying degrees of relief from pain and inflammation, all patients with muscle pain experienced relief. A total of fifty-six patients were followed with questionnaires. The authors recommend that the patients take no more than 0.5-1 gram/day of powered ginger. There is approximately 1 gram in a teaspoon. As it turned out, most patients took between 1-2 grams/day and some took more. No adverse side effects were noticed during the 3 month to 2.5 year period of intake. For example, an 80 year old woman with one kidney was able to consume ginger for three years without side effects. For the first six months she took 6 grams/day and the following two and half years she took 2 grams/day. The literature does not mention any adverse side effects associated with the consumption of ginger.

Much like ginger, turmeric has been used historically when patients suffer from pain and inflammation. Curcumin is derived from turmeric, a perennial herb of the ginger family. The exact mechanism of action of curcumin is not known. As indicated above, and in the section on LTB-4, it is thought that it may inhibit cyclooxygenase and lipoxygenase. Two human trials have examined the effectiveness of curcumin in the treatment of inflammation. One trial studied the use of curcumin in RA patients for 10 weeks[111], and the other studied patients with postoperative pain during a 6 day supplementation period[388]. Both trials demonstrated the effectiveness of curcumin in reducing inflammation and tenderness. In each trial, patients were given 400 mg t.i.d. of curcumin. Bucci[51-p.214] suggests that 1 to 2 grams per day is

safe for short term use. He indicates that during the many hundreds of years in which curcumin was used as an anti-inflammatory agent, there have been no known reports of toxicity.

There is also some evidence that bromelain may inhibit the arachidonic-prostaglandin cascade[443, 462]. The precise mechanisms are not well-understood. Taussig[443] suggests that although bromelain only partially inhibits PGE-2 production, it may be able to stimulate the production of the anti-inflammatory PGE-1.

Anti-inflammatory nature of EPA/DHA (fish oil)

Several authors maintain that fish oil supplementation can reduce arachidonic acid activity[275, 350, 380, 385]. Many other authors have also described the anti-inflammatory effects of eicosapentanoic acid (EPA)[45, 46, 58, 64, 68, 122, 201, 214, 248, 259, 260, 289, 375, 380, 417, 419, 445]. EPA and DHA (docosahexaenoic acid), are thought to function by inhibiting the formation of cyclooxygenase (ie., PGE-2) products that are derived from arachidonic acid[68].

Higgs states that EPA displacement of arachidonic acid may result in decreased PGE-2 synthesis. The mechanism by which this occurs is not straightforward. As EPA is known to be the precursor of PGE-3[45], one might be led to think that EPA consumption will lead to the production of PGE-3, which is anti-inflammatory compared with PGE-2. However, EPA is known to be a poor substrate for the cyclooxygenase enzyme[45, 445]. This means that the modest amount of PGE-3 that is produced[427a] from EPA, does *not* sufficiently explain the manner in which EPA exerts its anti-inflammatory effect. Rather, EPA's anti-inflammatory effect is probably derived from its ability to competitively inhibit the formation of arachidonic acid-derived prostanoids, i.e., PGE-2, PGI-2, PGF-2α, TXA-2[45, 445]. In other words, the presence of EPA (and DHA[68]) will reduce the chance for arachidonic to be acted on by cyclooxygenase. It is likely that DHA and EPA have some anti-inflammatory functions that are similar[46], although EPA is the fatty acid that is most commonly discussed in regards to these functions.

Whereas EPA is a poor substrate for cyclooxygenase, it is a good substrate for lipoxygenase which converts EPA into LTB-5[45, 461]. DHA is also a substrate for lypoxygenase, and therefore can be converted into LTB-5[46]. The thick dark arrow in *Figure 8-3* is there to emphasize these facts about EPA and its relationship to PGE-3 and LTB-5 (the same probably holds true for DHA, however this relationship is not illustrated). The details of leukotriene activity will be discussed in the next section; however, at this point it should be understood that LTB-5 from EPA is at least 30 times *less* inflammatory than LTB-4 from arachidonic acid[45]. EPA is also thought to reduce the production of IL-1 and TNF[46, 122, 350]. The pro-inflammatory effects of IL-1 and TNF will be discussed in more detail at the end of this chapter

Is it better to supplement with alpha-linolenic acid or EPA?

Several studies indicate that the conversion of alpha-linolenic acid to EPA is slow and thus, the most effective way to get EPA into the system is to take EPA directly[128, 129, 259, 385, 420]. A dysfunctional delta-6-desaturase (D-6-D) enzyme is often thought to be the problem with linolenic acid conversion to EPA.

D-6-D dysfunction may develop for many reasons. First, it is known that D-6-D is dependent on several nutrients, namely niacin, pyridoxine, magnesium and zinc[209, 55]. Secondly, "the delta-6-desaturase is inhibited by aging, fasting, diabetes mellitus, glucose, alcohol, deficiency of protein, saturated and trans fatty acids, adrenaline, thyroxin, glucocorticoids, oncogenic viruses and ionizing radiation"[420]. Unfortunately, the precise mechanisms of inhibition were not described in this paper.

More recent research suggests that alpha-linolenic acid is readily converted into EPA. This study demonstrated that flaxseed oil consumption (as an oil and spread) as a source alpha-linolenic acid resulted in an eightfold increase in serum phospholipid alpha-linolenic acid and a 2.5-fold increase in EPA concentrations. These authors suggest that the earlier studies [mentioned above] on alpha-linolenic consumption were misleading because the baseline diets were high in linoleic

acid which reduced the likelihood that alpha-linolenic acid would be converted to PGE-3.

"In this study, EPA concentrations resulting from flaxseed oil consumption in conjunction with a background diet low in n-6 fatty acids reached almost half those achieved with fish-oil consumption (nine fish-oil capsules per day for 4 wk.) over the same period of time. Although EPA supplied in the form of encapsulated fish oil is an efficient method of increasing EPA concentrations, the possibility exists that long-term domestic use of flaxseed oil in place of other cooking oils and spreads could also lead to significant increases in EPA."[284]

Although EPA levels increased during this research trial, the authors found that there was no increase in DHA levels. This outcome was consistent with other similar studies. However, because vegetarians do have modest amounts of DHA in their tissue, the authors suggest that the trial period was not sufficient to observe a conversion from alpha-linolenic acid to DHA. Despite this possibility, as so many factors can modify fatty acid synthesis, it is probably a better choice to consume EPA and DHA, instead of waiting for them to be produced from alpha-linolenic acid. Furthermore, because our goal is to promote an anti-inflammatory state, we need to quickly and efficiently incorporate EPA and DHA into our cell membranes, and it is agreed that the direct consumption of EPA and DHA is the best approach to achieve that goal[129, 485].

Kremer's chapter in *Textbook of Rheumatology* provides useful clinical information about EPA from both a dietary and a supplemental perspective[248]. Some of this information will serve as a review of the material already discussed in Chapter 5. Alpha-linolenic acid is commonly found in chloroplasts of green leaves and in some plant oils including flaxseed oil and canola oil. It is unlikely that we efficiently convert alpha-linolenic acid into EPA/DHA. Humans have probably always depended on foods that contain preformed EPA/DHA. Our hunter-gatherer ancestors easily obtained sufficient amounts of EPA/DHA from fat in wild game (these animals consume green plants and grasses), which contained 9% EPA. Unfortunately, the domestic livestock that we consume today contains almost undetectable amounts of EPA. Because domestic livestock is a main dietary staple, our current fatty acid intake pattern has been dramatically altered from that to which humans have adapted over thousands of years. To approach the fatty acid intake pattern of our ancestors, we must obtain our EPA/DHA from fish and/or from supplements.

Kremer studied the effects of fish oil supplementation in patients with rheumatoid arthritis (RA)[248]. In a pilot study, patients were provided with a daily supplement of 1.8 grams of EPA and 0.9 grams of DHA (which is about the equivalent to taking 6 fish oil capsules), while controls received no supplement. After 12 weeks there was a significant improvement in the number of tender joints in the supplementation group. The improvements disappeared after supplementation was discontinued. In a subsequent blinded cross-over study, RA patients received 2.8 grams of EPA and 1.8 grams of DHA (about the equivalent to taking 9 capsules of most EPA/DHA supplements) or olive oil for 14 weeks before switching to the opposite oil. The results indicated that only those patients receiving EPA/DHA experienced a statistically significant reduction in the number of tender joints.

In another study it was shown that patients with RA had an 8:1 ratio of arachidonic acid to EPA in their neutrophil membranes, which vividly demonstrates the pro-inflammatory nature of RA. Supplementation with 20 grams of EPA/DHA resulted in the development of a 3:1 ratio[192]. More recently, Kremer et al. supplemented RA patients with 130 mg/kg/day of fish oil. Some patients were able to discontinue NSAID use without experiencing a disease flare[693]. The beneficial effects of EPA/DHA supplementation are listed below:

1. EPA will directly compete with arachidonic acid as the substrate for cyclooxygenase and inhibit its metabolism into eicosanoids[248]

2. EPA consumption will increase anti-inflammatory LTB-5 production by neutrophils and reduce pro-inflammatory LTB-4 production[248]

3. EPA reduces neutrophil chemotaxis[248]

4. EPA reduces the production of platelet activating factor (PAF)[248]

5. EPA reduces interleukin-1 production[192a, 248] and tumor necrosis factor[192a]

6. EPA inhibits platelet-derived growth factor-like protein by endothelial cells[192a]

7. EPA suppresses human synovial cell proliferation[192a]

8. EPA improves rheologic status secondary to increased erythrocyte deformability[248]

9. EPA decreases plasma viscosity[248]

10. EPA promotes a more favorable response to ischemia[248]

11. EPA reduces the vasospastic response to catecholamines and angiotensin[248]

12. EPA increases levels of plasminogen activator[248]

13. EPA increases the endothelial-dependent relaxation of arteries in response to bradykinin, serotonin, adenine diphosphate and thrombin[248]

An important to remember about supplementation with EPA/DHA is that pain and tenderness eventually return when patients stop taking the oil. The most likely explanation for this is that the base diet is probably pro-inflammatory from the perspectives discussed in Chapter 5. For this reason, all patients need to improve their diets and this should be the focus of patient care. Recall the work of Kjeldsen-Kragh et al.[237], which was discussed several times in Chapter 5. This team of researchers saw dramatic improvements in RA patients in as little as four weeks of dietary modification and no supplements.

A combination of fish oil supplementation and dietary modification (i.e., a reduction in seed oils and an increase in green leafy vegetables and cold-water fish) appears to be the most logical way to restore appropriate fatty acid balance.

Anti-inflammatory nature of GLA

Several authors have described the anti-inflammatory nature of PGE-1 [46, 69, 209, 350, 390, 441, 506]. *Figure 8-3* illustrates how linoleic acid is desaturated into gamma-linolenic acid (GLA), and elongated into dihomo-gamma-linolenic acid (DGLA), and subsequently converted into anti-inflammatory PGE-1 by cyclooxygenase. As mentioned earlier, D-6-D dysfunction may impede appropriate fatty acid conversions. If this were the case, linoleic acid would not be efficiently converted into GLA, DGLA and ultimately, there would be a reduced production of PGE-1. By supplementing with GLA-rich oils such as evening primrose oil, black current seed oil, and borage seed oil, the problem with D-6-D dysfunction may be avoided.

Callegari [69] and Horrobin [209] suggest that DGLA is not readily converted to arachidonic acid by delta-5-desaturase (D-5-D). We should also balance this information with research suggesting that both D-6-D and D-5-D may operate fine in vegetarian subjects [384].

Several authors maintain that DGLA will compete with arachidonic acid for the cyclooxygenase enzyme [441, 69, 46, 350]. DGLA is not acted upon by 5-lipoxygenase and thus, DGLA is not converted into leukotrienes [46, 69, 350, 441, 468]. Moreover, DGLA is converted into hydroperoxy-DGLA which inhibits 5-lipoxygenase [69, 468].

One paper that discusses evening primrose oil states that, "the recommended adult dose is 4-6, 500mg capsules daily or as required. In conditions such as PMS or rheumatoid arthritis (RA), the drug may need to be taken for three months before benefits are seen." [390] This quote illustrates the two main problems that exist when it comes to nutritional supplementation. First, nutritional supplements, such as oils from food, are often incorrectly referred to as drugs. Secondly, we are told that it can take up to three months before RA symptoms improve. Compare this outcome with that of Kjeldsen-Kragh et al., who saw significant improvement in RA indices within 4 weeks. Clearly, dietary changes are the key, and supplements should be viewed as what they are, i.e., just supplements to a good diet. This study with evening primrose oil demonstrates why nutritional supplements cannot be used by themselves to effectively modify a disease process.

Nutritional supplementation:

Generally speaking, aspirin and NSAIDs are rapidly and completely absorbed. Each varies in their duration of activity, some lasting several hours [325]. The reader should understand that the anti-inflammatory medications give rapid relief, usually within hours. Dietary modifications and nutritional supplements (bioflavonoids, ginger, turmeric, antioxidants, EPA or GLA) usually take longer. Pain is sometimes reduced within a day or two, but it usually takes a week or two for the average patient. The reason for this should be clear; nutrients do not provide pharmacological effects and the degree to which various nutrients may inhibit eicosanoid synthesis is not clear. When it comes to fatty acid supplementation, I believe that EPA should be favored over GLA because of the overconsumption of linoleic acid from our diets.

Based on what was presented in this discussion about prostaglandins, the following supplements should be considered:

1. EPA

2. Anti-inflammatory botanical

3. Multiple vitamin/mineral

4. Bioflavonoids

The suggested amount of supplemental vitamins/minerals and flavonoids has already been discussed in the lactic acid section. This discussion will focus on EPA and an anti-inflammatory botanical.

1. *EPA*: No one knows the precise amount of EPA/DHA that people should take. Levels of

optimal intake will invariably differ from individual to individual. In the meantime, because we do not get omega-3 fatty acids in our diet, it behooves us to provide a steady flow of EPA/DHA to our cells. The initial supplemental amount will vary depending on the severity of the condition and the state of the diet. For example a recent article explained that intensive treatment of various forms of hyperlipidemia and for creating an antithrombotic state, fish oils need to be used in addition to the consumption of fish. Dosage may range from 6 to 15 grams per day, titrated to the desired endpoint[586].

For primary prevention of heart disease, 2-3 grams of fish oil per day is desireable[586], particularly for people who do not consume fish or shellfish.

The amount of n-3 fatty acids in fish oil supplements will depend on the choice of supplement. Fish oil supplements typically contain 1,000 mg of fish oil per capsule. Standard amounts of EPA will either be 180 mg or 330 mg, while DHA levels will be either 120 mg or 220 mg per capsule. The key is obviously the amount of n-3 fatty acids in the fish oil and not the total amount of "fish oil."

Kremer has studied the effects of n-3 supplementation on rheumatoid patients for many years. The number of tender joints on physical examination and the amount of morning stiffness is consistently reduced in patients who take n-3 supplements.

> "In these cases, supplements were consumed daily in addition to background medications and the clinical benefits of the n-3 fatty acids were not apparent until they were consumed for > or =12 wk. It appears that a minimum daily dose of 3 g eicosapentaenoic and docosahexaenoic acids is necessary to derive the expected benefits."

For those who count pills, this represents a minimum of 10 fish oil capsules per day if one were to take the common variety that contains 180 mg of EPA and 120 mg of DHA. Fortunately, there are virtually no reports of toxicity in the dose range used to treat rheumatoid arthritis, and the oil is generally very well tolerated. In one study the subjects ingested 6 grams of EPA/DHA per day for 7 years with no reported side-effects Based on the available literature, it would be reasonable to suggest supplementing the diet with 1-3 grams

of omega-3 fatty acids per day as both a therapeutic and preventive measure.

2. Anti-inflammatory botanical: Powdered ginger is probably the easiest and least expensive way to consume an anti-inflammatory botanical. Powdered ginger comes in capsules, and each usually contains 500 mg of ginger. Anywhere from 4 to 12 capsules can be taken each day in divided doses. See Srivastava and Mustafa[429] for an excellent review on the utility of powdered ginger.

An alternative way to increase ginger consumption is to take a 2 inch piece of raw ginger root and shave off the skin. Then chop the ginger into little pieces. Boil some water. After the water boils, turn off the stove. Place the ginger pieces into a pot and cover with a lid. Let the tea steep for about 20-30 minutes, then remove the ginger pieces and place them in a small dish. Now you can drink the tea and eat the ginger.

Ginger can also be added to homemade vegetable and fruit juice. Ginger can be juiced the same way that carrots, beets and other vegetables are juiced. A nice vegetable recipe includes carrots, beets, celery, and ginger. To this mix you can add an apple if you want a sweeter tasting juice, or you can add kale and garlic if you want a stronger vegetable taste. A spicy fruit juice could include apples, pineapple and ginger, or apples, lemons and ginger (this tastes like spicy lemonade). By the way, juicing is an excellent way to get nutrients and important phytochemicals into picky children.

LEUKOTRIENE B-4

As described earlier and as seen in *Figure 8-3*, arachidonic acid is the precursor for Leukotriene B-4 (LTB-4) and EPA is the precursor for LTB-5. Only neutrophils, eosinophils, basophils, mast cells, monocytes and macrophages are thought to produce LTB-4[2, 170, 253, 447, 401].

Although LTB-4 was not discovered until 1983, a slow-reacting substance of anaphylaxis (SRS-A) was first described in 1938. SRS-A is now thought to consist of a mixture of LTC-4 and LTD-4[316].

LTB-4 is a very pro-inflammatory molecule. I use the word "very" because it is involved in many aspects of inflammation. Some properties of inflammation include neutrophil chemotaxis and aggregation, increased vascular permeability, lysosomal enzyme release, superoxide generation, thromboxane A-2 release from platelets, increased vascular permeability, vasodilation, and nociception[152, 170].

LTB-4 appears to act as a sensitizing agent of nociceptors[34, 137, 262]. The exact mechanism of such sensitization is not understood. Authors state that LTB-4 will produce hyperalgesia only in the presence of neutrophils[34, 137, 267]. Recent papers maintain that leukotriene B-4 is involved in nociceptor sensitization; however, neither author describes a mechanism[187, 349].

Leukotriene A-4 is the precursor for both LTB-4 and LTC-4 (*see Figure 8-3*). The production of leukotrienes are linked to numerous diseases. LTB-4 is involved in asthma, psoriasis, gout, rheumatoid arthritis, ulcerative colitis and Crohn's disease. LTC-4 is involved in allergic rhinitis and adult respiratory distress syndrome[271].

The following nutrients are thought to inhibit lipoxygenase activity:

- Boswellia[17, 249, 379], ginger[149, 218, 431], turmeric[148], bioflavonoids[51-p.206, 194,496]

Boswellia is a very interesting botanical that should be mentioned. The Boswellia species consist of shrubs to small trees. The sap or gum resin from Boswellia plants is called frankincense. Between 60-70% of the resin consists of boswellic acid. Boswellia has proven to be helpful in reducing pain and inflammation in both animal and human studies[17, 249, 379].

Nutritional supplementation:

Same as prostaglandin E-2.

HISTAMINE

General information

Histamine was originally called beta-aminoethylimidazole. It was studied intensely in 1910 and it was demonstrated to stimulate a host of smooth muscles and promote vasodepressor activity. It was not until 1927 when aminoethylimidazole was found to be a natural constituent of various body tissues, after which it was given the name histamine. In the same year

other researchers discovered that histamine could be released from skin cells by injurious stimuli[119].

Like most of the other chemical mediators discussed thus far, histamine is generally thought of as a bad molecule. This makes sense because antihistamines (H1 receptor blockers) are a widely advertised medication for allergies. Antihistamines (H2 receptor blockers) are also used to inhibit hydrochloric acid production in patients who are suspected of having an ulcer.

The bad press that histamine has received often overshadows its importance in normal physiology. For example, there are several non-mast cell sites of histamine formation or storage. These include the human epidermis, neurons within the CNS, cells of the gastric mucosa, and cells in regenerating or rapidly growing tissues. In these sites, histamine is continuously released rather than stored[119]. Histamine is formed by the decarboxylation of the essential amino L-histidine. This conversion is catalyzed by vitamin B6-dependent histidine decarboxylase[61].

As alluded to above, histamine has specific types of receptors. The effects of the interaction between histamine and its H1 receptor include microcirculation vasodilation permeability, venular permeability, intestinal and bronchial smooth muscle contraction, and mucus secretion. H2 receptor stimulation results in stomach acid secretion by parietal cells. H3 receptors are involved in neurotransmitter release and histamine formation within the central and peripheral nervous systems[401].

Although histamine is found in many different tissues, most tissue histamine is found within the granules of mast cells, sometimes referred to as tissue basophils. Mast cells are concentrated at sites of potential tissue injury, where they function as "emergency repair kits"[61]. Histamine release at an injured site causes microcirculation vasodilation, increased venule permeability and activates nociceptors[177-p.192, 291, 119]. H1 receptors are present in nociceptors[119]. Histamine release in the gastrointestinal tract can increase gut permeability[370-p.19.13]. Altered gut permeability may contribute to an extra-intestinal pro-inflammatory state by permitting antigen absorption.

Mast cells

Mast cells are highly specialized secretory cells of mucosa and connective tissue. Mast cells release their mediators in response to antibodies [IgE, IgG, IgM], trauma[61], and substance P[268]. It should be understood that some mast cell mediators are pro-inflammatory and others are anti-inflammatory. As stated above, substance P causes mediator release from mast cells. Recall that substance P is released from activated nociceptive terminals and, in turn, causes mast cells to release histamine, serotonin, and leukotrienes[268].

Mast cells contain granule-bound mediators and non-granule mediators. Each is a released through different mechanisms which is described below under nutritional considerations.

Mast cell secretory granules store histamine, heparin, chondroitin sulfate E, and various neutral proteases including chymase, carboxypeptidase, cathepsin G-like, and tryptase[401]. Human tryptase has fibrinolytic activity, kininogenase activity (inhibits kinin production), and activates prostromelysin (activates latent collagenase). Tryptase may also activate complement (C3)[310, 370-p.19.13, 401]. Chymase provides chymotrypsin-like activity, and one of its functions is the inactivation of bradykinin.

Non-granule mast cell mediators include cytokines and eicosanoids. Mast cells are known to produce at least two cytokines, those being TNF and IL-4. Mast cells also release various arachidonic acid-derived eicosanoids, including LTB-4, SRS-A, TXA-2, PGD-2[401]. There is disagreement as to whether or not mast cells actually release platelet activating factor[370-p.19.12, 401].

Nutritional factors which modulate histamine release

Generally speaking, granule and non-granule mediator release occurs as a consequence of mast cell plasma membrane perturbation by one of the three triggers mentioned earlier (antibodies, trauma, substance P). There are two main affects of such plasma membrane receptor stimulation. The activation of ion channels and the other being the activation of phospholipase C and A-2.

The activation of ion channels permits calcium entry into the mast cell. Calcium entry triggers, in particular, the degranulation process[370]. The activation of phospholipase C and A-2 results in eicosanoid synthesis[401]. There are also interrelationships between these two mechanisms which are too involved to describe in this book.

Most of the nutritional factors appear to involve the biochemical stabilization of mast cell plasma membranes. Magnesium[252], zinc[286], bioflavonoids[194, 346, 311, 51-p.206], and vitamin E[51-p.73] are all thought to have such a function. Apparently, membrane stabilization reduces both granule and non-granule mediator release.

Ascorbic acid does not directly affect mast cell function; rather, vitamin C is known to inactivate the imidazole ring of histamine[436]. Animal experiments suggest that curcumin has anti-histaminic properties, although the precise mechanism is not described[78].

Nutritional supplementation:

Based on what was presented in this discussion about prostaglandins the following supplements should be considered :

1. Multiple vitamin/mineral

2. Magnesium

3. Bioflavonoids

The suggested amount of supplemental vitamins/minerals, flavonoids and magnesium has already been discussed in the lactic acid section.

5-HYDROXYTRYPTAMINE

General information

For over 100 years, scientists have been aware of the fact that blood contained a vasoconstrictor substance. It went by many names, including vasotonin. In 1948, researchers isolated the molecule and named it serotonin. Shortly thereafter (in 1949), an examination of the serotonin molecule revealed its chemical structure to be 5-hydroxytryptamine (5-HT)[119].

In the 1930's researchers set out to examine the nature of the biomolecules associated with the enterochromaffin cells of the gastrointestinal mucosa. The experiments led to the discovery of a gut stimulating factor (now known to stimulate smooth muscle contraction), which was named enteramine. In 1952, researchers identified enteramine as 5-HT. Then, in 1953, 5-HT was discovered in the brain[119].

There is approximately 10 grams of 5-HT in the human body. About 90% is located in the enterochromaffin cells of the stomach and small intestine[119]. Most of the remaining 5-HT is present in the CNS (raphe nuclei of the brain stem), mast cells, and platelets. Only 1-2% of total 5-HT is found in the raphe neurons[91-p.339]. The enterochromaffin cells and the raphe neurons synthesize 5-HT from tryptophan in situ, whereas platelets take up enterochromaffin cell-produced 5-HT as they pass through intestinal blood vessels[119].

Function of 5-HT

The activity of 5-HT depends upon its location because different tissues have different types of 5-HT receptors. As of 1991, a total of eight different receptor subtypes had been isolated[91-p.354].

In the nervous system, 5-HT has varied and seemingly paradoxical effects. In the CNS, 5-HT can influence behavior and reduce nociceptive activity; however, in the periphery, 5-HT functions as a nociceptor irritant and a pro-inflammatory molecule.

The following quote describes serotonin's affect on behavior:

"Altered function of serotonergic systems has been reported in several psychopathological conditions, including affective illness, hyper-aggressive states, and schizophrenia. There is mounting evidence for impaired serotonergic function in major depressive illness' and suicidal behavior. In this connection, it is interesting that several effective antidepressant drugs appear to act by enhancing serotonergic transmission."[91-p.37]

Tricyclic antidepressants inhibit membrane re-uptake of both 5-HT and catecholamines, and monoamine oxidase inhibitors block enzymatic degradation of both serotonin and catecholamines. Newer medications referred to as serotonin re-uptake inhibitors, such as Prozac and Zoloft, specifically inhibit 5-HT re-uptake. The purpose for reducing re-uptake and degradation is to extend the synaptic activity of 5-HT in the hope of reducing the untoward effects of reduced serotonergic activity.

Another CNS action of 5-HT is pain modulation. Numerous authorities agree that the descending serotonergic system, emanating from the caudal raphe nuclei (i.e., nucleus raphe magnus), is involved in anti-nociception. It is thought that descending serotonergic neurons can directly inhibit nociceptive transmission at the level of the spinal cord, and can indirectly inhibit nociception by exciting inhibitory interneurons which contain transmitters such as enkephalin or GABA[31a, 47, 137, 176, 488, 491, 495]. It is not uncommon for the antidepressant medications mentioned earlier to help reduce pain. Naturally, enhanced serotonergic activity is thought to be the mechanism of action of these medications. Before the amino acid tryptophan was banned from the market in the late 1980's, it was often used as a natural aid to enhance serotonin activity in the treatment of pain[231].

In the periphery, 5-HT has very different functions. As mentioned above, peripheral 5-HT is known to excite nociceptors[47, 137, 228, 491] and promote inflammation. Recall that most of the systemic 5-HT is sequestered in blood platelets. The remainder of this section on 5-HT will address platelet function.

Platelets

Platelets were discussed in some detail in Chapter 3. Before continuing, I would recommend reviewing the sections in Chapter 3 devoted to platelets and fibroblasts.

As you have just re-read, platelet mediators are involved in nociception (5-HT) and fibroblast activation (PDGF, TGF-β, TG-β). Platelets also release mediators which promote fibrin deposition such as fibrinogen and thrombin, and other mediators which inhibit fibrinolytic activity including antiproteinases such as α1-antitrypsin, α2-macroglobulin, and factors which inhibit plasmin activity such as α2-antiplasmin and plasminogen activator inhibitor-1[455]. It seems likely that these four factors, i.e., nociception, excessive fibroblast activity, increased fibrin deposition and reduced fibrin degradation, all probably contribute to the pathogenesis of joint complex dysfunction. This proposition is based on logical physiological deductions; however, as of yet, little if any chiropractic literature exists on this subject.

Several papers demonstrate that platelets are involved in musculoskeletal tissue damage. Awad uses the term "interstitial myofibrositis" when discussing muscle pain due to injury.

"Myofibrositis is usually defined as chronic inflammation of the fibrous connective tissue in muscle giving rise to pain and stiffness. The diagnosis is usually made on the basis of the presence of circumscribed tender areas which were thought to be muscle to vasoconstriction and localized edema in the muscle...Trauma leads to extravasation of platelets which release serotonin leading to vasoconstriction and localized edema in the muscle."[22] [Tissue biopsy revealed platelet clots between muscle fibers.]

Platelets are also known to be involved in joint inflammation. Research has demonstrated that platelets participate in the inflammatory process associated with rheumatoid arthritis (RA)[276, 455]. Little states that platelet serotonin release may contribute to joint inflammation[276].

Jones indicates that immune complex-induced platelet aggregation is known to occur in patients with RA, as well as in patients with arthralgia and/or joint swelling[225]. An interesting finding was that platelet aggregating complexes were detectable several months before RA could be diagnosed, and that the resolution of arthralgia in the non-RA group appeared to coincide with a decrease in platelet aggregation.

An important point to remember is that platelet mediator release occurs as a consequence of platelet aggregation. Thus, our main practical concern in this section is to discuss those factors which promote and inhibit platelet aggregation.

Promoters of platelet aggregation

Numerous factors appear to promote platelet aggregation. Interestingly enough, these factors are life-style choices. Active and passive smoking, stress-induced secretion of epinephrine, skipping breakfast, sucrose intake, saturated fat intake, an imbalance in prostaglandin precursors and food antigens, all appear to increase the aggregability of platelets. Each topic will be discussed in the following paragraphs.

Research suggests that both active and passive smoking can increase the tendency of platelet aggregation[105]. Despite this information, die-hard smokers will probably not quit on your recommendation. In patients such as these, I would emphasize the extraordinary importance of dietary modification and nutritional supplementation to help counteract some of the detrimental effects of smoking.

In experimental situations, ADP, collagen and epinephrine are used to induce platelet aggregation[74]. These and many other aggregating factors are also thought to be involved in vivo[455]. In the early 1970's, animal studies revealed that stress-induced catecholamine release enhanced platelet stickiness and induce platelet aggregation[179]. It was hypothesized that this mechanism is probably the link between stress and acute myocardial infarction. A recent paper suggested that, "because the concentrations of epinephrine required to initiate aggregation are higher than those achieved in vivo, it is likely that the physiologic role of epinephrine is to potentiate the activity of other agonists"[29]. Clearly, stress management should be a component of any treatment plan.

It is known that myocardial infarction (MI) occurs more commonly in the morning hours compared to other times during the day. Especially high risk hours for MI exist between 6 a.m. and noon, and a less significant risk period exists between 4 and 8 p.m.[323]. The morning hours are associated with a surge in systemic arterial pressure of 20-30 mm Hg, increased cardiovascular tone, increased platelet aggregation and decreased fibrinolytic activity[323]. These are all thought to be normal physiological processes in the morning. Interestingly enough, research suggests that eating breakfast may reduce morning heart attack risk[358]. This is probably because skipping breakfast would induce a hypoglycemic counter-regulatory response that would cause additional epinephrine release.

In the past several years there has been an on going debate about whether or not sucrose causes disease. In recent years, authorities have conceded that there is a direct link between sucrose intake and dental carries formation; however, it is still maintained that other such cause and effect relationships are not clear at this time. Such a position contradicts the work of John Yudkin, MD, Ph.D., who in 1957 stated that, "it is not surprising then that international statistics show a relationship of coronary mortality with sugar consumption as well as with fat consumption; in fact, the former relationship [with sugar] is somewhat better"[499]. Twenty years later Yudkin writes:

"The addition of sucrose to the diets of human subjects and experimental animals results in the production of a number of features that have been found to be present in individuals who have chronic heart disease (CHD), or are especially at risk to develop CHD. These 'risk factors' produced by dietary sucrose include an increase in the blood concentration of cholesterol, triglycerides, insulin and corticosteroids; a decrease in glucose tolerance and an increase in adhesiveness and rate of aggregation of the blood platelets[500]."

It certainly seems like we have not been given the full story on sucrose. It makes a great deal of sense to consume as little sucrose as possible.

Numerous authors agree that saturated fat intake is associated with increased platelet aggregation[158, 334, 335, 365, 386]. Unsaturated fatty acids are thought to have a less pronounced effect. However, it should be understood that hyperlipemia in general promotes platelet aggregation. This is because a pro-aggregatory state probably has to do with essential fatty conversion into prostaglandin precursors. Platelets are less prone to aggregation when they contain dihomo-gama-linolenic acid (DGLA) and eicosapentaenoic acid (EPA) over arachidonic acid[357, 386]. As described in the section of prostaglandins and leukotrienes, DGLA is the immediate precursor of anti-inflammatory PGE-1, and EPA is the immediate precursor of anti-inflammatory PGE-3, TXA-3, PGI-3 and LTB-5.

Food antigens also appear to induce platelet aggregation and serotonin release. This was demonstrated in a group of RA patients who developed joint inflammation after the ingestion of certain foods. The paper suggests that 5-HT release may occur when immune complexes, containing either IgG1 or IgG3, are bound to the platelet membrane[276].

Nutritional factors which may inhibit platelet aggregation:

Several nutritional factors appear to reduce the likelihood of platelet aggregation. As we go through these factors, please keep in mind that a confluence of factors promotes aggregation and that a confluence of nutritional factors probably reduces platelet aggregation.

As mentioned earlier several times in this text, the United States population consumes insufficient amounts of fruits and vegetables to maintain an appropriate antioxidant status[36]. Research suggests that low antioxidant status and a high fat intake promotes lipid peroxidation, the capacity of platelets to aggregate and to produce TXA-2 (and probably their other mediators), and in vivo platelet activation[381]. This study demonstrated that antioxidant supplementation helps to reduce these tendencies. As flavonoids are known to possess antioxidant properties, flavonoid supplementation may also provide similar benefits.

Bordia and Verma[50] fed healthy males 75 grams of butter, which significantly increased platelet adhesiveness and aggregation at the end of four hours. This response was prevented when 1 gram of ascorbic acid was added to the fatty meal. These researchers also demonstrated that providing 1 gram of ascorbic acid every eight hours to coronary artery patients, resulted in a significant reduction in platelet adhesiveness and aggregation. A mechanism of action was not discussed.

Several papers suggest that vitamin E can reduce platelet adhesiveness and/or aggregation. It is thought that vitamin E reduces platelet adhesiveness by increasing membrane fluidity[274], which is thought to be more of a physiochemical effect rather than an antioxidant effect[98]. One study showed that 1600 IU per day given to six subjects for seven days reduced thromboxane synthesis and arachidonic-induced platelet aggregation[51-p.74, 274]. Whether this was due to an antioxidant effect or a physicochemical stabilization is not clear. Perhaps both mechanisms were involved.

In Machlin's review of vitamin E[279], he indicates that in normal subjects, as little as 400 IU/day can significantly reduce adhesion of platelets to collagen. Machlin also cites research that demonstrated how 300-600 IU/day for at least six months in patients with intermittent claudication appeared to enhance blood flow and permit longer walking periods without pain. Lin's review of the literature suggests that vitamin E supplementation of 400 IU to 800 IU per day in so-called healthy humans may significantly reduce platelet adhesion and lipid peroxidation, and to a lesser degree, reduce platelet aggregation[274]. Supplementation with about 400 IU/day of vitamin E may be a good preventive measure.

A very interesting article described how low dose EPA raised vitamin E levels in platelets. For two months eight subjects took 100 mg/day. Results demonstrated that EPA concentrations in platelets did not change, nor did plasma levels of vitamin E; however, platelet vitamin E levels increased significantly[100]. It was suggested that EPA-induced increases in platelet vitamin E levels may be responsible for the reduction in platelet aggregation.

A sufficient amount of EPA consumption is known to inhibit platelet aggregation in a direct manner[5, 127, 169, 239, 354, 415, 467], which differs from the indirect fashion described in the previous paragraph. In platelets, EPA serves as a precursor for thromboxane A3 (TXA-3) and 3-series prostacyclin (PGI3), both of which are anti-aggregatory compared to the arachidonic acid counterparts, namely TXA2.

As little as 500 mg of EPA per day (in fish meals) for 3 months reduced platelet arachidonic acid concentration, increased EPA concentration and reduced platelet aggregation activity. Other groups in this study consumed 600 mg and 1.1 g/day respectively, which resulted in more marked changes compared with the 500 mg/day group[5].

Olive oil was once thought of as an inert oil as it relates to eicosanoid synthesis. Research now suggests that olive oil consumption can reduce platelet aggregation and TXA2 synthesis[26]. Adding 21 g/day of olive oil to an average diet for a period of eight weeks resulted in a significant increase in oleic acid incorporation in platelet membranes and a significant reduction in arachidonic acid. The incorporation of oleic acid from olive oil may also have changed the fluidity of the platelet membrane and it is thought that oleic acid may be able to suppress phospholipase activity. One subject withdrew from the study because of abdominal discomfort and heartburn. The seven who finished the trial reported occasional abdominal discomfort and occasional increases in bowel movements with soft stools. Approximately 1.5 tablespoons of olive oil per day is equal to 20 grams and 180 calories[348-p.63].

The water soluble fraction in the flesh of fresh melon contains adenosine, a substance known to strongly inhibit platelet aggregation "in vitro"[16]. The authors do not comment on whether or not consumption of fresh melon will have a similar effect.

Preliminary research suggests that the consumption of onions, garlic and ginger in the diet may reduce platelet aggregation by inhibiting thromboxane synthesis[429]. I do not know how much is needed in the diet to provide such effects. Until such information is known, I would consume these foods on a daily basis if the social setting permits. Curcumin from turmeric (the herb that gives Indian curry its yellow color) is also known to inhibit platelet aggregation[430]. These substances have been used for ages to aide in the treatment of pain and inflammation. A discussion about ginger and curcumin supplementation can be found in the discussion of prostaglandin E-2.

As early as at least 1966, it was known that magnesium deficiency could induce platelet aggregation[212]. The data in several recent papers suggest that magnesium supplementation may help reduce platelet aggregation[13, 21, 185, 208, 292, 328, 329, 341, 361, 367, 393, 407, 501]. The mechanism of action is unlike any discussed thus far. Magnesium appears to reduce platelet aggregation via stabilization of ion channels[13, 21, 185, 212, 292, 341, 361, 393, 407, 501]. In essence, magnesium acts as nature's calcium channel blocker[13, 21] by inhibiting inappropriate calcium influx[185, 292, 341]. Another theory is that magnesium is needed for ATP synthesis, and ATP is needed to extrude calcium out of the cell[393]. It is known that extracellular calcium entry into platelets (and into cells in general) can activate phospholipase A2 and C, both of which may release arachidonic acid from the platelet membrane. Platelets convert arachidonic acid into TXA-2, which cause vasoconstriction and is a potent activator of platelet aggregation.

Zinc is also thought to stabilize membranes. Although the exact mechanism is not known, it is thought that zinc may have a similar affect on ion channels as magnesium. Zinc may interact and displace calcium ions[83], which might result in calcium influx. The amount of in vivo zinc needed to cause such an effect is not described. In actuality, it is probably not known. Future research may demonstrate that zinc adequacy helps to stabilize platelet membranes. In the mean time, we should make sure that we are getting enough zinc, because numerous Americans are known to be marginally deficient[275-p.229].

Supplemental bromelain is known to inhibit platelet aggregation. This was first demonstrated back in 1972[196]. The precise mechanism by which bromelain inhibits aggregation is unknown. One hypothesis is that bromelain inhibits TXA-2 synthesis and facilitates prostacyclin (PGI2) production[443]. It should be remembered that arachidonic acid is the precursor of both TXA-2 and PGI-2, both of which have antagonistic actions. Whereas TXA-2 causes vasoconstriction and platelet aggregation, PGI-2 causes vasodilation and does not promote aggregation[443].

Flavonoids also appear to inhibit platelet aggregation by inhibiting cyclooxygenase which leads to a reduction in thrombotic tendencies[114]. Fruits and vegetables are the best sources of flavonoids. Red wine is also rich in flavonoids, and it is thought that the cardio-protective effect of red wine is exerted through the flavonoids from grapes[114].

Nutritional supplementation to reduce platelet aggregation:

Based on what was presented in this discussion about platelet aggregation, the following supplements should be considered.

1. EPA

2. Anti-inflammatory botanical

3. Multiple vitamin/mineral

4. Bioflavonoids

5. Magnesium

5. Vitamin E (400 IU/day)

The suggested amount of supplemental vitamins/minerals, flavonoids, magnesium, EPA, and anti-inflammatory botanicals has already been discussed in the lactic acid, magnesium, and prostaglandin E-2 sections respectively.

Platelets and fibrin deposition

Fibrin deposition is required for normal healing to take place (see section on vascular response-platelets and fibroblasts); however, excess fibrin deposition and insufficient degradation of fibrin is pathological. Fibrin is the final product of the coagulation cascade of which platelets play an inextricable role[368].

The precursor of fibrin is fibrinogen, which when acted on by thrombin is converted to fibrin and a soft clot forms. Clotting factor XIII, also call fibrin stabilizing factor, converts the soft clot into a hard clot[466-p.1091]. Fibrinogen, which represents 2-3% of the plasma proteins is made by liver cells and then enters the circulation. Platelets pick up fibrinogen via pinocytosis. Fibrinogen is known to be an acute phase reactant and is released after acute injury and inflammation[368].

It appears that injury and inflammation is associated with an upregulation of fibrinogen synthesis and a down regulation of fibrinolysis, both of which promote fibrin deposition. High plasma fibrinogen levels are associated with increased risks of ischemic heart disease, stroke, and arterial disease in the legs[153]. Many patients with osteoarthritis[164, 337], rheumatoid arthritis[193, 347], systemic lupus erythematosus, anticardiolipin syndrome and scleroderma[193] have demonstrated reduced fibrinolytic activity.

Most germane to the chiropractic practice is the fact that numerous studies have demonstrated that certain patients with low back pain have documented defects in fibrinolytic activity[90, 178, 213, 220, 221, 352]. In this regard, the 1992 Volvo Award in Experimental Studies was issued to a group that correlated a poor surgical outcome with reductions in endogenous production of fibrinolytic agents[178]. Their research supports the contention that, "hypofibrinolysis favors fibrin deposition, which in turn may serve as a matrix for connective tissue invasion and consequently, failure of surgery and chronic low back pain[178]."

The degree to which decreased fibrinolysis plays a role in the pathogenesis of joint complex dysfunction is unknown. It most likely is involved with certain patients at varying levels. Although this could be a fruitful area for chiropractic research, we should not wait for research outcomes before developing protocols to prevent fibrinolytic deficiencies from developing, as such deficiencies promote many serious diseases.

Factors that reduce fibrinolytic activity

At least as early as 1957, it was suspected that tissue injury reduced fibrinolysis. Researchers theorized that inflammatory mediators could inhibit plasmin activity. We are told that, "if an inflammatory peptide inhibits plasmin locally, deposition of fibrin in the protein network of the capillary wall would not be counteracted by a fibrinolytic action"[290]. Recent papers state that tissue injury can temporarily reduce fibrinolysis[90]. "Impaired fibrinolysis is found for a period of approximately 1 week after a variety of acute injuries"[352]. "In response to injury there is a temporary decrease in fibrinolytic enzyme activity that will gradually return to normal during the course of a few weeks"[221]. As tissue injury, and the many serious diseases mentioned earlier, are associated with a reduced fibrinolytic capacity, it would be prudent to treat all of our patients as if they have fibrinolytic defects.

As fibrinogen is the precursor of fibrin,

increasing circulating fibrinogen levels is likely to promote fibrin deposition. Consider the following quote which discusses factors that influence fibrinogen levels:

> "In population surveys, cigarette smoking has been related to fibrinogen concentrations, and after smoking cessation the concentration falls. Other factors that may influence fibrinogen concentrations include age, social class [implication here is associated life-styles], obesity, serum cholesterol, diabetes mellitus, alcohol consumption, intake of cereal fiber, use of oral contraceptives, and menopause."[153]

Although the authors do not state specifically, it appears that numerous life-style choices can be pro-inflammatory because they raise fibrinogen levels.

Smoking[90, 178, 220, 221, 352], physical inactivity[178] and high triglyceride levels[178] are thought to reduce fibrinolytic activity. High fat diets increase the production of clotting factor VII, which is thought to be a marker of hypercoagulability of the blood[313]. A recent paper devoted to obesity stated: "It seems possible to link diabetes, hypertriglyceridemia, reduced fibrinolysis, and hypertension to elevated portal free fatty acid concentrations because of an increased visceral adipose tissue depot"[421].

Nutritional factors that increase fibrinolytic activity

Atherosclerosis triggers endogenous plasminogen activators to increase fibrinolytic capacity. In recent years, endogenous tissue-type plasminogen activator is used as a marker for patients at risk of future myocardial infarction[366]. In certain situations, the body appears to fight a hypofibrinolytic state by increasing the endogenous production of fibrinolytic activators. Fortunately, we can utilize several therapies which assist in this process and thereby help to prevent a hypofibrinolytic state.

At the most basic level, life-style modification is of the utmost importance. Exercise, eating properly and cessation of smoking are known to help restore fibrinolytic activity to the body. Several papers discuss how regular exercise is known for its ability to increase fibrinolysis[178, 106, 397]. Dietary fiber and other constituents of a healthy diet may influence fibrinolytic activity. Whereas guar gum decreased plasminogen activator inhibitor-1 (PAI-1), plasma fibrinogen levels remained the same[254]. The authors indicate that the net effect is improved fibrinolytic activity. In the presence of PAI-1, plasminogen will not be converted into plasmin, the proteolytic enzyme that degrades fibrin. Previous studies did not consistently demonstrate that dietary fiber could reduce PAI-1. "PAI-1 activity is, however, lower in subjects consuming large amounts of fruits and vegetables"[254].

Chiropractic care may also help to increase fibrinolysis. Two old osteopathic articles indicate that osteopathic manipulation can increase fibrinolytic activity of the blood[138, 76]. One paper states that soft tissue manipulation increased fibrinolytic activity and decreased fibrinogen concentrations of the plasma[138]. Neither paper makes it clear whether the manipulations were osseous adjustments or myofascial work.

Certain nutritional supplements, such as vitamin C, EPA and proteolytic enzymes, have demonstrated an ability to improve fibrinolysis. Over a period of 6 months, patients with a past history of myocardial infarction were provided with 2 g/day of vitamin C (b.i.d.) which maintains fibrinolytic activity about 50% above control levels[48]. Marine oils are known to decrease plasma fibrinogen levels[26].

Proteolytic enzymes such as bromelain are thought to stimulate plasmin production which is needed to degrade fibrin. Indeed, many authors indicate that bromelain is thought to activate the body's fibrinolytic system in this manner[8, 84, 86, 142, 217, 314, 426, 443, 471]. Clinical trials have demonstrated the efficacy of bromelain supplementation in the reduction of inflammation and pain associated with musculoskeletal injuries[51, 84, 107], surgery[51, 84, 497], and rheumatoid arthritis[86].

Nutritional supplementation to enhance fibrinolysis:

The suggested amounts of supplemental flavonoids has already been discussed in the lactic

acid and platelet aggregation sections, respectively.

1. Bioflavonoids

2. Bromelain

Regarding bromelain supplementation, the studies on proteolytic enzyme use indicate that no apparent side effects were seen. Bucci states that, "in many thousands of subjects, oral protease supplementation has not been associated with any side effects"[51-p.173]. However, it should be understood that the effects of long-term enzyme use is not well known. Anecdotal reports demonstrate that long term use of enzymes can result in digestion of human proteins, such as those associated with the teeth. Therefore, it is not recommended that enzymes be used on a long term basis for their anti-inflammatory effects.

For an anti-inflammatory effect, enzymes should be taken 4 times/day on an empty stomach. Bucci[51-p.174] recommends taking 2-8 tablets 3-5 times daily, and that this should be continued for 1 week or until improvement is noted. I would not recommend using proteolytic enzymes for more than 10 days. However, long term use is not a problem if the enzymes are taken with meals as a digestive aid, which is a reasonable practice so long as the patient shows an indication for such use.

BRADYKININ

General information

In 1909 researchers demonstrated that the injection of urine into dogs resulted in a lowering of blood pressure. In 1928, researchers confirmed that urine contains a hypotensive agent. They also found that this substance could be obtained from saliva, plasma and a variety of other tissues such as the pancreas. An old Greek synonym for the pancreas is kallikreas, and thus, this substance was named kallikrein[120].

In 1937, researchers discovered that kallikrein was not the active substance. Instead, it acted as an enzyme which cleaves off the pharmacologically active substance from an inactive precursor present in plasma. In 1948, this active substance was named kallidin and the inactive precursor molecule was called kallidinogen[120].

In 1949, it was discovered that a new substance was isolated from plasma that had hypotensive effects and caused a slowly developing contraction in the gut. Hence, the substance was called bradykinin. Bradykinin is a Greek word meaning, "slow" (bradys) "to move" (kinein).

Soon it became clear that bradykinin and kallidin were very similar molecules; they were formed under similar conditions and had similar actions. In 1960, the structures of both kallidin and bradykinin were delineated. Bradykinin (BK) is referred to as a nonapeptide and kallidin is referred to as a decapeptide[120]. Several other kinins have been identified including Met-Lys-bradykinin, T-kinin, BK(1-8), and BK(1-7), all of which are thought to have similar actions as bradykinin and kallidin[433]. Collectively, these six peptides are referred to as kinin peptides or kinins.

It does not appear that the activities of T-kinin, BK(1-8) and BK(1-7) are as well understood as bradykinin, kallidin, and Met-Lys-bradykinin. In Stewarts review[433], he often uses bradykinin in the generic sense to refer to bradykinin, kallidin and Met-Lys-bradykinin.

Kinins are involved in numerous and diverse functions in the body, some of which include the clotting cascade, immune function, glandular secretion, ion transport, glucose uptake in exercising muscles, renal function, blood pressure, and cell growth[433]. This clearly demonstrates that, like all other mediators of inflammation, bradykinin is not a bad molecule.

Problems with bradykinin occur when there is excessive production. Bradykinin plays a role in circulatory shock (endotoxic, hemorrhagic, acute pancreatitis). Bradykinin activates phospholipase-A2 which in turn stimulates leukotriene generation from leukocytes. Leukotrienes are thought to be responsible for the bronchoconstrictor reactivity seen in asthma and other allergic bronchial pathologies. Through this mechanism, kinins are thought to exert powerful bronchoconstrictor activity[433]. Kinins also induce histamine release from mast cells and thus, kinins are thought to be responsible for allergic rhinitis and cold-evoked rhinitis[433].

A common misconception is that lactic acid causes ischemic pain. Another common misconception is that lactic acid is the molecule that builds up in muscles and prohibits further exercise. In fact, it is bradykinin that causes ischemic pain and inhibits further exercise[433]. Serotonin released from platelets is probably an important synergist of bradykinin in ischemic pain[433].

Bradykinin also plays a preeminent role in the inflammatory process. It is known that bradykinin itself can cause the four cardinal signs of inflammation, those being dolor/pain, calor/fever, rubor/redness and tumor/swelling[433]. Kinins are typically released in the initial moments of inflammation and then trigger the release of all the other mediators of inflammation[433]. Authors agree that bradykinin is the most potent nociceptor irritant[137-p.31, 433]. Chiropractors should consider this information in light of the fact that research has demonstrated the presence of kinins in synovial fluid of all patients whether they had gout, rheumatoid arthritis or psoriatic arthritis of unknown etiology[307].

Recent research has demonstrated that kinins appear to be intimately involved in the pathophysiology associated with rheumatoid arthritis[33, 411, 433] and osteoarthritis[33]. The activation of bradykinin receptors, i.e., B_1 and B_2, may be involved in the release of prostaglandins, prostacyclin, leukotrienes, histamine, PAF, IL-1 and TNF which are derived mainly from neutrophils, macrophages, endothelial cells and synovial tissue[411].

Biochemistry of bradykinin

The liver synthesizes two principle kininogens, which are protein precursors of the kinin peptides. One is a high-molecular-weight-kininogen (HMWK) and the other is a low-molecular-weight-kininogen (LMWK). Kininogens travel in the circulatory system and enter tissue spaces throughout the body; they are ubiquitous[433].

Several enzymes liberate kinins, the most well known being plasma kallikrein, tissue kallikrein and elastase. The kallikreins are also ubiquitous. Whereas plasma kallikrein cleaves bonds in HMWK and LMWK to yield bradykinin, tissue kallikrein cleaves bonds in HMWK and LMWK to yield kallidin and Met-Lys-bradykinin[43]. Prekallikrein must first be converted into kallikrein before kinins can be generated. Kallikrein production is catalyzed by several factors including tissue injury. Injury exposes negatively charged molecules of tissues, such as collagen, which activates the Hageman factor of the coagulation cascade. So-called Hageman fragments are known to powerfully activate kallikrein. Complement activation and the resulting cell lysis can also ultimately activate bradykinin[120].

There are two other factors which can activate kinins and both appear to involve nutritional factors (tissue acidity and food intolerance). Although the specific details are not well understood, it is thought that tissue acidification may be a major mechanism of kinin production[433]. Lactic acid production and acidic lysosomal enzyme are thought to activate kallikrein. Activated macrophages are also known to release acidic products. Local acidity also inactivates the enzyme kininase I, that deactivates bradykinin, which may then allow bradykinin concentration to increase even more rapidly[433].

Thus far in this book several different nutritional factors were described that relate to tissue pH. First, review the section on the pro-inflammatory state that is devoted to tissue acidity and then review the nutrients needed to drive ATP production. It may turn out that these nutritional factors are of preeminent importance since it is known that the tissue kinin system is more difficult to inhibit than the plasma system[433].

Food intolerance may in some way activate kinin production. People with food sensitivities have symptoms that are very similar to symptoms associated with excess kinins such as flushing, nausea, dyspnea, fatigue, irritability, throbbing headache, local pain and many more. It is also known that the symptoms of patients with hyperbradykininism syndrome become worse after meals[27]. See Chapter 2 for a discussion about food allergies.

Physiological inhibition of bradykinin

There are two major kinin degrading enzymes: carboxypeptidase N and angiotensin I converting enzyme. Carboxypeptidase N is also known as kininase I. It is found in plasma and permits a half life for bradykinin of no more than 15 seconds[433].

Angiotensin I converting enzyme (ACE) is also known as kininase II. It turns out that bradykinin is a better substrate for ACE/kininase II than angiotensin I. Kininase II is found in the vascular endothelium and, not surprisingly, the pulmonary vascular bed has high concentrations. Together, both enzymes permit very little kinin release from the local tissues where it was produced.

Nutritional inhibition of bradykinin

Several papers discuss how proteolytic enzymes, such as bromelain, are able to deplete plasma kininogen and/or antagonize the activity of bradykinin[39, 356-p.91, 391, 437, 471, 502]. Thus, it is possible that bromelain may work as a fibrinolytic agent, as well as a bradykinin inhibitor. Some of the effects of bradykinin, such as increased vascular permeability, may be antagonized by flavonoids. Hesperidin methyl-chalcone is thought to function in this fashion[159].

Remember, it is not recommended to use proteolytic enzymes for their anti-inflammatory effects for more than a week. See the section on 5-Hydroxytryptamine where enzyme supplementation is discussed.

Nutritional supplementation:

1. Multiple vitamin/mineral

2. Bioflavonoids

3. Bromelain

The suggested amount of supplements has already been discussed in the lactic acid and fibrin deposition sections.

CYTOKINES

Cytokines is the generic term which refers to molecules of cell communication. such as interleukins (IL), interferon (INF), growth factors, and colony-stimulating factors are all considered to be cytokines. Cytokines function as local mediators of intercellular communication when cells are healthy and when cells are diseased. Cytokines work in an autocrine, paracrine, and endocrine fashion. Lymphokines and monokines refer to cytokines derived from lymphocytes and monocytes respectively[19].

Cytokine research is a relatively new field. Whereas preliminary work began 50 years ago, most advances in understanding have occurred in the past 10-20 years. It was only recently, in 1979, that the term interleukin-1 (IL-1) was coined, and numerous additional cytokines have been discovered since that time. For a general overview of the subject see Robson[369] and for more in depth discussions see Arend[19] and Gallin[160].

An in depth understanding of cytokines is difficult to achieve, unless one specializes in such research. Developing a basic working concept about the subject should be our goal. It is important to understand that cytokines do not have minds of their own; their production and actions depend upon the needs of a cell at a given time. In other words, it is not possible to characterize in vivo cytokine function unless the tissue milieu is also characterized.

A classic example of a tissue environment that augments the activity of the cytokine system is viral and bacterial invasion. In fact, cytokine function is typically discussed from the perspective innate and acquired immune responses against invading microbes[532]. While this aspect of cytokine function is obviously important for our survival, this altered tissue milieu is not typically encountered or treated by chiropractors. However, cytokine activity is augmented by factors other than microbial invasion which do apply to chiropractic practice.

It seems clear that cytokines are driven into action by inflammatory states, such as that associated with rheumatoid arthritis (RA). In fact, researchers agree that cytokines play a major role in promoting the tissue damage and chronic inflammation associated with rheumatoid arthritis[19, 192]. Recall, in the discussion about platelets (see Chapter 3), that platelet activating factor (PAF) stimulates monocytes to release IL-1 and TNF, both of which are known to contribute to joint injury and bone resorption.

Cytokines are also known to be involved in the

pathogenesis of atherosclerosis [see review by Ross[780]]. Meydani suggests that an unregulated, over production of cytokines contributes to the pathogenesis of acute and chronic inflammatory, autoimmune, atherosclerotic, and neoplastic diseases[729]. A more recent review by Luster suggests that many common diseases are driven, in part, by chemotactic cytokines (i.e., chemokineses) that mediate inflammation, including asthma, sarcoidosis, glomerular nephritis, rheumatoid arthritis, osteoarthritis, atherosclerosis, ulcerative colitis, Crohn's disease, psoriasis, and meningitis[710].

The paragraphs that follow briefly outline the activity of certain cytokines which are known to be produced by monocytes/macrophages, including IL-1, TNF-α, IL-6 and IL-8. Colony stimulating factors will also be mentioned.

Interleukin-1 (IL-1)

To some degree, nearly all cells can produce IL-1, however, monocytes and macrophages are the main producers. Macrophage production of IL-1 can have systemic and local effects. Some general systemic effects include fever, decreased appetite, muscle proteolysis, synthesis of acute-phase proteins, and increased granulocyte/macrophage-CSF production. Some local effects include prostaglandin E_2, collagenase, and neutral protease production by fibroblasts, chondrocytes and synovial cells; chemotaxis of neutrophils, lymphocytes and monocytes; adherence of leukocytes to endothelial cells; fibroblast production; increased production of collagen and an inhibitor of neutral proteases; and stimulation of T and B lymphocytes[19].

An aspect of IL-1 function that is not well-known has to do with its affects on articular cartilage. IL-1 can dramatically alter the character of articular cartilage. Consider the following quote:

"IL-1 alters collagen production in chondrocytes, reducing production of type II collagen and enhancing synthesis of types I and III collagen. Because type II collagen is the predominant form in articular cartilage, this effect of IL-1 may result in a further weakening of the joint...IL-1 has complex effects on proteoglycans in cartilage, inhibiting synthesis and enhancing degradation." [19]

More recent research suggest that IL-1 may play a role in nociceptor activation and sensitization, by acting in concert with bradykinin. Indomethacin was shown to reverse IL-1 sensitization, which suggests that pro-inflammatory eicosanoids may also be involved in cytokine-mediated nociception [766].

Tumor necrosis factor-α (TNF-α)

In 1984 TNF-α was cloned and expressed. It was originally described as a monocyte product that caused tumor lysis in experimental animals and cachexia in mice [19]. Cachexia is defined as a state of ill health, malnutrition and waisting [440-p.265]. The original name for TNF-α was cachectin.

Monocytes and macrophages are thought to be the main TNF-a producers [19]. However, TNF-α can be synthesized and released by several cells in response to inflammation and tissue injury, including macrophages, mast cells, Schwann cells, fibroblasts, and endothelial cells [856]. Many effects of TNF-α overlap those of IL-1. Experimentally, TNF-α seems to augment the inflammatory damage caused by IL-1. TNF-α stimulates collagenase and prostaglandin E_2 production by fibroblasts, and may play a role in synovial inflammation [19]. TNF-α has also been shown to stimulate bone resorption and proteoglycan degradation [75]. Additionally, both animal and human studies suggest that TNF plays a role in nociceptor activation [815, 856].

Interleukin-6 (IL-6)

IL-6 is produced by monocytes, T lymphocytes and fibroblasts. IL-6 production is induced by IL-1, TNF-α, and PDGF [455]. IL-6 induces hepatocytes to produce some of the acute phase proteins including haptoglobin, fibrinogen, and 1-antitrypsin [273].

Interleukin-8 (IL-8)

IL-8 is produced by monocytes, tissue macrophages, endothelial cells, fibroblasts and other cells as well. IL-1 and TNF-α stimulate IL-8 production in all of these cells. IL-8 causes neutrophil chemotaxis, increased expression of

Leu-CAMS, release of lysosomal enzymes, and generation of free radicals [19].

Colony stimulating factors (CSF)

In general, CSFs have two main functions including induction of growth and proliferation of hematopoietic progenitor cells in the bone marrow and activation of granulocytes and monocytes. Granulocyte-macrophage CSF (GM-CSF), G-CSF and M-CSF are produced by macrophages and fibroblasts and endothelial cells that have been stimulated by IL-1 and TNF-α [19].

Cytokine modulation by drugs

At the present time, efforts are being made to create drugs which influence cytokine function [19, 456]. Consider how one author characterizes cytokine function:

"Cytokines have overlapping, redundant, and synergistic effects so that multiple factors are usually involved in any particular biologic response. Cytokines exhibit both enhancing and inhibiting effects on immune and inflammatory cells. It is important to note that the cytokine network is, in large part, self-regulating through the simultaneous presence of factors with opposing properties, feedback inhibition of production, and induction of specific cytokine-binding proteins or receptor antagonists." [19]

The cytokine system is designed with numerous checks and balances. Altering cytokine activity with medications might prove to be more damaging than helpful. Except for in life threatening situations, it appears that a dietary reduction of the pro-inflammatory state may be the most logical way to influence cytokine activity, for it seems that cytokine activity becomes dysregulated mostly during chronic inflammation.

Nutritional factors

Regarding patient care, Grimble states that, "prior as well as concurrent nutrient intake are of importance in the outcome of the inflammatory response" [636]. He explains that n-6 fatty acids promote TNF and IL-1 production. However, an exception to this rule seems to be evening primrose oil, a rich source of the n-6 gamma-linolenic acid, which also seems to reduce cytokine activity[636]. In fact, in patients with colorectal cancer, gamma-linolenic acid had a suppressive effect on the production of pro-inflammatory cytokines, including IL-1, IL-2, IL-4, IL-6, TNF, and interferon-gamma[636].

Additional nutrients can also suppress TNF and IL-1 production and activity including monounsaturated fatty acids, n-3 fatty acids, and antioxidants[636]. A recent human trial suggests that olive oil rich diets, i.e., the monounsaturated fat component, may also suppress cell adhesion molecule expression and reduce inflammatory disease progression[859]. These same authors mentioned that animal experiments demonstrated that monounsaturated fat intake reduced interleukin-2 activity[859].

Several recent articles have reviewed the suppressive effect on cytokine production by omega-3 fatty acids[572, 636, 637, 729].

> "IL-1 and TNF are principal mediators of inflammation. Recent work also suggests involvement of these cytokines in the pathogenesis of atherosclerosis. Eicosanoids such as LTB4, PGE2, and TXB2 have also been indicated as contributory factors to the development of inflammatory and atherosclerotic diseases. Therefore, decreased production of these cytokines and eicosanoids following consumption of (n-3) PUFA may reduce pathogenesis of these diseases. Epidemiological, clinical, and animal studies support this notion."[729]

Supplementation with omega-3 fatty acids (eicosapentanoic acid from fish oil) leads to an inhibition of a PDGF-like protein from endothelial cells, suppression of IL-1 and TNF by mononuclear cells, suppression of human synovial cell proliferation, and a reduction in neutrophil LTB-4 production[248]. When supplementing with fish oil, Meydani states that it is important to insure adequate antioxidant intake, particularly vitamin E, to reduce the likelihood of peroxidation of the omega-3 fatty acids[729]. See the Prostaglandin E-2 section of this chapter for a thorough list of anti-inflammatory benefits of omega-3 fatty acid supplementation.

Conner and Gisham state, "It is becoming increasingly apparent that in addition to promoting cytotoxicity, reactive oxygen metabolites may also initiate and/or amplify inflammation via the upregulation of several different genes involved in the inflammatory process, such as those that code for pro-inflammatory cytokines and adhesion molecules"[589]. Research suggests that antioxidant nutrients, such as vitamins E and C can inhibit this pro-inflammatory process[589]. Vitamin C has been shown to reduce TNF-induced HIV expression in AIDS patients[651]. Grimble states that, "low antioxidant results in enhanced cytokine production and effects"[636]. He discusses the importance of the cellular antioxidant defense system with a particular emphasis on trace element-supported systems including metallothionein (An), ceruloplasmin (Cu), superoxide dismutase (Cu, Se, Zn) and glutathione peroxidase (Se)[636]. In a similar article, Grimble emphasizes the importance of in vivo production of glutathione in antioxidant defense[637]. See Chapter 5 for a review of an antioxidant defense system involving glutathione and other antioxidants.

Finally, with respect to overall dietary modifications, recall the work of Kjeldsen-Kragh et al.[237]. When 27 patients with rheumatoid arthritis consumed a vegetarian based diet, all experienced significant improvements in inflammatory indicators, while the 26 controls continued to suffer. Although cytokines were not assessed in this trial, it is very likely that pro-inflammatory cytokine activity was reduced by this dietary intervention.

Nutritional supplementation:

Based on what was presented in this discussion about cytokines, the following supplements should be considered :

1. Multiple vitamin/mineral

2. Bioflavonoids

3. Omega-3 fatty acids

The suggested amount of supplements has already been discussed in the lactic acid and prostaglandin sections.

Chapter 9

GLYCOSAMINOGLYCANS AND TISSUE HEALING

CONNECTIVE TISSUE REPAIR

The responsibility of the "repair phase" of inflammation is to insure that adequate glycosaminoglycans (GAGS), proteoglycans, and collagen is provided to repair injured tissues. The synthesis of connective tissue is an involved process, requiring adequate motion and specific nutrients. Additionally, certain hormonal factors can influence the tissue repair process.

Chiropractors often make the mistake of assuming that connective tissue repair only requires restoring mobility to an injured area. A look at the nature of connective tissue and the manner in which the body produces collagen and proteoglycans will demonstrate that this view is shortsighted.

Connective tissue consists of a cellular component and the extracellular matrix. The cellular component consists of resident cells (fibroblasts, osteoblasts, chondroblasts) which synthesize the extracellular matrix, and circulating cells (lymphocytes and macrophages) which defend against infections and clean up debris[336]. The extracellular matrix of connective tissue consists of a fibrous and a nonfibrous component. Collagen and elastin make up the fibrous component which forms the connective tissue structure. Proteoglycans and glycoproteins make up the nonfibrous component which is more commonly referred to as ground substance.

Collagen Production

Collagen is the most abundant protein in the human body, making up approximately 30% of total proteins. Connective tissues are 70-90% collagen by weight and collagen makes up about 6% of the total body weight[51, p.10]. The tensile strength of collagen approaches that of steel[336].

There are eleven different types of collagen. Types I and II are abundant in musculoskeletal structures. Type I is found in structures that are subjected to tension and compression (ligaments, joint capsules, annulus fibrosis). Type II is found in tissues that are habitually exposed to pressure (nucleus pulposus and articular cartilage)[41, p.17-19].

Most of what is known about collagen synthesis has been discovered by studying how fibroblasts synthesize type I collagen. It is thought that the same basic mechanisms are involved when other cell types (osteoblasts and chondroblasts) synthesize other molecular varieties of collagen[166].

Several steps are involved in the synthesis of collagen (see *Figure 9-1*)[660], the first being DNA transcription of various RNA molecules[11, p.204]. These RNA molecules are synthesized by RNA polymerase enzymes, which make an RNA copy of the DNA sequence [11, p.202]. [DNA and RNA polymerases are thought to be zinc dependent[275, p.227; 264, p.208].] Messenger RNA (mRNA) contains the code for the collagen that is to be synthesized. Transfer RNA (tRNA) has a structural role, in that it determines where amino acids are added during collagen synthesis. Ribosomal RNA (rRNA) catalyzes collagen synthesis within a respective ribosome. Ribosomes consist mostly of rRNA molecules and protein to which mRNA and tRNA are added.

There are two different types of ribosomes. Free ribosomes are found in the cytoplasm and membrane-bound ribosomes are attached to the endoplasmic reticulum. Several free ribosomes usually attach to an mRNA molecule to form a

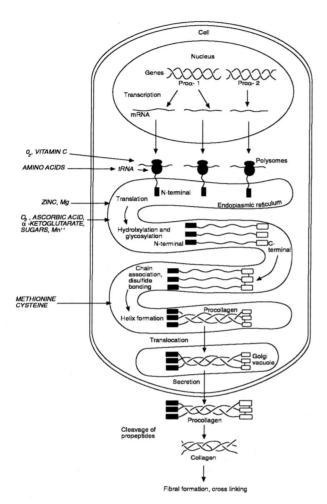

Figure 9-1

polyribosome and collagen synthesis begins, which causes the polyribosome to attach to the endoplasmic reticulum[166; 474, p.39]. Polyribosomes produce molecules known as pro-alpha chains, which are single strand precursors to the triple helix configuration of mature collagen. Enzymes in the endoplasmic reticulum hydroxylate the pro-alpha chains with proline and lysine. The hydroxylation process requires oxygen, alpha-ketoglutarate, ferrous iron (Fe^{++}), and ascorbic acid[51, p.12; 166; 451, p.117]. The pro-alpha chains are also glycosylated in the endoplasmic reticulum with oligosaccharides such as galactose, mannose and N-acetylglucosamine. Bucci[51, p.12] indicates that the associated glycosyltransferase enzymes require manganese and perhaps vitamin A. Similarly, Linder states that manganese is required for the

activity of galactose transferase and other glycosyltransferase enzymes[275, p.238].

Within the endoplasmic reticulum, three pro-alpha chains are combined via covalent and non-covalent bonding to form a pro-collagen molecule that is shipped to the golgi apparatus. The golgi complex packages the pro-collagen in a secretory vesicle which travels to the plasma membrane of the fibroblast. The vesicle fuses with the membrane and releases pro-collagen into the extracellular space where it is then converted into a collagen fiber[166]. Bucci indicates that zinc and vitamin A are required for the secretion of pro-collagen into the extracellular space[51, p.12].

When pro-collagen enters the extracellular space, it is acted on by pro-collagen peptidase enzymes which cleave off molecules known as propeptides, that specifically lie on either end of the pro-collagen molecule. The newly formed molecule is called tropocollagen, the building block of mature collagen. Collagen microfibrils are formed as tropocollagen molecules aggregate, or self assemble, which occurs spontaneously and via the direction of the already cleaved propeptides[11, p.812; 451, p.118].

Microfibrils have little tensile strength until covalent bonds or "cross-links" form between adjacent tropocollagen molecules within a microfibril (intramolecular cross-links), and when such "cross-links" form between adjacent microfibrils (intermolecular cross-links)[451, p.118]. Cross-linking occurs as a consequence of the activity of the Cu^{++}-dependent lysyl oxidase enzyme[275, p.145] that acts on specific lysine residues to form aldehydes[451, p.118]. The aldehydes initiate the cross-linking process that involves the already mentioned covalent bonding[451, p.118; 324, p.634].

Microfibrils are made thicker by adding layers of tropocollagen chains which forms a large collagen fibril. When several large fibrils aggregate a collagen fiber is formed[41, p.17].

Chiropractic considerations regarding collagen production

It should be understood that the cross-linking within collagen molecules is required for the development of tensile strength; however, when joints are immobilized, excessive cross-linking occurs which can reduce tissue strength and predispose associated structures to an increased risk of injury.

When we think of *immobilization,* a cast often comes to mind; however, immobilization "may be self imposed as a reaction to pain and inflammation[336, p.87]." Norkin[336, p.88] provides us with the following information regarding self-imposed immobilization:

> "An injured joint or joint subjected to in-flammation and swelling will assume a loose-packed position in which the pres-sure within the joint space is minimized. This position may be referred to as the position of comfort because pain is de-creased in this position. Each joint has a position of minimum pressure...If the joint is immobilized for a few weeks in the posi-tion of comfort, contractures will develop in the surrounding soft tissues and as a consequence a normal range of joint mo-tion will be impossible."

Biochemical observations from immobilized joints provide specific details about the nature of some of the changes that take place in articular and periarticular structures. The knee joints of rabbits are most commonly used for such experimental observations. Akeson found that articular cartilage and meniscus show a reduction in GAG production of 24 percent and 31 percent, respectively. In periarticular tissues there was a 30% reduction of chondroitin-4 and 6 sulfate, 40% reduction of hyaluronic acid, and there was a 4-6% reduction in water content[7]. The rate of collagen turnover, degradation and synthesis are all increased; the cumulative result being about a 10% reduction in collagen mass[131].

The net effect of these biochemical changes is a relative loss of the proteoglycan/water to collagen fiber ratio within joint structures. The half-life of GAGs is about 1.7-7 days versus that of collagen which is about 300 to 500 days, which is consistent with observed preferential loss of GAGS over collagen[7]. Such an imbalance is thought to drive inappropriate intermolecular cross-linking between collagen microfibrils.

It is thought that GAGs and water allow for separation and lubrication of collagen microfibrils within a given structure. Appropriate fibril-fibril distance permits microfibrils to glide past one another without making direct contact. A loss of GAGs results in reduced lubrication and separation of microfibril. This promotes fibril-fibril friction and the potential for inappropriate cross-linking (also referred to as adhesions) between adjacent preexisting microfibrils and newly synthesized microfibrils, which can restrict normal joint motion[7].

Clinically, the restricted joint motion induced by cross-linking, as well as the restricted joint motion induced by muscle spasm and sympathetic hyperactivity, is what chiropractors attempt to palpate and subsequently adjust. Indeed, researchers suggest that a group of chronic pain patients were, in part, suffering from chronic adhesions within connective tissue structures in the low back. They hypothesized that the spinal adjustments could reduce such adhesions and restore motion[233]. Johnson[224] suggests that improved mobility, as a consequence of soft tissue manipulation, may be the result of one or more of the following factors:

- An alteration in of the scar tissue matrix

- A redistribution of interstitial fluids

- The stimulation of GAG synthesis re-storing normal or improved lubrica-tion and hydration

- The breaking of restrictive intermo-lecular cross-links

- The mechanical and viscoelastic elon-gation of existing collagenous tissues through the phenomena of creep and hysteresis

- A neuroreflexive response that may alter vascular, muscular, and biochemical fac-tors related to immobility

As spinal adjustments are thought to be superior to other forms of therapy in the treatment of certain spinal pain syndromes[242; 282], we can infer that chiropractic care may be the most effective method to improve joint mobility and enhance local tissue function. The implications here are great. As described above, the biochemical manifestations of joint immobility are increased degradation and synthesis of the extracellular matrix which results in a net loss of the said matrix. These changes parallel the changes seen in osteoarthritic joints.

The osteoarthritic process is characterized by a mixture of degradation, attempted repair and mild inflammation[175, p.200; 299]. Grieve[175, p.200] provides a diagram that illustrates increased extracellular matrix breakdown and increased matrix synthesis. In a review of the immobilization literature by Videman[464], he states that the evidence, "shows beyond reasonable doubt that immobilization is not only a cause of osteoarthritis, but it delays the healing process."

If we were to appropriately characterize ourselves as the doctors most suited to restore joint mobility, then the future of chiropractic could be quite bright. We should appreciate that osteoarthritis is the most common type of joint disease for which billions of dollars are spent annually in its treatment and for lost days of work[93, p.1247]. Perhaps in the future, chiropractors will be regarded as the doctors of choice for patients with joint dysfunction.

Nutritional considerations for collagen production

As mentioned earlier in this book, doctors rarely emphasize nutritional recommendations as part of a treatment plan. Medical doctors typically treat arthritis and joint injuries with anti-inflammatory medications and perhaps exercise. Chiropractors typically treat the same problems with joint adjusting and perhaps exercise. A dietary analysis of patients with osteoarthritis (OA) and rheumatoid arthritis (RA) demonstrated the folly of such limited approaches. Researchers demonstrated that a large percentage of patients with OA and RA were ingesting less than 67% of the RDA for vitamins E, C, A, B-12, B-6, folic acid, pantothenic acid and the minerals zinc, magnesium, iron, and calcium[167; 247]. A more recent study on 48 RA patients in New Zealand (13 men, 35 women; mean age, 64.5) indicated that significant deficiencies existed. The percentage of patients who did not achieve the

recommended dietary intake (RDI) was 67% for calcium, 54% for folic acid, 71% for vitamin E, 90% for zinc, and 94% for selenium[822].

It is impossible for joints to repair if patients are deficient in nutrients that are essential for joint tissue function. The several nutrients thought to be involved in collagen production include zinc, proline, lysine, oxygen, alpha-ketoglutarate, iron, vitamin C, manganese, and vitamin A. Although the precise mechanisms have yet to be elucidated, silicon is also known to be involved in collagen formation[275, p.246]. Once collagen is formed it must be protected against damage.

One way to help protect collagen may involve the ingestion of bioflavonoids. Bioflavonoids fortify connective tissue by inhibiting cyclooxygenase/prostaglandin-induced elastase activity, and by stimulating collagen cross-linking[194].

The diet-induced pro-inflammatory state may also play a role in promoting a net loss in extracellular matrix. As described earlier, cytokines (IL-1, TNF, etc.) are involved in chronic inflammation of joints[19]. Their activity results in a loss of extracellular matrix[19; 93; p.1247; 456]. Several nutritional factors may be related to enhanced cytokine function such as deficiencies in antioxidants and fatty acid imbalances (see Chapter 8 for details).

Proteoglycan production

Glycosaminoglycans (GAGs) are the building blocks for proteoglycans (see *Figure 9-2*). In essence, GAGs are polysaccharides, or a chain of repeating disaccharide units. Each sugar molecule is derived from the glycolytic pathway and then connected to make a GAG. *Figure 9-2* illustrates how chondroitin-6-sulfate and chondroitin-4-sulfate are constructed[318, p.325].

A chondroitin sulfate subunit, or disaccharide unit, consists of N-acetyl-D-galactosamine and D-glucuronic acid. The typical chondroitin sulfate chain consists of numerous repeating disaccharide units. Depending upon the type of tissue and location, Bucci indicates that each disaccharide unit can be repeated from several dozen to several hundred times[51, p.8]. Murray and Keeley state that each chain contains some 40 disaccharide units[324].

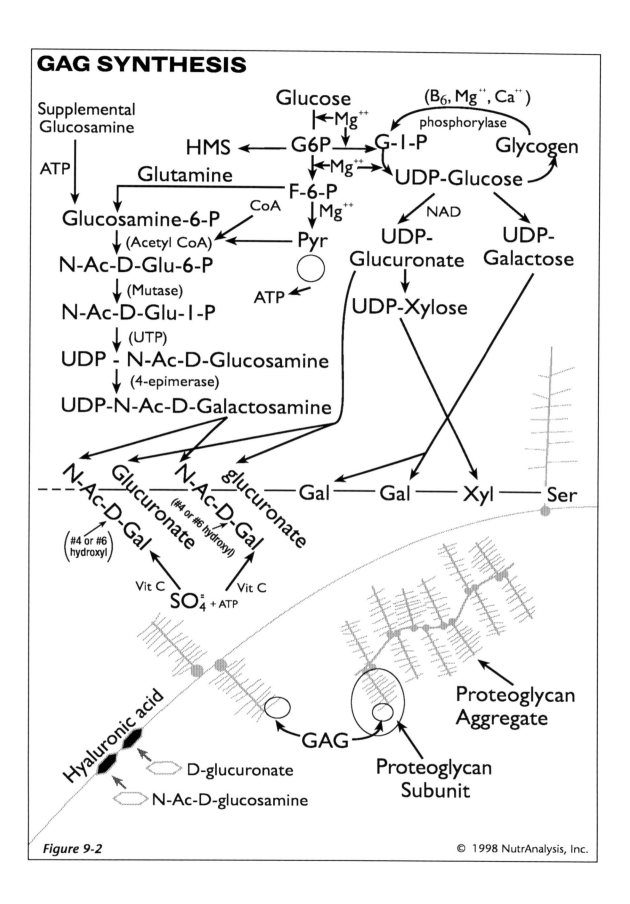

Figure 9-2

© 1998 NutrAnalysis, Inc.

Other GAGs include hyaluronic acid, keratan sulfate, dermatan sulfate, heparan sulfate, and heparin (*Figure 9-3*).

Figure 9-2 demonstrates where xylose and galactose are incorporated into the GAG. The enzymes that drive the production of these molecules, as well as glucuronate, require magnesium and niacin (NAD)[318, p.325; 482]. *Figure 9-2* also shows where glucuronate and N-acetyl-D-galactosamine are incorporated into the GAG.

The production of N-acetyl-D-galactosamine requires magnesium, glutamine and the acetyl CoA. Recall that acetyl CoA is also needed to drive the Krebs Cycle. Pyruvate and CoA join to create acetyl CoA via the activity of the pyruvate dehydrogenase enzyme complex which requires several nutrients including B1, B2, B3, B5, magnesium, manganese, glutathione (GSH), and calcium[318, p.325; 343; 482]. The nucleotide known as UTP (uridine triphosphate) is also required for N-acetyl-D-galactosamine production[318, p.325]. UTP synthesis depends upon the presence of magnesium and NADPH which is produced by the hexose monophosphate shunt [HMS] [482]. The various sugars are then specifically connected to one another to form the appropriate GAG, a function which is controlled by manganese-dependent glycosyltransferase enzymes located in the golgi apparatus[51, p.141-42; 275, p.238].

Depending on whether a chondroitin-4 or 6

Glycosaminoglycans

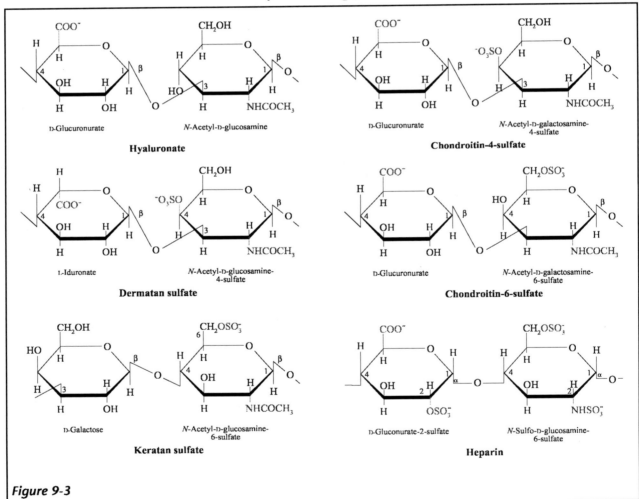

Figure 9-3

sulfate is being produced, a sulfate molecule is esterified to the 4-hydroxyl or the 6-hydroxyl group of the N-acetyl-D-galactosamine residue in each disaccharide unit[317, p.370]. This incorporation requires a pH that is not too acidic[339], ATP[317] and its nutrient precursors, vitamin C[275, p.144], and manganese-dependent sulfonotransferase enzymes[51, p.141-42]. Linder[275, p.246] states that silicon is also needed for GAG synthesis, although she does not mention its mechanism.

After GAGs are formed they are attached to a core protein to make a proteoglycan subunit[41]. Varying numbers of subunits are then attached by a link protein to a hyaluronic acid molecule to create a proteoglycan aggregate[41].

GAGs contain numerous carboxyl (COO-) and sulfate ($SO_4^=$) anions. Their high density of negative charges attracts a cloud of cations, such as Na^+, that are osmotically active and cause large amounts of water to be drawn into the matrix. This creates a swelling pressure, or turgor, that enables the matrix to withstand compressive forces (in contrast to collagen fibrils, which resist stretching forces)[11, p.804]. In solution, proteoglycans occupy a volume approximately 1000 times larger than in the dry state[466, p.258].

Chiropractic considerations in proteoglycan production

A key point that should be repeated here is that the restoration of joint mobility may stimulate GAG synthesis which can help restore lubrication and hydration within the extracellular matrix. Another glycosaminoglycan that should be mentioned in some detail is hyaluronic acid, which acts as the backbone for proteoglycans and also stands as the major component of the synovial fluid. Synovial fluid is produced by the synovial membrane or synovium that lines the inner surface of the joint capsule[336, p.62]. Synovial fluid is also present in synovial tendon sheaths and synovial bursae[382, p.6].

The synovium lines the joint capsule but not the articular cartilage surfaces. It is a loosely textured sheet of vascular connective tissue made up of collagen fibers, ground substance, capillaries, lymphatic vessels, and nerve fibers[222a]. The synovium houses two types of cells. Type A synoviocytes function as macrophages and clear the joint cavity of waste material. Type B synoviocytes synthesize hyaluronic acid, the component in synovial fluid responsible for providing joint lubrication that allows for almost frictionless movement[382, p.6]. Indeed, the coefficient of friction of a lubricated synovial joint is only one-fifth of that between two pieces of ice[382, p.2]. Whereas the coefficient of friction of ice-on-ice is about .03, a lubricated cartilaginous interface has a coefficient of friction of .002[450]. Quite astonishing! Remember that hyaluronic acid is formed by the union of D-glucuronate and N-acetyl-D-glucosamine (see *Figure 9-2*). Save for the nutrients involved in sulfate incorporation, hyaluronic acid synthesis utilizes the same biochemical pathways and nutrient cofactors that are involved in the production of chondroitin sulfate.

Triano indicates that the composition of synovial fluid is nearly identical to blood plasma. Plasma consists of water, electrolytes, metabolites, nutrients, proteins, and hormones [188], whereas whole blood consists of plasma and the various blood cells (i.e., RBCs, WBCs, and platelets)[112, p.60]. The difference between plasma and synovial fluid, is that synovial fluid has a decreased total protein content and a higher concentration of hyaluronic acid[450]. In essence, protein is semi-dialyzed from plasma to make synovial fluid. Thus, synovial fluid is referred to as a dialysate of plasma, which contains albumin and globulin, but none of the clotting protein fibrinogen[382, p.6]. Serum is also nearly identical to plasma, except that serum, like synovial fluid, does not contain fibrinogen[112, p.60].

The reason for discussing the relationship among synovial fluid, serum and plasma, is to demonstrate their similarities. An additional similarity to emphasize is that the *pH of synovial fluid parallels that of blood serum*[472]. This is important to remember because *an acidic environment reduces GAG synthesis*[339]. Recall that pH is modulated largely by the concentrations of bicarbonate ions and carbon dioxide, both of which are greatly influenced by diet and respiration. Thus, it appears that our diet will influence the pH of synovial fluid and impact upon the vitality and inflammatory potential of articular structures.

The function of synovial fluid is two-fold, those

being joint surface lubrication and nutrition of articular cartilage chondrocytes. As articular cartilage is avascular[451,p.17], the synovial fluid is the only means of nutrition. Articular cartilage consists of four different zones[257; 451, p.14-29]. Zone IV is calcified cartilage that is continuous with the subchondral bone. Zone III is referred to as the deep or radial zone. It contains collagen fibers that are oriented perpendicular, or vertical, to the articular surface and subchondral bone. Zone III contains functional chondrocytes. Zone II also contains functional chondrocytes. Zone II is referred to as the transitional zone because the collagen fibers are oriented in a manner that is more or less oblique to the vertical fibers of the deep zone and the horizontal fibers of Zone I. Zone I contains a tangential zone and a gliding zone. The tangential zone contains collagen fibers that are oriented parallel to the articular surface. Chondrocytes here resemble inactive fibrocytes. The gliding zone contains only collagen fibers. An important fact to know is that articular cartilage is only a few millimeters thick.

The nutrient rich synovial fluid is transferred to the metabolically active chondrocytes in Zones II and III via diffusion and imbibition that occurs during joint motion which causes intermittent compression and distraction of articular surfaces[257]. Hettinga does a nice job of characterizing the chondrocytes of articular cartilage:

> "Chondrocytes are metabolically very active cells, continuously utilizing both aerobic and anaerobic pathways. The chondrocytes from zones II and III of articular cartilage have extensive networks of rough-surfaced endoplasmic reticulum, dilated cisternae, vacuoles, and Golgi apparatus—suggesting that they actively synthesize protein, polysaccharides, collagen, and other components of the matrix. Metabolic studies using radioisotopes demonstrate that the chondrocyte cell synthesizes the components of macromolecules of proteoglycans and collagen, assembles them intracellularly, and then rapidly extrudes them into the surrounding matrix."

In addition to facilitating nutrient delivery to chondrocytes, mobility also allows for the clearance of enzymes and exudate from the joint. On the contrary, abnormal pressure and immobilization will inhibit synovial fluid entry into articular cartilage, resulting in degeneration[300].

In summary, joint motion provides articular structures with important nutrients that are needed to synthesize gags and collagen which, in turn, help stabilize the joint and allow for uncompromised movement. As described above, connective tissue structures of joints require mobility and appropriate nutrients to maintain normal function. Biomechanics and biochemistry cannot be separated, for each is mutually dependent on the other.

Nutritional considerations in proteoglycan production

The nutrients involved in the biochemical pathways associated with GAG synthesis include: B1, B2, B3, B5, magnesium, manganese, cysteine, calcium, iron, vitamin C, silicon and bioflavonoids/antioxidants [see *Figure 9-2*]. Bioflavonoids can protect hyaluronic acid and collagen from free radical damage. Bioflavonoids also stabilize capillary membranes[51, p.206].

In the past, many of us have been told that to help rebuild damaged connective tissues, we should give patients manganese. Such a recommendation is a little short-sighted when we consider the pathways and nutrients involved in GAG synthesis. Today, the popular and somewhat short-sighted recommendation is to supplement patients with chondroitin sulfate or glucosamine sulfate. While it seems evident that these products help patients recover from various musculoskeletal problems, I am concerned about the rationale for providing these nutrients and the potential problems that patients may develop in the long run.

Based on the numerous pathways involved in collagen and proteoglycan synthesis (see *Figure 9-2*), it should be clear that the human body is designed to produce collagen, GAGs, and proteoglycans on its own. Thus, our primary goal should be to insure the nutritional integrity of these pathways. In this regard, it appears that supplemental glucosamine bypasses part of body's synthetic machinery. Exogenous glucosamine is phosphorylated by ATP into glucosamine-6-phosphate, which then enters directly into GAG synthesis[51, p.196]. Even though supplementation with purified chondroitin sulfate and glucosamine salts have been used to increase connective tissue healing and reduce pain and inflammation[51, p.177-203], it should be understood that we cannot possibly support proteoglycan biochemistry with these supplements alone. Indeed, supplemental glucosamine still requires ATP before it can enter into GAG synthesis.

In the long run, after patients complete a supplementation program with chondroitin/glucosamine sulfate as the only supplement, they are left with the same aberrant biochemical status that helped to promote their initial injury, i.e., a biochemical status that is pro-inflammatory and incapable of generating thorough tissue repair and healing. Once again, diet modification is the key intervention, and then various nutrients can be supplemented.

For an excellent review on the utility of chondroitin sulfate and glucosamine salts, see Bucci[51, p.177-203]. For recent articles see de Camara[591], Gottlieb[632], Kelly[683], McCarty[719], and Talent[827]. Gottlieb also reviewed the side effects associated with NSAID use and compared the efficacy of NSAIDs versus glucosamine in the treatment of osteoarthritis[632].

CONNECTIVE TISSUE REPAIR - HORMONAL AND NUTRITIONAL FACTORS

Hormonal factors

Chapter 6 discussed many of the biochemical and metabolic factors related to glycemic regulation. Recall that the stress hormone cortisol can negatively impact upon connective tissue function. Cortisol can reduce bone formation and collagen synthesis[31]

Fibroblasts are also insulin-sensitive cells[503,

p.406; 848], and *Figure 9-2* demonstrates that glycosaminoglycan synthesis is dependent, in part, upon the cell's glycolytic machinery, which might lead one to think that NIDDM might alter glucose utilization in fibroblasts and chondrocytes, and thereby significantly diminish GAG synthesis. Recent research has demonstrated that the discs of NIDDM patients do exhibit less disaccharide units than normal discs; however, the significant difference between normal and diabetic discs involves sulfate incorporation. The discs from normal patients have 15 times the rate of sulfate incorporation into GAG molecules compared to the discs of NIDDM patients[776]. These findings help to explain why NIDDM patients have a higher risk of disc prolapse then their normal counterparts[776]. Recall from Chapter 6 that numerous factors promote insulin resistance, hyperinsulinemia and subsequently, the development of non-insulin-dependent diabetes mellitus (NIDDM).

Collagen synthesis can also be affected by glycemic dysregulation. Weiss recently stated that insulin is essential for production of collagen by fibroblasts[848]. However, research has also demonstrated that supplemental vitamin A can restore collagen production and tensile strength in steptozotocin-induced diabetic rats in the presence of hyperglycemia, glycosuria, polydipsia, and polyuria[266]. Supplemental vitamin C has a similar effect on collagen production[266].

Nutritional factors

Figures 9-1 and *9-2* demonstrated that many nutrients are required to insure adequate connective tissue synthesis. Dietary modification is obviously the most important intervention; however, it may often be useful to supplement the diet with the nutrients required to drive connective tissue synthesis. Supplementing with a multiple vitamin/mineral, vitamin C and bioflavonoids, and magnesium may be useful. The suggested amounts for supplementation has already been discussed in Chapter 8. Additionally, supplementation with chondroitin sulfate and glucosamine salts may be advisable.

Bucci suggests at least 1 gram of chondroitin

sulfate per day is required to facilitate connective tissue repair[51, p.184]. For glucosamine salts, daily doses of 1500 mg, divided into two or three doses is suggested. However, the minimum effective dose is not known and some patients may need to take more to derive a positive clinical effect. Fortunately, doses as high as 3 to 6 g/day appear to be quite safe[51, p.202]. It should be noted that glucosamine sulfate seems to get the most attention; however, other salts such as glucosamine-HCL, N-acetylglucosamine, glucosamine chlorhydrate are equally effective[51, p.202].

In recent years, many practitioners have claimed that gelatin provides a similar effect as chondroitin/glucosamine supplements, and subsequently recommend its use because it is less expensive than the supplements. I do not know if this is true; however, research is available that reviews the health promoting effects of supplemental gelatin [see *Gelatin in Nutrition and Medicine.* Grayslake (IL): Grayslake Gelatin Co, 1945].

GAGS/Proteoglycans as promoters of nociception and inflammation

The suggestion that GAGs can irritate nociceptors seems a little strange at first glance because it is well-known that GAGs allow for normal joint function to take place. For several years, Carrick[71] has promoted the notion that glycosaminoglycans, specifically the polyanionic glycosaminoglycans, are released from pathomechanical joints and directly depolarize nociceptors. I have yet to find a resource that supports this contention. The following quote describes how GAGS are probably involved in nociception:

> "A high concentration of hydrogen ions in the tissues is a cause of pain. The mucoprotein gel contains a variety of glycosaminoglycans, some of which are acid and lately believed capable of causing the pain associated with degenerative disc disease."[175, p.47]

If glycosaminoglycans in the disc can activate nociceptors, then the possibility exists that glycosaminoglycans in joint capsules and ligaments may also activate nociceptors. As far as I know, there is very little research that discusses this topic. It is possible that GAG breakdown, due to direct joint injury and joint restriction, adds to the acidity of the so-called "inflammatory soup." The degree to which this occurs is unknown, and there is probably a more integrated way to view GAG breakdown and its role in nociception. For example, proteoglycans have three main functions[336, p.74-75]: 1) they imbibe water which allows joints and discs to withstand compressive forces, 2) they form a supporting substance for both cells (fibroblasts, osteoblasts and chondroblasts) and fibrous components (collagen, elastin), and 3) they also play an important role in the protection of the connective tissue structure by contributing to the overall strength of the structure. As described in the section on collagen, a loss of proteoglycans [from a joint or disc] would reduce the integrity of the tissue and predispose the associated structures to injury and the subsequent release of inflammatory mediators would be responsible for nociceptor irritation.

While there is little information about connective tissue breakdown and nociception, there is data suggesting that proteoglycans released from damaged joints may promote immune-mediated inflammation. Macromolecules of hyaline cartilage, including proteoglycans, glycoproteins and collage, provoke cell-mediated humoral immune responses in experimental animals and they may supply an autoantigen depot in man. Research suggests that antigenic components (i.e., proteoglycans) released by an inflammatory process or trauma may trigger a vicious circle of chronic inflammation and joint destruction[165]. This pathological process echoes that of rheumatoid arthritis and is probably an uncommon occurrence in the great majority of acute and chronic pain patients.

Bogduk provides a similar explanation and indicates that, "it has been demonstrated that disc material contains potent inflammatory chemicals, and when disc material ruptures into the epidural space, it seems to elicit an autoimmune inflammatory reaction that can affect not only the roots, but the dura as well[41, p.157]." Early researchers in this area referred to this situation as chemical radiculitis. It was thought to occur because the glycoproteins in the disc were found to be inflammatory[288]. It was also proposed that disc material could act as an antigen[40]. A more recent paper suggests how nuclear material may be inflammatory as it contains increased levels of IgG and IgM[428].

Chapter 10

NUTRITIONAL RECOMMENDATIONS

One of the main problems encountered in clinical nutrition practice centers around ineffective methods of application during patient care. An unfocused approach to nutrition during patient care only adds to the confusion that patients are routinely exposed to by the media, the "experts" who work in health food stores, and the various "fad" approaches to diet and nutrition. Confusion leads to a lack of motivation and subsequently, patients tend to become indifferent and avoid making important nutritional modifications. When patients do not follow instructions, doctors usually place all of the blame on patients, often suggesting that "patients just don't care." In my experience, this statement proves to be quite revealing.

Why would a patient not care that their eating habits are actively promoting their current condition, i.e., pain, inflammation, fatigue, fibromyalgia, heart disease, cancer, and numerous other diseases? The suggestion that the average patient is happy to eat him/herself into a state of physical disability is difficult to fathom. Albeit, there are patients who will not modify their nutritional habits no matter what, but this is not the average patient; this patient is the exception. The typical patient just needs to be effectively motivated to make appropriate dietary changes. In this regard, Haber recently stated:

> "Even when people have available to them sound and persuasive scientific evidence, they still will not change their eating habits unless they find personal reasons for doing so"[645].

It should be mentioned that these personal reasons must be present time concerns because people do not think about their lives 20 or 30 years into the future and simultaneously consider the need to prevent cancer and heart disease. Believe it or not, it is easy to provide personal "present time" reasons to help motivate many people to change their dietary habits and take nutritional supplements. In actual fact, every patient who enters your office *provides their own reasons*. For example, pain, fatigue, mental lethargy, and depression are some of the most common complaints heard from patients, and each of these conditions can be promoted by a faulty diet. The problem is that patients do not know that these conditions are diet related! Unfortunately, even after patients leave a doctor's office, most still do not know about these important nutritional relationships. In this regard, doctors, nutritionists, and dietitians would do well to look in the mirror and honestly question whether their nutritional efforts are sufficient, efficient, and appropriate.

Many patients leave a doctor's office without sound nutritional advice and instead are told that dietary "moderation" is the key to good nutrition. I have met many practitioners who actually promote this myth to their patients. This represents a tragedy as the concept of "moderation" in nutrition has no practical meaning and utility, and certainly cannot promote health and prevent disease. In no other walk of life is "moderation" considered to be the key to success, so how could "moderation" be the key to a healthy diet and lifestyle?

The purpose of Chapter 10 is to outline a basic approach to practical clinical nutrition which involves the application of the concepts described in this text. Contrary to what one might think, applying this information in clinical practice is quite straightforward. Four basic steps should be considered when incorporating this material into your practice. Each will be discussed separately. These four steps include:

1. Patient education

2. Nutritional Evaluation

3. Visual eating guidelines for patients

4. Nutritional supplements

PATIENT EDUCATION

Effective patient education is of critical importance if patients are to ever change their nutritional habits. Thus, a basic understanding of how learning takes place can help us to develop education methods and tools.

The more our brain is exposed to new information, the more readily it remembers what it has learned. Researchers maintain that learning is a nervous system-dependent process involving increased synaptic activity within brain tissue. Neuronal plasticity is the term used to describe such activity. Recall that the term plasticity was used in Chapter 2 to describe central nociceptive sensitization.

In general, plasticity refers to morphological and functional changes in neuronal function that occur due to internal and external environmental stimuli.

> "The characteristics of a neuron at any given time depend on its genetic program and on past and present interactions with its milieu, i.e. other cells, the extracellular matrix, ions, growth factors, hormones, and transmitters. Neurons are thus endowed with structural and functional plasticity."[125-p.44]

The basic neurological components of learning include synaptic activity, upregulation of NMDA receptors, and morphological changes in the postsynaptic cell. Synaptic activity, the initiator of the learning process, occurs whenever there is environmental stimulation.

The hippocampus is vital for memory consolidation[387-p.169]. The hippocampus is particularly abundant in *N*-methyl-D-aspartate (NMDA) receptors and non-NMDA receptors, both of which are glutamate receptors. Glutamate, an amino acid, is a major excitatory neurotransmitter in the brain. The NMDA receptor controls ion channels which are permeable to Ca^{++}, Na^+ and K^+. However, the channel does not conduct ions efficiently when activated by glutamate, unless membrane depolarization is large enough[228-p.158].

Since glutamate is an excitatory amino acid, it produces excitatory post synaptic potentials (EPSPs). In other words, when glutamate is released from an axon terminal, it traverses the synapse and excites the postsynaptic cell. As mentioned above, non-NMDA receptors, located on the postsynaptic cell, are readily activated by glutamate. In the early phase of EPSP development, only the non-NMDA receptors are activated. The more the neuron is depolarized by the activation of non-NMDA receptors, the more NMDA-activated receptor channels open. The delayed opening of the NMDA-activated channels characterizes the late phase of EPSP development[228-p.159]. It is thought that Ca^{++} entry through the NMDA-activated channels is responsible for initiating Ca^{++}-dependent second messenger pathways, which contribute to long-lasting postsynaptic changes involved in memory and learning[228-p.160, 1020].

NMDA receptor activation, Ca^{++} entry, and the subsequent second messenger cascade serve to trigger immediate early genes (IEGs) which induce protein synthesis within the nucleus of the postsynaptic cell. Through a number of steps, the IEGs ultimately induce the expression of more conventional late phase genes, which can modify synaptic structure and function[372]. "Thus the IEGs are an essential link between synapse and nucleus, and their activation is a key step in the molecular cascade of memory formation."[372]

The term long-term potentiation (LTP) is used to describe the plastic changes that are induced by NMDA activity[228-p.1009]. In other words, when we see or hear "LTP," we should think of synaptic activity, NMDA receptor upregulation, and morphological changes in the postsynaptic cell. Of great importance to those of us who educate patients is the fact that, "LTP is induced by repeatedly stimulating the afferents leading to the synapse under study"[446].

Clearly, the best way to educate patients is to repetitively stimulate them with information. A doctors office should be learning resource centers for patients. Of critical importance is that educational information must be consistent. Whenever you use charts, posters, videos, audios, slides and pamphlets, the information must be consistent. Contradictory information reduces interest, motivation and confidence which is detrimental to the learning process. To get some ideas for explaining nutrition to your patients, see Appendix A which contains a sample narrative for a slide presentation.

Additionally, it should be emphasized that a wide variety of educational tools will facilitate learning. Each of our primary sensory systems should be stimulated to promote thorough and effective learning.

"Critical components of neuronal circuits that encode internal representations are assumed to be stored in cortical areas bordering with appropriate primary sensory areas: visual memories in the inferotemporal, auditory memories in the superior-temporal, somatic memories in the posterior-parietal, olfactory and gustatory memories in the orbital-prefrontal cortex. All memories have access to each other via cortic-cortical and subcortical pathways...In all cases, the prefrontal cortex can integrate and use the internal representations for the *adhoc* guidance of behavior, and probably for generating 'higher-order' representations in processes of implicit learning."[125-p.249]

NUTRITIONAL EVALUATION

Evaluations are a key aspect of clinical nutrition, for without nutritional assessments, clinical nutrition becomes guess work. McGanity et al. explain the importance diet assessment in the care of pregnant patients[722]. Naturally, this information also applies to males and non-pregnant females.

"The physician in solo practice must be able to identify available personnel in the community who can provide a detailed nutritional assessment. Such individuals may be within the hospital setting as a part of its dietary department, they may associated with the local health clinic and/or WIC program, or they may be in private practice."[722]

There are many methods of assessment available to clinicians, including 24-hour recalls, food frequency recalls, weighed food diary, and an estimated diet diary. The estimated diet diary is thought to be one of the more accurate and effective methods of assessment.

In addition to a standard physical examination, a detailed nutritional assessment is recommended when treating pregnant patients. In part, the assessment should include, "A dietary food intake assessment based on either a food frequency utilization or a dietary history of a 3-, 5-, or 7-day food intake"[722].

"To assess the diet of an individual, a 7-day record is recommended to include both weekdays and the weekend. In practice, however, 3-4-day records are kept to minimize the time and costs of the analysis. Dietary records and diaries are the most objective methods available for evaluating dietary patterns."[830]

Schoenthaler states that, "identification of a malnourished condition could also be improved upon by using multiple measures of malnutrition – a 7 day diet analysis, physical examinations, history taking, and clinical tests"[790].

"Despite problems of the underreporting in overweight individuals in 20% of this sample, weighed records remained the most accurate method of dietary assessment, and *only an estimated 7-day diet diary* was able to approach this accuracy"[558]. "It is concluded that the diet diary technique is the *method of choice* for investigations of the ingestive behavior of free-living humans"[594].

There are two basic ways to incorporate such assessments in clinical practice. Several different companies provide computer programs that can be used in the office. In this case patients fill out diet diaries and upon completion they are returned to the office. An assistant or the practitioner must then enter the foods into the computer. Upon completing the necessary data entry, the computer program will print out the average daily intake of calories, protein, fats, carbohydrates, vitamins and minerals, which can then be compared to the RDAs for that person's age and sex. *Figure 10-1* is an example of the information that can be derived from a diet diary.

Lee recently reviewed eight different software programs available to practitioners[699]. This is an excellent article to help get better acquainted with the various programs. Another way to perform assessments in the office is to work with a company that does the data entry and reporting as a service to the practitioner[798].

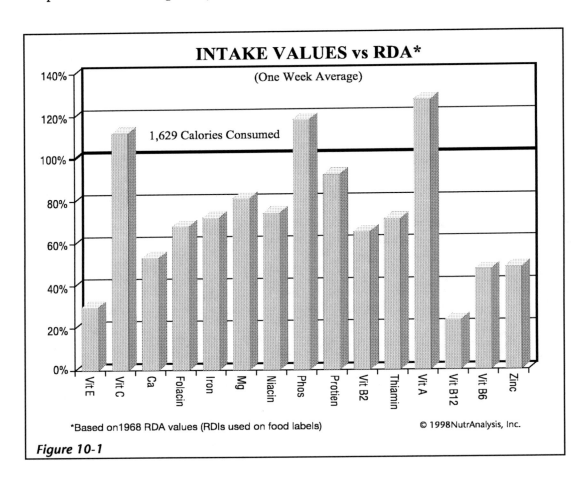

INTAKE VALUES vs RDA*
(One Week Average)

1,629 Calories Consumed

*Based on 1968 RDA values (RDIs used on food labels)   © 1998 NutrAnalysis, Inc.

Figure 10-1

VISUAL EATING GUIDELINES FOR PATIENTS

The following 5 pages consist of visual and written eating guidelines for patients. The directions are very simple.

Figure 10-2 demonstrates that each meal (plate of food) should consist of approximately 25% protein and 75% vegetable, and if desired, a moderate grain portion. This will roughly approach a 2:1 carbohydrate to protein ratio, resulting in overall caloric balance of about 40:20:40 from carbohydrates, proteins, and fats respectively.

Table 10-1 lists numerous types of foods. These foods can be used to fill up a plate with the proper 25% and 75% portions. Salads are to be placed in a separate plate/bowl (remember to use extra virgin olive oil in the dressing).

Table 10-2 lists examples of meals for breakfast, lunch, and dinner. Sample snacks, desserts and salad dressing are also listed.

Table 10-3 provides a handful of cooking ideas for dinner. Eating in this fashion is very satisfying and often reduces the desire for desserts.

Table 10-4 provides the glycemic index (GI) for a variety of foods. Make sure to have patients focus on low GI foods.

Eating meals in the fashion outlined in this section will provide the following:

1. Sufficient vegetable, fruit, and olive oil consumption to insure an adequate intake of anti-inflammatory nutrients.

2. An adequate balance among carbohydrates, protein and fat to insure proper glycemic regulation.

3. A diet that focuses on low glycemic index foods

These recommendations are similar to nutritional recommendations that have been put forth by various authorities over the years[25, 36, 412, 400, 453, 454]. The main difference is that the recommendations in this book suggest that we do not focus on grain products, but instead try to minimize their consumption. The rationale for that recommendation was discussed in Chapters 6 and 7.

Patients should also be urged to get a couple of books that will help them to better appreciate the foods they are eating. *The Omega Plan* lists the n:6-n-3 balance for a great variety of foods[811]. It would also be a good idea to have your patients get a copy of *Food Values of Portions Commonly Consumed* (16th ed. Pennington J. Philadelphia: JB Lippincott, 1994), which lists the carb/pro/fat balance and the nutrient content of nearly every food a patient might consume.

Additionally, patients should be urged to get a small scale so they can weigh their food portions. I do not think patients should weigh every meal; however, initially, such a practice will better familiarize a patient with portion sizes and their related nutrient content. These scales cost a couple of dollars and can be purchased in most department stores. Many patients state that weighing their foods and checking for nutrient content is fun and very educational.

MEAL PLATE

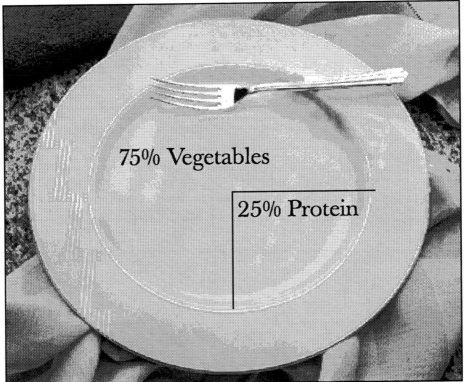

Reprinted with permission: Adobe Photoshop,
Classroom in a Book (1st ed.), p.79, Hayden Books,
Carmel, IN 1993

Figure 10-2

SNACK PLATE

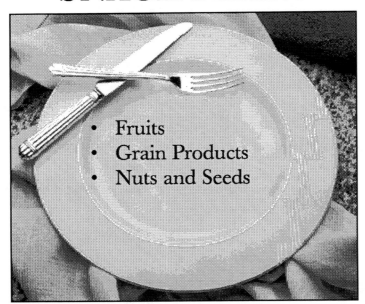

Reprinted with permission: Adobe
Photoshop, Classroom in a Book (1st ed.),
p.79, Hayden Books, Carmel, IN 1993

Figure 10-3

EXAMPLES OF IDEAL FOODS

SEASONINGS
Herbamare
Spike
Onion Magic
Veg-It

STANDARD HERBS AND SPICES
Sea Salt
Basil
Cayenne Pepper
Cinnamon
Cumin
Garlic
Nutmeg
Oregano
Tarragon
Thyme

OILS
Cold Pressed, Green, Extra Virgin Olive Oil
Cold Pressed Sesame Oil
Cold Pressed Flaxseed/Linseed Oil
Canola Oil
Butter

PROTEINS
Beans w/ Corn or Rice:
    Adzuki, Kidney, Lima
    Pinto & Mung
Eggs
Fish: esp. Salmon
    Red Snapper
    Scrod
    Cod
    Haddock
    Tuna
    Sardines (unsmoked)
    Herring
Lentils/Peas w/corn or rice
Organic Lamb, Beef
Organic Chicken
Organic Turkey
Dairy: Yogurt
    Cheese

VEGETABLES
Arugula
Artichoke
Asparagus
Avocado
Beets
Beet Greens
Bok Choy
Broccoli
Broccoli Rabe
Brussel Sprouts
Cabbage: red, white
Carrots
Cauliflower
Celery
Collard Greens
Coriander-aka cilantro
Eggplant
Endive
Escarole
Fennel
Green Pepper
Jerusalem Artichoke
Kale
Kohlrabi
Leeks
Mustard Greens
Okra
Onions: red, white, Vidalia
Parsley
Parsnip
Peas
Pumpkin
Rhubarb
Romaine Lettuce
Scallions
Shallots
Snow Peas
Spinach
Sprouts: Alfalfa, Buckwheat
    Lentil, Mung Bean
    Pea, Sunflower
Squash: Acorn, Butternut
    Spaghetti, Zucchini
String Beans
Swiss Chard
Tomato
Turnip
Turnip Greens
Watercress

FRUITS
Apple
Apricot
Banana
Blackberries
Blueberries
Boysenberries
Cantaloupe
Cherry
Cranberries
Dates
Figs
Grapes
Grapefruit
Kiwi
Lemon
Lime
Mango
Melons
Nectarine
Orange
Papaya
Peach
Pear
Pomegranate
Pineapple
Plum
Prune
Raspberries
Raisins
Strawberries
Tangerine
Watermelon

GRAINS/CARBOHYDRATES
Corn Meal
Corn Grits
Millet, Quinoa
Oats, Rye, Wheat
Rice: Basmati
    Brown
    Wild
100% whole grain pastas
Potatoes: red, white
    sweet, yams

SWEETNERS
Tupelo Honey
Grade B Maple Syrup
Stevia

NUTS & SEEDS (raw butters)
Almonds
Cashews
Walnuts
Pumpkin Seeds
Sesame Seeds
Sunflower Seeds

Table 10-1

Examples of Meals

Breakfast:

1. Fruit and cottage cheese or yogurt
2. Cooked grains (oats, corn meal,grits etc.) with fruit and yogurt
3. Eggs and sprouted grain bread
4. Vegetable omelet with grain, grain bread or hash browns

Lunch and Dinner:

1. Vegetable omelet
2. Protein and salad
   Example salad: Romaine lettuce, watercress, coriander, arugula, endive, red bell peppers, raddichio, sprouts, vine-ripened tomatoes, avocado, onions, garlic
3. Protein, vegetable (stir fried or lightly steamed) and a salad
4. Protein, sweet or red potatoes, assortment of vegetables (stir fried or lightly steamed)
5. Protein, whole grains, vegetables, and a salad

Snacks:

1. Fresh fruit
2. Raw vegetables
3. Raw nuts
4. Grain products
5. Yogurt
6. Cheese

Salad Dressing:

1. Olive oil, lemon, salt (with dry or fresh herbs, spices to taste)
2. Tahini Dressing (sesame seed)
3. Vinigrette Dressing: Squeeze fresh lemons, add salt, pepper, chopped shallots, fresh tarragon or basil; stir in olive oil in a 3:1 ratio, Olive oil : Lemon mixture.
4. Olive oil, Balsamic vinegar, mustard

Desserts: (wait at least 2 hours after meal.)

1. Blend frozen bananas and frozen strawberries, or other fruit
2. Soak pumpkin seeds in water for at least 1 day . Blend in soy milk to make a cream. Pour over fruit (kiwi, berries, mango, papaya).

Table 10-2

Cooking Ideas

1. In a skillet or wok saute onions, chopped garlic, chopped ginger root, red bell peppers, broccoli, and other vegetables of your choice in olive oil. When the vegetables are cooked, but still firm and bright in color, remove from the pan and set aside. Add a protein of your choice such as organic chicken strips, cubes or strips of lamb or beef. Saute the protein until cooked to your liking, add the vegetables back into the pan and season slightly with tamari or soy sauce. If you wish, eat as is, or serve over a small grain portion of your choice, i.e. millet, brown rice, quinoa, etc.

2. Saute vegetables as mentioned above. Instead of using chopped ginger, add freshly chopped parsley and oregano (use dried herbs if you don't have fresh herbs). Cook a protein portion of your choice and mix in the vegetables. While cooking the protein, add several chopped fresh or canned organic tomatoes. If you wish, eat as is, or serve over a small pasta protion. Try to use vegetable pastas, whole grain or artichoke pastas.

3. If you like to cook outdoors, try grilling your vegetables and protein. Marinate the veggies and protein in an olive oil, salt and garlic mixture, then brush the items with the olive oil mixture while cooking. Try not to overcook any of the items. It is best to cook the veggies in strips or large pieces and then slice them up when cooked. You can even grill whole tomatoes and chop them into the mixture as well. You can eat as is, or mix all the vegetables and protein together and serve over a small portion of pasta, rice, millet, etc.

4. Any of the above dishes can be changed around with different grains, vegetables, proteins, etc. Instead of adding the proteins mentioned above, try grilling, baking or sauteing fish (i.e. salmon, tuna, snapper) and serving this with your meal.

5. Soak the bean of your choice for at least 24 hours. Boil the beans with a seasoning of vegetable broth and soy sauce. Saute your favorite vegetables as described earlier and serve the beans and vegetables with a small portion of your favorite grain.

6. It is often possible to purchase organic or free range meats at your grocery store or health food store. If so, ask them to grind up turkey, chicken, lamb, beef, etc. to make burgers. Mix the ground protein with chopped onions, garlic, parsley and a little olive oil to help hold it all together. Saute or grill your burgers and serve with a selection of sauted/steamed or grilled vegetables.

7. Bake a potato or sweet potato and serve this with your protein and vegetable combination of choice.

Table 10-3

GLYCEMIC INDICES OF FOODS

FOOD	GLYCEMIC INDEX	FOOD	GLYCEMIC INDEX
Breads		**Legumes**	
Rye (crispbread)	95	Baked beans (canned)	70
Rye (whole meal)	89	Bengal gram dal	12
Rye (whole grain, i.e. pumpernickel)	68	Butter beans	46
Wheat (white)	100	Chickpeas (dried)	47
Wheat (wholemeal)	100	Chick-peas (canned)	60
		Frozen peas	74
Pasta		Garden peas (frozen)	65
Macaroni (white, boiled 5 min)	64	Green peas (canned)	50
Spaghetti (brown, boiled 15 min)	61	Green peas (dried)	65
Spaghetti (white, boiled 15 min)	67	Haricot beans (white, dried)	54
Star pasta (white, boiled 5 min)	54	Kidney beans (dried)	43
		Kidney beans (canned)	74
Cereal Grains		Lentils (green, dried)	36
Barley (pearled)	36	Lentils (green, canned)	74
Buckwheat	78	Lentils (red, dried)	38
Bulgur	65	Pinto beans (dried)	80
Millet	103	Pinto beans (canned)	64
Rice (brown)	81	Peanuts	15
Rice (instant, boiled 1 min)	65	Soya beans (dried)	20
Rice (parboiled, boiled 5 min)	54	Soya beans (canned)	22
Rice (parboiled, boiled 15 min)	68		
Rice (polished, boiled 5 min)	58	**Fruit**	
Rice (polished, boiled 10 - 25 min)	81	Apple	52
Rye kernels	47	Apple juice	45
Sweet corn	80	Banana	84
Wheat kernels	63	Grapes	62
		Grapefruit	36
Breakfast Cereals		Orange	59
"All Bran"	74	Orange juice	71
Cornflakes	121	Peach	40
Muesli	96	Pear	47
Porridge oats	89	Plum	34
Puffed rice	132	Raisins	93
Puffed wheat	110		
Shredded wheat	97	**Sugars**	
"Weetebix"	108	Fructose	26
		Glucose	138
Cookies		Honey	126
Digestive	82	Lactose	57
Oatmeal	78	Maltose	152
Plain crackers (water biscuits)	100	Sucrose	83
"Rich Tea"	80		
Shortbread cookies	88	**Dairy Products**	
		Custard	59
Root Vegetables		Ice cream	69
Potato (instant)	120	Skim milk	46
Potato (mashed)	98	Whole milk	44
Potato (new/white boiled)	80	Yogurt	52
Potato (Russet, baked)	118		
Potato (sweet)	70	**Snack Foods**	
Yam	74	Corn chips	99
		Potato chips	77

Table 10-4

NUTRITIONAL SUPPLEMENTS

The topic of nutritional supplements is shrouded in emotionalism. So-called experts often suggest that billions of dollars are wasted on unnecessary supplements. Indeed, the pro-supplementation consumers are often accused of being duped by the supplement sellers. The degree to which this is true is unknown. The degree to which bureaucrats are working to inappropriately regulate supplements is also unknown; however, this type of meddling is suspected by millions of people.

At different times throughout this book, particularly in Chapters 5, 7, and 8, research was presented which indicates that many people are, at least, marginally deficient in a variety of nutrients. Can eating more nutritious food reduce deficiencies? It is hard to say for sure because the micronutrient status of our soils is also an unknown. Considering the fact that toxicity levels for most nutrients is far in excess of the RDAs, it makes sense that nutritional supplements should be taken to make up for potential deficiencies.

Supplements should also be taken to help reduce the pro-inflammatory potential of our tissues. The following list are the main supplements that should be considered:

1. Multiple vitamin/mineral

2. Magnesium

3. Bioflavonoids/antioxidants

4. Coenzyme Q10

5. Ginger

6. Fish oil

7. Chondroitin/glucosamine product or gelatin

8. Bromelain

9. Vitamin E (particularly when taking fish oil)

Suggested amounts of supplements were discussed in Chapter 8. Some patients may do well with just a multiple and some need more. It is really an individual-specific situation with each patient.

There are numerous supplement companies in the marketplace. Whether there is a "best company" and a "best product" is difficult to say. Of course, each company says that it is the best. I would recommend investigating various companies and their products.

REFERENCES

1. Abraham G, Flechas, G. Management of fibromyalgia: Rationale for the use of magnesium and malic acid. J Nutr Med 1992;3(1):49-59

2. Adams, D. Macrophages as destructive cells in host defense. In: Gallin, Goldstein & Snyderman. eds. Inflammation: Basic Principles and Clinical Correlates. 2nd ed. New York: Raven Press, 1992: p.637-62

3. Adebajo A, Hazelman B. Incidence, nature and economic effects of soft tissue injury. In McLatchie, G. et al., The Soft Tissues: Trauma and Sports Injuries Oxford: Buterworth Heinemann, 1993: p.3-29

4. Advertisement. For Chronic Arthritis, Expect Nothing Less. Hospital Medicine 1992;28(10):6-7

5. Agren J, et al. Dose responses in platelet fatty acid composition, aggregation and prostanoid metabolism during moderate freshwater fish diet. Thromb Res 1990;57:565-75

6. Aguayo S. Neuropeptides in inflammation and tissue repair. In Henson & Murphy eds. Mediators of the Inflammatory Process, Handbook of Inflammation. New York: Elsevier, 1989: p.219-44

7. Akeson W, et al. Immobility effects on synovial joints and the pathomechanics of joint contracture. Biorheology 1980;17:95-110

8. Ako H, et al. Isolation of a fibrinolysis enzyme activator from commercial bromelain. Arch Int Pharmacodyn 1981;254:157-67

9. Alam S. Adenylate cyclase activity, membrane fluidity and fatty acid composition of the rat heart in essential fatty acid deficiency. J Mol Cell Cardiol 1987;19:465-75

10. Albert S. & Mulder G. eds. Issue on Wound Healing. Clin Podiatric Med Surg 1991;8:4

11. Alberts B, et al. Molecular Biology of the Cell (2nd ed). New York: Garland Publishing; 1989

12. Albritton J. Complications of wound healing. In Albert S. & Mulder G. eds. Issue on Wound Healing. Clin Podiatric Med Surg 1991;8(4):773-85

13. Alfrey A. Disorders of magnesium metabolism. In Seldin D. ed. The Kidney: Physiology and Pathophysiology (2nd ed). New York: Raven Press; 1992: p.2357-73

14. Allen R. Free radicals and differentiation: The interrelationship of development and aging. In Yu B. ed. Free Radicals in Aging. Boca Raton: CRC Press, 1993: p.11-37

15. Alter M. Science of Stretching. Champaign, IL: Human Kinetics Publishing; 1988

16. Altman R, et al. Identification of platelet inhibitor present in the melon (Cucurbitacea Cucumis Melo). Thromb Haemostasis 1985;53(3):312-13

17. Ammon H, et al. Inhibition of leukotriene B-4 formation in rat peritoneal neutrophils by a ethanolic extract of the gum resin exudate of Boswellia serrata. Planta Med 1991;57:203-07

18. Applewhite T. Trans-isomer, serum lipids and cardiovascular disease: Another point of view. Nutr Rev 1994;51(11):344-45

19. Arend W. Cytokines and growth factors. In Kelley W, et al. eds. Textbook of Rheumatology (4th ed). Philadelphia: W. B. Saunders; 1993: p.227-47

20. Aspergen D. Treating the athlete's back: The ultimate challenge. Chiro Sports Med 1992;6(2):49-56

21. Atar D, et al. Effects of magnesium supplementation in a porcine model of myocardial ischemia and reperfusion. J Cardiovasc Pharmacol 1994;24(4):603-11

22. Awad E. Interstitial myofibrositis: Hypothesis of the mechanism. Arch Phys Med Rehabil 1973;54:449-53

23. Babior B. Function of neutrophils and mononuclear phagocytes. In Wyngaardenn, Smith and Bennett, eds. Cecil Textbook of Medicine (19th ed). Philadelphia: W. B. Saunders; 1992: p.898-904

24. Ballou S, Kusher I. Laboratory evaluation of inflammation. In Kelley W, et al. eds. Textbook of Rheumatology (4th ed). Philadelphia :W. B. Saunders; 1993: p.671-79

25. Barnard N. The Power of Your Plate. Summertown, TN: Book Publishing Co.; 1990

26. Barradas M, et al. The effect of olive oil supplementation on human platelet function, serum cholesterol-related variables and plasma fibrinogen concentrations: A pilot study. Nutr Res 1990;10:430-11

27. Bell I. A kinin model for food and chemical sensitivities: Biobehavioral implications. Ann Allergy 1975;35:206-15

28. Bengtsson A, Henriksson K. The muscle in fibromyalgia – A review of Swedish studies. J Rheumatol 1989;16(suppl 19):144-49

29. Bennett J. Mechanisms of platelet adhesion and aggregation: An update. Hosp Pract 4/15/92, p.124-34

30. Bennett R. Fibromyalgia and the facts: Sense or nonsense. Rheum Dis Clin N Am 199;319(1):45-59

31. Berne R, Matthew L. Physiology (3rd ed), St. Louis: Mosby Year Book; 1993: p.949-79

31a. Berne R, Matthew L. Physiology (3rd ed). St. Louis: Mosby Year Book; 1993

32. Berton G, et al. Inhibition by quercetin of activation of polymorphonuclear leukocyte function: Stimulus-specific effects. Biochim Biophys Acta 1980;595:47-55

33. Bhoola K, et al. Kinins-Key mediators in inflammatory arthritis. Bri J Rheumatol 1992;31:509-518

34. Bisgaard H, Kristensen J. Leukotriene B-4 produces hyperalgesia in humans Prostaglandins 1985;30(5):791-97

35. Bjarnason I. Intestinal permeability and inflammation in rheumatoid arthritis: effects of non-steroidal anti-inflammatory drugs. Lancet Nov. 24, 1984;1171-74

36. Block G. Dietary guidelines and the results of food consumption surveys. Am J Clin Nutr 1991;53:356S-57S

37. Block G. The data support a role for antioxidants in reducing cancer risk. Nutr Rev 1992;50(7):207-13

38. Blond J, et al. Effect of 18:3 n-3 geometrical isomers of heated linseed oil on the biosynthesis of arachidonic acid. Nutr Res 1990;10:69-79

39. Bodi T. Modifications of tissue permeability by orally administered proteolytic enzymes in man. Exp Med Surg (Suppl) 1965;51-62

40. Boden S, et al. The Aging Spine. Philadelpia: W.B. Saunders; 1991: p.28

41. Bogduk N, Twomey L. Clinical Anatomy of the Lumbar Spine (2nd ed). Churchill New York :Livingstone; 1991: p.14-16

42. Bogduk N. Innervation patterns of the cervical spine. In Grant R. Physical Therapy of the Cervical and Thoracic Spine, (2nd ed). New York: Churchill Livingstone; 1994: p.65-76

43. Bogduk N, Valencia F. Innervation patterns of the thoracic spine. In Grant R. Physical Therapy of the Cervical and Thoracic Spine (2nd ed). New York: Churchill Livingstone; 1994: p.77-87

44. Bogduk N. Innervation, pain patterns, and mechanisms of pain production. In Twomey L, Taylor J. Physical Therapy of Low Back. New York: Churchill Livingstone; 1994: p.93-109

45. Bollet A. Nutrition and diet in rheumatic disorders. In Shils M, Young V. eds. Modern Nutrition in Health and Disease (7th). Philadelphia: Lea & Febiger; 1988: p.1471-81

46. Bollet A. Nutrition and diet in rheumatic diseases. In Shils M, et al. eds. Modern Nutrition in Health and Disease (8th), Philadelphia: Lea & Febiger; 1994: p.1362-1390

47. Bonica J. The Management of Pain. Philadelphia: Lea & Febiger; 1990: p.28-121

48. Bonica J. Clinical importance of hyperalgesia. In Willis W. ed. Hyperalgesia and Allodynia. New York: Raven Press; 1992: p.17-43

49. Bordia A. The effect of vitamin C on blood lipids, fibrinolytic activity and platelet adhesiveness in patients with coronary artery disease. Atherosclerosis 1980;35:181-187

50. Bordia A, Verma S. Effect of vitamin C on platelet adhesiveness and platelet aggregation in coronary artery disease patients. ClinCardiol 1985;8:552-54

51. Bucci L. Nutrition Applied to Injury Rehabilitation and Sports Medicine. Boca Raton: CRC Press, FL; 1995

52. Borenstein D. Medical therapy for low back pain. Drug Therapy 1992;22(10):93-102

53. Boron E. Chemistry of buffer equilibria in blood plasma.In Seldin D, Giebisch G. eds. The Regulation of Acid-Base Balance. New York: Raven Press; 1989: p.3-32

54. Bourne G. Nutrition and wound healing. In Glynn, Houck & Weismann, eds. Handbook of Inflammation, Vol 3, Tissue Repair and Regeneration. New York: Elsevier; 1981: p.211-42

55. Brenner R. The oxidative desaturation of unsaturated fatty acids in animals. Mol Cell Biochem 1974:3(1):41-52

56. Brodal A. Neurological Anatomy in Relation to Clinical Medicine (3rd ed). New York: Oxford Univ Press; 1981

57. Brodsky I, Devlin J. Hormone and nutrient interactions. In Shils M, et al. Modern Nutrition in Health and Disease (8th ed). Philadelphia: Lea & Febier; 1994: p.603-22

58. Bronsgeest-Schoute H, et al. The effect of various intakes of n-3 fatty acids on the blood lipid composition in healthy human subjects. Am J Clin Nutr 1981;34:1752-57

59. Brown R, et al. Angiogenic factors from synovial fluid resembling that from tumors. Lancet 1980;(Mar 29):682-85

60. Brown R, Weiss J. Neovascularization and its role in the osteoarthritic process. Ann Rheum Dis 1988;47:881-85

61. Buckwalter A, Frick O. Histamine, serotonin, & ergot alkaloids. In Basic and Clinical Pharmacology (3rd ed). Norwalk, CT: Appleton & Lange; 1987: p.183-200

62. Buckwalter J, Woo S. Ligaments, In DeLee J, Drez, D. eds. Orthopedic Sports Medicine: Principles and Practice. Philadelphia: W.B. Saunders; 1994: p.46-59

63. Buckwalter J, Woo S. Effects of repetitive loading and motion on the musculoskeletal tissues, in DeLee, J, Drez D. eds. Orthopedic Sports Medicine: Principles and Practice. Philadelphia: W.B. Saunders; 1994: p.60-72

64. Budowski P, Crawford M. μ-linolenic acid as regulator of the metabolism of arachidonic acid: dietary implications of the ratio, n-6:n:3 fatty acids. Proc Nutr Soc 1985;44:221-29

65. Buisseret P. Prostaglandin-synthesis inhibitors in the prophylaxis of food intolerance Lancet 1978;(Apr 29):906-908

66. Bullock B. Pathophysiology: Adaptations and Alterations in Function. Boston: Scott, Foresman & Co.; 1988

67. Busse W, et al. Flavonoid modulation of human neutrophil function. J All Clin Immunol 1984;73(6):801-9

68. Callegari P. Botanical lipids: Potential role in modulation of immunologic responses and inflammatory reactions. Rheum Dis Clin N Am 1991;17(2):415-25

69. Campbell J, et al. Sympathetically maintained pain: A unifying hypothesis. In Willis W. ed. Hyperalgesia and Allodynia. New York: Raven Press; 1992: p.141-49

70. Capron A. Platelets as effectors of hypersensitivity reactions. In Kay A. ed. Allergy and Inflammation. New York: Academic Press; 1987 p.125-38

71. Carrick F. Diplomate Course in Chiropractic Neurology, Logan College, Chesterfield, MO

72. Carroll H, Oh M. Water, Electolyte and Acid-Base Metabolism: Diagnosis and Management (2nd ed). Philadelphia: J. B. Lippincott; 1989

73. Casey K. Nociceptors and their sensitization. In Willis W. ed. Hyperalgesia and Allodynia. New York: Raven Press; 1992: p.13-15

74. Cassaro G, et al. Human plasma kallikrein: Effect on the induced platelet aggregation. Thromb Res 1987;48:81-87

75. Cathcart E, Gonnerman W. Fish oil fatty acids and experimental arthritis. Rheum Dis Clin N Am 1991;17(2):235-42

76. Celander E, et al. Effect of osteopathic manipulative therapy on autonomic tone as evidenced by blood pressure changes and activity of the fibrinolytic system. J Am Osteo Assoc 1968;67:1037-38

77. Chamberlain G. Cyriax's friction massage: A review. J Ortho Sports Phys Ther 1982;4(1):16-22

78. Chandra D, Gupta S. Anti-inflammatory ad anti-arthritic activity of volatile oil of Curcuma longa (Haldi). INdian J Med Res 1972;60:138-42

79. Chandra R. Food Allergy. In Shills M, Young M. eds. Modern Nutrition in Health and Disease (7th ed). Philadelphia :Lea & Febiger; 1988: p.1298-1305

79a. Chandra R. Nutrition, immunity, and infection: Present knowledge and future directions. Lancet 1983;(Mar 26):688-91

80. Charney A, Fledman G. Internal exchanges of hydrogen ions: Gastrointestinal tract. In Seldin D. & Giebisch G. eds. The Regulation of Acid-Base Balance. New York: Raven Press; 1989: p.89-105

81. Cherkin D, MacCornack F. Patient evaluations of low back pain care from family physicians and chiropractor. West Med J 1989;150:351-55

82. Chiu D et al. Lipid peroxidation in human red blood cells. Sem Hematol 1989;26(4):257-76

83. Chvapil M, et al. Inhibitory effect of zinc ions on platelet aggregation and serotonin release reaction. Life Sci 1976;16(4):561-72

84. Cirelli M. Five years of clinical experience with bromelains in therapy of edema and inflammation in postoperative tissue reaction, skin infections and trauma. Clinical Med 1967;(Jun):55-59

85. Ciprandi G, Canonica G. Incidence of digestive diseases in patients with adverse reactions to foods. Ann Allergy 1988;61:334-36

86. Cohen A, Goldman J. Bromelains therapy in rheumatoid arthritis. Penn Med J 1964;(Jun):27-30

87. Cohen, Diegelmann, & Lindblad, eds. Wound Healing: Biochemical and Clinical Aspects. Philadelphia: W.B. Saunders; 1992

87a. Combs G. The Vitamins: Fundamental Aspects in Nutrition and Health. New York :Academic Press; 1992

88.   Cooke T. Studies in the pathogenesis of rheumatoid arthritis. 1. Immunogenetic associations. Brit J Rheumatol 1989;28:243-50

89.   Cooper N. The complement system. Stites D. Basic & Clinical Immunology (6th ed). Norwalk: Appleton & Lange; 1987: p.114-27

90.   Cooper R. The role of epidural fibrosis and defective fibrinolysis in the persistence of postlaminectomy back pain. Spine 1991;16(9):1044-48

91.   Cooper J, Bloom F, Roth R. The Biochemical Basis of Neuropharmacology (6th ed). New York : Oxford Univ. Press; 1991

92.   Cotran, Kumar & Robbins. Robbins' Pathologic Basis of Disease (4th ed). Philadelphia: W.B. Saunders; 1989

93.   Cotran R et al. Robbins Pathologic Basis of Disease (5th ed). Philadelphia: W.B. Saunders; 1994

94.   Cotran R. Endothelial cells. In Kelley W et al. eds. Textbook of Rheumatology (4th ed). Philadelphia: W. B. Saunders; 1993: p.327-36

95.   Cox I. Red blood cell magnesium and chronic fatigue syndrome. Lancet 1991;337:757-60

96.   Cranton E. Free-radical patholgy in age-associated disease: Treatment with EDTA chelation, nutrition and antioxidants. J Hol Med 1984;6(1):6-37

97.   Crawford M. Essential fatty acids and their prostanoid derivatives Brit Med Bull 1983;39(3):210-13

98.   Creter D et al.,Effect of vitamin E on platelet aggregation in diabetic retinopathy. Acta Haematol 1979 ;62:74-77

99.   Croft A. & Foreman S. Whiplash Injuries Baltimore: Williams & Wilkins; 1988

100. Croset M et al. Functions and tocopherol content of blood platelets from elderly people after low intake of purified eicosapentanoic acid. Thromb Res 1990;57:1-12

101. Curtis P, Bove G. Family physicians, chiropractors, and back pain. J Fam Pract 1992;35(5):551-56

102. Cush J. Cellular basis for rheumatoid inflammation. Clin Ortho Rel Res 1991;265:9-22

103. Cutler R. Antioxidants and aging. Am J Clin Nutr 1991;53:373S-79S,

104. Davidson J. Wound repair. In Gallin, Goldstein & Snyderman eds. Inflammation: Basic Principles and Clinical Correlates (2nd ed). New York: Raven Press; 1992: p.809-19

105. Davis J et al. Passive smoking affects endothelium and platelets. Arch Int Med 1989;149:386-89

106. de Geus E et al. Effects of exercise training on plasminogen activator inhibitor activity. Med Sci Sports Exer 1992;24(11):1210-19

107. Deitrick R. Oral proteolytic enzymes in the treatment of athletic injuries: A double-blind study. Penn Med J 1965;(Oct):35-37

108. Del Maestro R. An approach to free radicals in medicine and biology. Acta Physiol Scand 1980;492(Suppl):153-68

109. Demopoulos H. Control of free radicals in biologic systems. Fed Proc 1973;32:1903-08

110. Demopoulos H. The development of secondary pathology with free radical reactions as a threshold mechanism J Am Coll Toxicol 1983;2:173-84

111. Deodhar S et al. Preliminary studies on antirheumatic activity of curcumin (diferuloyl methane). Ind J Med Res 1980;71:632

112. Despopoulos A, Silbernagl S. Color Atlas of Physiology (4th ed). New York: Thieme Med Pub; 1991

113. Devlin J, Horton E. Hormone and nutrient interactions. In Shils M, Young M. eds. Modern Nutrition in Health and Disease (7th ed). Philadelphia :Lea & Febiger; 1988: p.570-84

114. Dietary flavonoids and risk of coronary heart disease. Nutr Rev 1994;52(2):59-61

115. Dilman V, Dean W. The Neuroendocrine Theory of Aging and Degenerative Disease. Pensacola, FL: Center for Biogerontology; 1992

116. Di Luzuio N. The employment of antioxidants in the prevention and treatment of experimentally induced liver injury. Prog Biochem Pharmacol 1967;3:325-42

117. Dinarello C. The Acute phase response. In Wyngaarden, Smith & Bennet eds. Cecil Textbook of Medicine (19th ed). Philadelphia :W. B. Saunders; 1992: p.1571-73

118. Dorland's Medical Dictionary (25th ed). Philadelphia : W.B. Saunders; 1974

119. Douglas W. Histamine and 5-hydroxytryptamine (serotonin) and their antagonists. In Gilman A et al. eds. Pharmacologic Basis of Disease (7th ed). New York: Macmillan; 1985: p.605-38

120. Douglas W. Polypeptides—Angiotensin, plasma kinins, and other. In Gilman A et al. The Pharmacological Basis of Therapeutics (7th ed). New York: MacMillan; 1985: p.639-59

121. Drash A. Nutrition and the etiology of insulin-dependent diabetes mellitus. Nutr & the MD 1993;19(2):1-3

121a. Dreosti I. Magnesium status and health. Nutr Rev 1995; 53(9):S23-S27

122. Drevon C. Marine oils and their effects. Nutr Rev 1992;50(4):38-45

123. Dubner R. Neuronal plasticity in the spinal and medullary dorsal horns: A Possible Role in Central Pain Mechanisms. In Casey K. ed. Pain and Central Nervous System Disease: The Central Pain Syndromes. New York: Raven Press; 1991: p.143-55

124. Dubner R, Ruda A. Activity-dependent neuronal plasticity follwoing tissue injury and inflammation. Trends Neuroscience 1992;15(3):96-103

125. Dudai Y. The Neurobiology of Memory. New York: Oxford Univ Press; 1989

126. Dupont J. Lipids. In Brown M ed. Present Knowledge in Nutrition (6th ed). Int Life Sci Inst Washington, DC: Nutrition Foundation; 1990: p.56-66

127. Dyerberg J et al. Eicosapentanoic acid and prevention of thrombosis and atherosclerosis? Lancet 1978;(Jul):117-119

128. Dyerberg J et al. μ-linolenic acid and eicosapentanoic acid, (letter to editor) Lancet 1980;(Jan):199

129. Dyerberg J. Linolenate-derived polyunsaturated fatty acids and prevention of atherosclerosis. Nutr Rev 1986;44(4):125-34

129a. Elin R. Magnesium: The fifth but forgotten electrolyte. Am J Clin Path 1994;102(5):616-22

130. Englemann B. Replacement of molecular species of phophotidylcholine: Influence on erythrocyte Na trasnport. Am J Physiol 1990;258:C682-91

131. Engles M. Tissue reponse. In Donatelli R & Wooden R. Orthopedic Physical Therapy (2nd ed). Churchill Livingstone; 1994: p.1-31

132. Ernst P et al. Immunity and mucosal tissues. In Stites D ed. Basic and Clinical Immunology (6th ed). Norwalk, CT: Appleton & Lange; 1987: p.159-66

133. Evans C. The role of proteinases in cartilage destruction. Agents Actions 1991;32:135-52

134. Everson G, Shrader R. Abnormal glucose tolerance in manganese-deficient guinea pigs. J Nutr 1968;94:89-94

135. Faye L. Personal communication with Dr. Faye. He first described the subluxation complex in 1976 while teaching at Canadian Memorial College of Chiropractic.

136. Faye L, Schafer R. Motion Palpation and Chiropractic Technic (2nd ed). Hunt. Beach, CA :MPI; 1990

136a. Feinstein B et al. Experiments on pain referred from deep somatic tissues. J Bone Joint Surg 1954; 36-A(5):981-97

137. Fields H. PAIN. New York: McGraw Hill; 1987: p.92,213

138. Fichera A, Celander D. Effect of osteopathic manipulative therapy on autonomic tone as evidenced by blood pressure changes and activity of the fibrinolytic system. J Am Osteo Assoc 1969;68:1036-38

139. Fick D. Resolving inflammation in active patients. Phys Sportsmed 1993;21(12):55-63

140. Filipovic I. Comparative studies on fatty acid synthesis in atherosclerotic and hypoxic human aorta. Atherosclerosis 1976;24:457-69

141. Firestein G. Mechanisms of tissue destruction and cellular activation in rheumatoid arthritis. Curr Opin Rheumatol 1992;4:348-54

142. Fisher J. Effects of an oral enzyme preparation, Chymoral, upon serum proteins associated with injury (acute phase reactants) in man. J Med 1974;5:258-73

143. Fisher A. Vestibular-proprioceptive processing and bilateral integration and sequencing deficits. In Fisher, Murray, Bundy eds. Sensory Integration: Theory and Practice. Philadelphia: F.A Davis; 1991: p.71-107

144. Fitz-Ritson D. The anatomy and physiology of the muscle spindle, and its role in posture and movement. J Can Chiro Assoc 1982;26(4):144-50

145. Fitz-Ritson D. The chiropractic management and rehabilitation of cervical trauma. JMPT 1990;13(1):17-25

146. Fleck S, Kraemer W. Designing Resistance Training Programs. Champaign, IL: Human Kinetics Pub; 1987: p.137

147. Floyd R. Basic free radical biochemistry. In Free Radicals in Aging. Yu B ed. Boca Raton: CRC Press; 1993: p.39-55

148. Flynn D, Rafferty M. Inhibition of 5-hydroxy-eicosatetraenoic acid (5-HEYE) formation in intact human neutrophils by naturally-ocurring diarylheptanoids: Inhibitory activities of curcuminoids and yakuchiones. Prost Leuk Med 1986;22:357-60

149. Flynn D, Rafferty M. Inhibition of human neutrophil 5-lipoxygenase activity by gingerdione, shogaol, capsaicin and related pungent compounds. Prost Leuk Med 1986;24:195-98

150. Folkman J, Klagsbrun M. Angiogenic factors. Science 1987;235:44247

151. Food and Nutrition Board, Recommended Daily Allowances (10th ed). National Academy Press. Washington, DC; 1989

152. Ford-Hutchinson A. Leukotrienes: their formation and role as inflammatory mediators. Fed Poc 1985;44:25-29

153. Fowkes F et al. Fibrinogen genotype and risk of peripheral atherosclerosis. Lancet 1992;339:693-96

154. Franson R et al. Human disc phospholipase A-2 is inflammatory. Spine 1992;17(6):S129-32

155. Freeman B, Crapo J. Biology of disease: Free radicals and tissue injury. Lab Invest 1982;47(5):412-26

156. Frick O. Immediate hypersensitivity. In Stites D. ed. Basic and Clinical Immunology (6th ed). Norwalk, Conn: Appleton & Lange; 1987: p.197-227

157. Fuller R. Target tissues for mediators in human allergic reactions. In Hogate S. Mast Cellls, Mediators and Disease. Boston: Kluwer Academic Publishers; 1988: p.241-58

158. Furhman B et al. Increased platelet aggregation during alimentary hyperlipidemia in normal and hypertriglyceridemic subjects. Ann Nutr Metab 30:250-60. 1986

159. Gabor. Pharmacologic effects of flavonoids on blood vessels. Angiologica 1972;9:355-74

160. Gallin, Goldstein, Snyderman eds. Inflammation: Basic Principles and Clinical Correlates (2nd ed) New York: Raven Press; 1992

161. Ganong W. Review of Medical Physiology (13th ed). Norwalk, CT: Appleton & Lange; 1987

162. Gerster H. Review: Antioxidant protection of the ageing macula. Age and Aging 20:60-69; 1991

163. Ghez C. Muscles: Effectors of the motor system. In Kandel E et al. Principles of Neural Science (3rd ed). New York: Elsevier; 1991: p.548-63

164. Ghosh P.The role of cartilage-derived antigens, pro-coagulant activity and fibrinolysis in the pathogenesis of osteoarthritis. Med Hypothesis 1993;41:190-94

165. Glant T.Immunopathologic role of proteoglycan antigens in rheumatoid joint disease. Scand J Immunol 1980;11:247-52

166. Goldberg B, Rabinovich M. Connective Tissue. In Weiss L. ed. Cell and Tissue Biology: A Textbook of Histology, Baltimore: Urban & Schwarzenberg; 1988: p.155-88

167. Good C. Osteoarthritis and nutritional support: A literature Review. Nutr Pers 1991;14(2):11-15

168. Goodson W. Traumatic injury. In Cohen I et al. Wound Healing: Biochemical and Clinical Aspects, Philadelphia: W.B. Saunders; 1992: p.316-25

169. Gorlin R. The biological actions and potential clinical significance of dietary n-3 fatty acids. Arch Int Med 1988;148:2043-48

170. Gorman R. Leukotriene B₄. In Henson, Murphy eds. Mediators of the Inflammatory Process, Handbook of Inflammation (Vol 6). New York: Elsevier; 1989: p.15-27

171. Goss R. Regeneration versus repair. In Cohen I et al. Wound Healing: Biochemical & Clinical Aspects. Philadelphia: W.B. Saunders; 1992; p.20-39

172. Gould J. Orthopedic and Sports Physical therapy (2nd ed). St. Louis: Mosby; 1990

173. Greene H, Roberto M. The gastrointestinal tract: Regulator of nutrient absorption. In Shils M, Olson J, Shike M eds. Modern Nutrition in Health and Disease (8th ed). Philadelphia: Lea & Febiger; 1994: p.54968

174. Grekin R. Ketoacidosis, hyperosmolar states, and lactic acidosis. In Kokko, Tannen eds. Fluids and Electorlytes. Philadelphia: W.B. Saunders; 1986: p.688-711

175. Grieve G. Common Vertebral Joint Problems (2nd ed). New York: Churchill Livingstone; 1988

175a. Gubler C. Thiamin. In Machlin L. Editor. Handbook of Vitamins. 2nd ed. New York: Marcel Dekker; 1991: p.233-81

176. Guyton A. Basic Neuroscience (2nd ed). Philadelphia: W.B. Saunders; 1991

177. Guyton A. Textbook of Medical Physiology (8th ed). Philadelphia: W.B. Saunders; 1991

178. Haaland A. Fibrinolytic activity as a predictor of the outcome of prolapsed intervertebral lumbar disc surgery with reference to back ground variables: Regions of a prospective cohort study. Spine 1992;17(9):1022-27

179. Haft J. Intravascular platelet aggregation in the heart induced by stress. Circulation 1973;XLVII:353-58

180. Haldeman S. The neurophysiology of spinal pain. In Haldeman S. ed. Principles and Practice of Chiropractic (2nd ed). Norwalk, CT: Appleton-Century-Crofts; 1992: p.165-84

181. Haller E, Bell K. Rehabilitation's relationship to inactivity. In Kottke F, Lehmann J. eds. Kruzen's Handbook of Physical Medicine and Rehabilitation (4th ed). Philadelphia: W.B. Saunders; 1990: p.1113-33

182. Halliwell B. Free radicals and antioxidants: A personal view. Nutr Rev 1994;52(8):253-65

183. Hambly M. Effect of smoking and pulsed electromagnetic fields on intradiscal pH in rabbits. Spine 1992;17(6 Suppl):S83-S85

184. Hammer W. Friction massage. In Hammer W. ed. Functional Soft Tissue Examination by Manual Methods. Gaithersburg, MD: Aspen; 1991: p.235-49

185. Hampton E. Intravenous magnesium therapy in acute myocardial infarction. Ann Pharmacother 1994;28:212-19

186. Handwerker H, Reech P. Nociceptors: Chemosensitivity and sensitization by chemical agents. In Willis W. ed. Allodynia and Hyperalgesia. New York: Raven Press; 1992: p.107-15

187. Hanesch U. et al. Nociception in normal and arthritic joints: Structural and functional aspects. In Willis W. ed. Allodynia and Hyperalgesia. Raven Press; 1992: p.81-106

188. Harfenist E, Murray R. Plasma proteins, immunogloblulins, and blood coagulation. In Murray R. et al. Harper's Biochemistry (23rd ed). Norwalk, CT: Appleton & Lange; 1993: p.665-87

189. Harlan D. A factor in food which impairs NA+/K+-ATPase in vitro. Am J Clin Nutr 1982;35:250-57

190. Harland B. et al. Calcium, phophorus, iron, iodine, and zinc in the "Total diet". J Am Diet Assoc 1980;77:16-20

191. Harman D. Free radical therory of aging: A hyposthesis on the pathogenesis of senile demetia of the Alzheimer's type. Age 1993;16:23-30

192. Harris E. Etiology and pathology of rheumatoid arthritis. In Kelley W. et al. eds. Textbook of Rheumatology (4th ed). Philadelphia: W. B. Saunders; 1993: p.833-73

192a. Harris E. Treatment of rheumatoid arthritis., in Kelley W. et al. eds. Textbook of Rheumatology (4th ed). Philadelphia:W. B. Saunders; 1993: p.912-23

193. Hart D, Fritzler M. Regulation of plasminogen activators and their inhibitors in rheumatic diseases: New understandings and the potential for new directions. J Rheumatol 1989;16:1184-91

194. Havsteen B. Flavonoids, A class of natural products of high pharmacologic potency. Bioch Pharmacol 1983;32(7):1141-48

195. Haynes R, Murad F. Adrenocorticotropic hormone; adrenocortical steroids and their synthetic analogs; inhibitors of adrenocortical steroid biosynthesis. In Gilman A. et al. The Pharmacological Basis of Therapeutics (7th ed). New York: McMillan; 1985: p.1459-89

196. Heinicke R. et al. Effect of bromelain (Ananase) on human platelet aggregation. Experientia 28:844: 1972

197. Henriksson K. Muscle pain with special reference to primary fibromyalgia. In Dubner R. ed. Proceedings of the Vth World Congress on Pain; New York: Elsevier; 1988: p.232-37

198. Hepper E. et al. Back school. In Kirkaldy-Willis W, Burton C. Managing Low Back Pain (3rd ed). New York: Churchill Livingstone; 1992: p.263-81

199. Hettinga D. Inflammatory response of synovial joint structures. In Gould J. ed. Orthopedic and Sports Physical Therapy (2nd ed). St. Louis: Mosby; 1990: p.87-117

200. Higgs G, Vane L. Inhibition of cyclo-oygenase and lipoxygenase. Brit Med Bull 1983;39(3):265-70

201. Higgs G. The effects of dietary intake of essential fatty acids on prostaglandin and leukotriene synthesis. Proc Nutr Soc 1985;44:181-87

202. Holman R. Aaes-Jorgensen E. Effects of *trans* fatty acid isomers upon essential fatty acid deficiency in rats. Proc Soc Exp Biol Med 1956;93:175-79

203. Holman R, Mahfouz M. *Cis* and *trans*-octadecenoic acids as precursors of polyunsaturated acids. Prog Lipid Res 1981;20:151-56

204. Holman R. Control of polyunsaturated acids in tissue phospholipids. J Am Coll Nutr 1986;5:183-211

205. Hooker D. Back rehabilitation. In Prentice W. ed. Rehabilitation Techniques in Sports Medicine (2nd ed). St. Louis: Mosby; 1994: p.277-302

206. Hooshmand H. Chronic Pain: Reflex Sympathetic Dystrophy, Prevention and Management. Boca Raton, FL: CRC Press; 1993: p.34

207. Hoppel C. et al. Deficiency of the reduced nicotinamide adenine dinucleotide dehydrogenase component of Complex I of mitochondrial electron transport. J clin Invest 1987;80:71-77

208. Horner S. Effficacy of intravenous magnesium in acute myocardial infarction reducing arrythmias and mortality: Meta-Analysis of magnesium in acute myocardial infarction. Circulation 1992;86:774-79

209. Horrobin D. The importance of gamma-linolenic acid and prostaglandin E-1 in human nutrition and medicine. J Hol Med 1981;3(2):118-139

210. Hubbard D, Berkoff G. Myofascial trigger points show spontaneous needle EMG activity. Spine 1993;18(13):1803-07

211. Huggins B. Trauma physiology Nurs Clin N Am 1990;25(1):1-10

212. Hughes A, Tonks R. Magnesium, adenosine diphophate, and blood platelets Nature 1966;210:106-7

213. Hurri H. Fibrinolytic defect in chronic back pain. Acta Orthop Scand 1991;62(5):407-09

214. Hwang D, Carroll A. Decreased formation of prostaglandins derived from arachidonic acid by dietary linoleate in rats. Am J Clin Nutr 1980;33:590-97

215. Ilyia E. of Diagnos-Techs. A Clinical and Research Laboratory. Kent, Wash. personal communication

215a. Inhibition of LDL oxidation by phenolic substances in red wine: A clue to the French paradox? Nutr Rev 1993;51(6):185-87

216. Injeyan H. Pathology of musculoskeletal soft tissues. In Hammer W. Functional Soft Tissue Examination and Treatment by Manual Methods. Gaithersburg, Maryland: Aspen Publishers; 1991: p.9-23

217. Innerfield I. Parenteral administration of trypsin. J Am Med Assoc 1953;152(7):597-605

218. Iwakami S. et al. Inhibition of arachidonate 5-lipoxygenase by phenolic compounds. Chem Pharm Bull 1986;34:3960-63

219. Is fibromyalgia caused by a glycolysis impairment?, Nutr Rev 1994;52(7):248-50

220. Jarvinen M. The effects of early mobilisation on the healing process following muscle injuries. Sports Medicine 1993;15(2):8-78-89

221. Jayson M. Chronic inflammation and fibrosis in back pain syndromes., in Jayson, M. ed. The Lumbar Spine and Back Pain (3rd ed). New York: Churchill Livingstone; 1987: p.411-18

222. Jayson M. The role of vascular damage and fibrosis in the pathogenesis of nerve root damage. Clin Ortho Rel Res 1992;279:4048

222a. Jee W. The skeletal tissues. In: Weiss L. ed. Cell and tissue biology: A textbook of histology. 6th ed. Baltimore:Urban & Schwarzenberg; 1988: p.211-54

223. Jenkins D. et al. Diet factors affecting absorption and metabolism. In Shils M. et al. eds. Modern Nutrition in Health and Disease (8th ed). Philadelphia: W. B. Saunders; 1994: p583-602

224. Johnson G. Soft Tissue Mobilization. In Donatelli R, Wooden M. eds. Orthopaedic Physical Therapy (2nd ed). New York: Churchill Livingstone; 1994: p.697-56

225. Jones V. et al. Immune complexes in early arthritis. I. Detection of immune complexes before rheumatoid arthritis. Clin Exp Immunol 1981;44:512-21

226. Joris I. Capillary leakage in inflammation: A study of vascular labeling. Am J Path 1990;137(6):1353-63

227. Kahn C, Catanese V. Secondary forms of diabetes mellitus. In Becker K. et al. eds. Principles and Practice of Endocrinology and Metabolism. Philadelphia: J.B. Lippincott Company; 1990: p.1087-93

228. Kandel, Schwartz & Jessel. Principles of Neural Science (3rd ed). New York :Elsevier; 1991

229. Kellet J. Acute soft tissue injuries —a review of the literature. Med Sci Sports Exer 1986;18(5):489-500

230. Khaw K, Barrett-Connor E. Dietary potassium and stroke-associated mortality. New Eng J Med 1987;316(5):235-40

231. King R. Pain and tryptophan. J Neurosurg 1980;53:44-52

232. Kirchgessner M, Roth H. Biochemical changes of hormones and metalloenzymes in zinc deficiency. In Zinc in the Environment. John Wiley & Sons; 1980: p.71-103

233. Kirkaldy-Willis W, Cassidy,J. Spinal manipulation in the treatment of low-back pain. Can Fam Phys 1985;31:536-40

234. Kirkaldy-Willis W. Pathology and pathogenesis of low back pain. In Kirkaldy-Willis W, Burton C. eds. Managing Low Back Pain (3rd ed). New York: Churchill Livingstone; 1992: p.49-79

235. Kisner C, Colby L. Therapeutic Exercise: Foundations and Techniques (2nd ed). Philadelphia: F.A. Davis; 1990: p.214-28

236. Kitsis E. The role of the neutrophil in rheumatoid arthritis. Clin Ortho Rel Res 1991;265:63-72

237. Kjeldsen-Kragh J. et al. Controlled trial of fasting and one-year vegetarian diet in rheumatoid arthritis. Lancet 1991;338:899-902

238. Kleiner I, Orten J. Human Biochemistry (5th ed). St. Louis: C.V. Mosby; 1958: p.355

239. Knapp H. et al. In vivo indexes of platelet and vascular function during fish-oil administration in patients with atherosclerosis. New Eng J Med 1986;314(15):937-42

240. Knochel J. Correlates of potassium exchange. In Seldin D, Giebisch G. eds. The Regulation of Potassium Balance. New York: Raven Press; 1989: p.31-55

241. Knochel J. Clinical expression of potassium disturbances. In Seldin D, Gievisch G. eds. The Regulation of Potassium Balance. New York: Raven Press; 1989: p.207-40

242. Koes B. et al. Randomized clinical trial of manipulative therapy and physiotherapy for persistant back and neck complaints: results of one yeara follow up. Brit J Med 1992;304:601-5

243. Korr I. The facilitated segment: A factor in injury to the body frame work. Osteopathic Annals 1973;1:10-12,17-18

244. Korr I. Proprioceptors and somatic dysfunction. J Am Osteo Assoc 1975;74:638-50

245. Korr I. Sustained sympathicotonia as a factor in disease. In Korr I. ed. The Neurobiologic Mechanisms in Manipulative Therapy. New York: Plenum Pub; 1978: p.229-68

246. Kottke F. Therapeutic exercise to maintain mobility. In Kottke F, Lehmann J. eds. Krusens' Handbook of Physical Medicine and Rehabilitation (4th ed). Philadelphia: W.B. Saunders; 1990: p.436-51

247. Kowsari B. et al. Assessment of the diet of patients with rheumatoid arthritis and osteoarthritis. J Am Diet Assoc 1983;82:657-59

248. Kremer J. Nutrition and rheumatic diseases. In Kelley W. et al. eds. Textbook of Rheumatology (4th ed). Philadelphia: WB Saunders; 1993: p.484-97

249. Kulkarni R. et al. Treatment of osteoarthritis with a herbomineral formualtion: A double-blind, placebo-controlled, cross-over study. J Ethnopharmacol 1991;33(1/2):91-95

250. Kunkel S. et al. Suppression of chronic inflammation by evening primrose oil. Prog Lip Res 1981;20:885-88

251. Kurtz I. et al. Effect of diet on plasma acid-base composition in normal humans. Kidney Int 1983;24:670-80

252. Lagunoff D. Agents that release histamine from mast cells. Ann Rev Pharmacol Toxicol 1983;23:331-51

253. Lam B, Austen K. Leukotrienes: Biosynthesis, release, and actions. In Gallin J. et al. Inflammation: Basic Principles and Clinical Correlates 92nd ed). New York: Raven Press; 1992: p.139-47

254. Landin K. et al. Guar gum improves insulin sensitivity, blood lipids, blood pressure, and fibrinolysis. Am J Clin Nutr 1992;56:1061-65

255. Lantz C. Immobilization degeneration & the fixation hypothesis of the chiropractic subluxation. Chiro Res 1988;1(1):21-46

256. Lantz C. The vertebral subluxation complex. ICA Int Rev Chiro 1989;Sep/Oct:37-61

256a. Lantz C. The Vertebral Subluxation Complex. In Gatterman M. ed. Foundation of Chiropractic: Subluxation. St. Louis: Mosby; 1995: p.149-174

257. Lawrence D, Bergmann, T., Joint anatomy and basic biomechanics, p.11-50, in Bergmann T. et al. Chiropractic Technique. New York: Churchill Livingstone; 1993

258. Leadbetter W. Cell-matrix response in tendon injury. Clin Sports Med 1992;11(3):533-78

259. Leaf A, Weber P. Cardiovascular effects of n-3 fatty acids. New Eng J Med 1988;318(9):549-56

260. Leaf A. Health Claims: Omega-3 fatty acids and cardiovascular disease. Nutr Rev 1992;50(5):150-54

261. Lee A, Lagner R. Shark cartilage contains inhibitors of tumor angiogenesis. Science 1983;221:1185-87

262. Lee D. The Pelvic Girdle. New York: Churchill Livingstone; 1989

263. Lee T. et al. Effect of quercetin on human polymorphonuclear leukocyte lysosomal enzyme release and phospholipid metabolism. Life Sci 1982;31:2765-74

264. Lehninger A. Principles of Biochemistry. New York: Worth Publishers; 1982

265. Leung A. Encyclopedia of Commmon Natural Ingredients Used in Food, Drugs and Cosmetics. New York: John Wiley & Sons; 1980

266. Levenson S, Demetriou A. Metabolic factors. In Cohen I. et al. eds. Wound Healing: Biochemical & Clinical Aspects. Philadelphia: W.B. Saunders; 1992: p.248-73

267. Levine J. et al. Leukotriene B-4 produces hyperalgesia that is dependent on polymorphonuclear leukocytes. Science 1984;225:743-45

268. Levine J. The peripheral nervous system and the inflammatory Process., in Dubner R. ed. Proceeding of the Vth World Congress on Pain. New York: Elsevier; 1988: p.33-43

269. Levine J. et al. Hyperalgesic pain: Inflammatory and neuropathic. In Willis W. ed. Hyperalgesia and Allodynia. New York: Raven Press; 1992: p.117-23

270. Levine S, Kidd P. Antioxidant Adaption: Its role in free radical pathology. San Leandro, CA: Biocurrents Division, Allergy Research Group; 1986

271. Lewis R. Leukotrienes and other products of the 5-lipoxygenase pathway. New Eng J Med 1990;323(10):645-55

271a. Lewit K. Manipulative therapy in rehabilitation of the locomotor system. 2nd ed. Boston: Butterworth Heineman, 1991: p.258

272. Liebenson C. Leads a certification program in Chiropractic Rehabilitation through Los Angeles College of Chiropractic, Phone # (310)470-2909

272a. Liebenson C. Rehabilitation of the spine: A practitioners manual. Baltimore: Williams & Wilkins; 1996

273. Lipsky P. T Cells and B Cells. In Kelley W. et al. eds. Textbook of Rheumatology (4th ed), Philadelphia: W. B. Saunders; 1993: p.108-54

274. Lin D. Review of vitamin E supplementation in healthy humans: effect on platelet activity, lipoprotein distribution, and oxidative damage. J Appl Nutr 1993;45(1):2-12

275. Linder M. Nutritional Biochemistry and Metabolism (2nd ed). New York: Elsevier; 1991

276. Little C. et al. Platelet serotonin release in rheumatorid arthritis: A study in food intolerant patients. Lancet 1981;(Aug 6):297-99

277. Lubek B, Mainwood G. Lactate and pyruvate production in isolated thiamine-deficient rat diaphragm strips. Can J Physiol Pharmacol 1984;62:277-281

278. Machlin L. Handbook of Vitamins (2nd ed). New York: Marcel Dekker; 1991

279. Machlin L. Vitamin E. In Machlin L. ed. Handbook of Vitamins (2nd ed). New York: Marcel Dekker; 1991: p.99-144

280. Mai J. High dose antioxidant supplementation to MS patients: Effects on glutathione peroxidase, clinical safety, and absorption of selenium. Biol Trace Elem REs 1990;24:109-17

281. Mainardi C. Fibroblast function and fibrosis. In Kelley W. et al. eds. Textbook of Rheumatology (4th ed). Philadelphia: W. B. Saunders; 1993: p.337-49

282. Manga. P. The Effectiveness and Cost-effectiveness of Chiropractic Management of Low-Back Pain. Richmond Hill, Ontario: Kenilworth Publishing; 1992

283. Manniche C. et al. Intensive dynamic back exercises for chronic low back pain: a clinical trial. Pain 1991:47:53-63

284. Mantzioris E. et al. Dietary substitution with an μ-linolenic acid-rich vegetable oil increases eicosapentanoic acid concentrations in tissues. Am J Clin Nutr 1994;59:1304-09

285. Marchesi V. Inflammation and healing. In Kissane J. ed. Anderson's Pathology (8th ed). St. Louis: Mosby; 1985: p.22-60

286. Marone G. et al. Physiological concentrations of zinc inhibit the release of histamine from human basophils and lung mast cells. Agents Actions 1986;18:103-6

287. Marsden C. Parkinson's disease. Lancet 1990;335:948-52

288. Marshall L. et al. Chemical radiculitis. Clin Ortho Rel Res 1977;129:61-67

289. Marshall L, Johnston P. Modulation of tissue prostaglandin synthesizing capacity by increased ratios of dietary alpha-linolenic acid to linoleic acid. Lipiids 1982;17(12):905-13

290. Martin G. Anti-inflammatory effect of trypsin. Ann NY Acad Sci 1957;68:70-88

291. Mascolo N. Flavonoids, leukocyte migration and eicosanoids. J Pharm Pharmacol 1988;40:293-95

292. Matz R. Magnesium: Deficiencies and therapeutic uses. Hosp Pract 1993;(Apr 30):79-92

293. Mayer T, Gatchel R. Functional Restoration for Spinal Disorders: The Sports Medicine Approach. Philadelphia: Lea & Febiger; 1988

294. Mayes P. Biosynthesis of fatty acids. In Murray R. et al. Harper's Biochemistry (23rd ed). Norwalk, CT: Appleton & Lange; 1993: p.212-19

295. Mayes P. Nutrition. In Murray R. et al. Harpers Biochemistry (23rd ed). Norwalk, CT: Appleton & Lange;1993: p.599-608

296. Mayes P. Digestion and absorption. In Murray R. et al. Harpers Biochemistry (23rd ed). Norwalk, CT: Appleton & Lange; 1993: p.609-21

297. Mayo Clinic Diet Manual (2nd ed). Philadelphia: W.B. Saunders; 1954: p.201-203

298. McArdle W. et al. Exercise Physiology (3rd ed). Philadelphia: Lea & Febiger; 1991

299. McCarthy C. et al. Osteoarthritis. In Wall P, Melzack R. eds. The Textbook of Pain (3rd ed). New York: Churchill Livingstone; 1994: p.387-96

300. McCarthy M. et al. The clincial use of continuous passive motion in physical therapy. Phys Ther 1992;15(3):132-40

301. McCord J. Oxygen-derived free radicals in postischemic tissue injury. New Eng J Med 1985;312(3):159-63

302. McCune D, Sprague R. Exercise for low back pain., In Basmajian J, Wolf S. Therapeutic Exercise (5th ed). Baltimore: Williams & Wilkins; 1990: p.299-321

302a. McGanity W et al. Nutrition in pregnancy and lactation. In Shils M et al. eds. Modern Nutrition in Health and Disease. 8th ed. Philadelphia: Lea & Febiger; 1994:705-27

303. McGreer P. Anti-inflammatory drugs and Alzheimer disease. Lancet 1990;335:1037

304. McLain R. Mechanoreceptor endings in human cervical facet joints. Spine 1994;19(5):495-501

305. McLatchie G, Lennox M. The Soft Tissues: Trauma and Sports Injuries. London: Butterworth-Heinemann; 1993

307. Melmon K. The presence of a kinin in inflammatory synovial effusions from arthritides of varying etiologies. Arth Rheum 1967;10(1):13-20

308. Mercy Guidelines - Guidelines for Chiropractic Quality Assurance and Practice Parameters. Haldeman S et al. eds. Aspen Publishing; 1993

309. Merry P. Oxidative damage to lipids with in the inflamed human joint provides evidence of radical mediated hypoxic-reperfusion injury. Am J Clin Nutr 1991;53:362S-69S

310. Metcalfe D. Mast Cells and Basophils. In Gallin, Goldstein, Snyderman eds. Inflammation: Basic Principles and Clinical Correlates (2nd ed). New York: Raven Press; 1992: p.709-25

311. Middleton E. Quercetin: An inhibitor of antigen-induced human basophil histamine release. J Immunol 1981;127:546-50

312. Miller B, Keane C. Encyclopedia and Dictionary of Medicine, Nursing, and Allied Health. Philadelphia: W.B. Saunders; 1987

313. Miller G. Does a high-fat diet promote clotting? paper presented at the American Heart Association's Twentieth Science Writers Forum. Monterey, California 1/17-20/93

314. Miller J. The increased proteolytic activity of human blood serum after the oral administration of bromelain. Exp Med Surg 1964;22:277-80

315. Moffroid M et al. Endurance training of trunk extensor muscles. Phys Ther 1993;73(1):33-10

316. Moncada, Flower, Vane. Prostaglandins, prostacyclin, thromboxane A-2, and leukotrienes. In Goodman & Gilman, eds. Pharmacoloic Basis of Disease (7th ed). New York: MacMillan; 1985: p.660-73

317. Montgomery R et al. Biochemistry: A Case Oriented Approach (4th ed)., , St. Louis: Mosby; 1983: p.246

318. Montgomery R et al. Biochemistry: A Case Oriented Approach. St. Louis; C. V. Mosby: 1990

319. Moreadith R. Deficiency of the iron-sulfur clusters of mitchondrial reduced nicotinamide-adenine dinucleotide-ubiquinone oxidoreductase (Complex I) in an infant with congential lactic acidosis. J Clin Invest 1984;74:685-97

320. Morgan K. Magnesium and calcium dietary intakes of the U.S. population, J Am Coll Nutr 1985;4:195-206

321. Moxley G, Ruddy S. Immune complexes and complement. Kelley W et al. Textbook of Rheumatology (4th ed). Philadelphia: W.B. Saunders; 1993: p.188-200

322. Muller-Eberhard H.Complement: Chemistry and Pathway. In Gallin, Goldstein, Snyderman eds. Inflammation: Basic Principles and Clinical Correlates (2nd ed). New York: Raven Press; 1992: p.33-61

323. Muller J. Morning increase of onset of myocardial infarction. Cardiology 1989;76:96-104

324. Murray R, Keeley F. The extracellular space. In Murray R et al. Harper's Biochemistry (23rd ed). Norwalk, CT: Appleton & Lange; 1993: p.634-46

325. Mutschler E et al. Drug Actions: Basic Principles and Therapeutics. Boca Raton, FL: CRC Press; 1995: p.163-72

326. Mygind N. Essential Allergy. Oxford: Blackwell Sci Pub; 1986: p.139

327. Nachemson A. Intradiscal measurements of pH in patients wit lumbar rhizopathies. Acta Ortho Scand 1969;40:23-42

328. Nadler J. Magnesium lowers blood pressure in Type II diabetes. Practical Cardiology 1990;16(10):4

329. Nadler J. Magnesium plays a key role in inhibiting platelet aggregation and release reaction. Arteriosclerosis Thromb 1991;11(5):156a

329a. Nansel D, Szlazak M. Somatic dysfunction and the phenomenon of visceral disease simulation: a probable explanation for the apparent effectiveness of somatic therapy in patients presumed to be suffering from true visceral disease. JMPT 1996;18(6):379-97

330. Netter F. The Ciba Collection of Medical Illustrations (Vol 8), Musculoskeletal System (Part i). Summit, New Jersey: Ciba-Geigy Corp; 1991: p.154

331. Newsholme E, Leech A. Biochemistry For The Medical Sciences. New York: John Wiley & Sons; 1983

332. Nielsen F. Ultratrace minerals. In Shils M et al. Modern Nutrition in Health and Disease (8th ed). Philadelphia: Lea & Febier; 1994: p.269-86

333. Nissley S. Growth factors. In Becker K et al. Principles and Practice of Endocrinology and Metabolism. Philadelphia: J. B. Lippincott; 1990: p.1315-21

334. Nordoy A et al. The effect of alimentary hyperlipaemia and primary hypertriglyceridemia on platelets in man. Scand J Haemat 1974;12:329-40

335. Nordoy A et al. Platelets during alimentary hyperlipaemia induced by cream and cod liver oil. Eur J Clin Invest 1984;14:339-45

336. Norkin C, Levangie P. Joint Structure and Function (2nd ed). Philadelphia: F.A. Davis; 1992: p.73-79

337. Norris C. Sports Injuries: Diagnosis and Management for Physiotherapists. Oxford: Butterworth-Heinemenn; 1993: p.21-48

338. Oakes B. Acute soft tissue injuries: Nature and management. Austr Fam Phys 1982;10(suppl):3-16

339. Ohshima H, Urban J. The effect of lactate and pH on proetoglycan and protein synthesis rates in the intervertebral disc. Spine 1992;17(9):1079-82

340. Orten J, Neuhaus O. Biochemistry (8th ed). St. Louis: C.V. Mosby; 1970: p.860

341. Ott P, Fenster P. Should magnesium be a part of the routine therapy for acute myocardial infarction? Am Heart J 1992;124(4):1113-17

342. Palmer D. The Science, Art and Philosophy of Chiropractic. Portland, OR: Portland Printing House Co; 1910: p.359

343. Pangborn J. Flow Chart - Amino Acid Metabolism. Lisle, IL: Bionostics Inc; 1981

344. Parkkola R, Kormano M. Lumbar disc and back muscle degeneration on MRI: Corrleation to age and body mass. J Spinal Disorders 1992;5(1):86-92

345. Patterson M. The spinal cord: Participant in disorder. Spinal Manipulation 1993;9(3):2-11

346. Pearce F. Mucosal mast cells III. Effect of quercetin and other flavonoids on the antigen-induced histamine secretion from rat intestinal mast cells. J Allergy Clin Immunol 1984;73:819-23

347. Pelletier J et al. Effects of tiaprofenic acid on plasminogen activators and inhibitors in human OA and RA synovium. Brit J Rheum 1992;31(suppl 1):19-26

348. Pennington, J., Church, N., Food Values (14th ed), p.63, Harper & Row, New York, 1985

349. Perl E. Alterations in the responsiveness of cutaneous nociceptors: Sensitization by noxious stimuli and the induction of adrenergic responsiveness by nerve injury. In Willis W. ed. Allodynia and Hyperalgesia. Raven Press; 1992: p.59-79

350. Pike M. Antiinflammatory effects of dietary lipid modification. J Rhematol 1989;16(6):718-20

351. Postlethwaite A, Kang A. Fibroblasts and matrix proteins. In Gallin J et al. Inflammation: Basic Principles and Clinical Correlates (2nd ed). New York: Raven Press; 1992: p.747-73

352. Pountain A. Impaired fibrinolytic activity in defined chronic back pain syndromes. Spine 1987;12(2):83-86

353. Powell W. Metabolism of arachidonic acid and other polyunsaturated fatty acids by blood vessels. Prog Lipid Res 1987;26:183-210

354. Prakash C et al. Decreased systemic thromboxane A-2 biosynthesis in normal human subjects fed a salmon-rich diet. Am J Clin Nutr 1994;60:369-73

355. Prentice W, Bell G. Pathophysiology of musculoskeletal injuries and the healing process. In Prentice W ed. Rehabilitation Techniques in Sports Medicine. St. Louis: Times Mirror/Mosby; 1990: p.1-23

356. Price D. Psychological and Neural Mechanisms of Pain. New York:Raven Press; 1988: p.100

357. Prisco D et al. Increased thromboxane A2 generation and altered membrane fatty acid composition in platelets with active angina pertoris. Thromb Res 1985;44:101-112

358. Raloff J. Breakfast may reduce morning heart attack risk. Sci News 1991;139:246-47

359. Raloff J. Margerine is anything but a marginal fat. Science News 1994;145:325

360. Rantanen J. The lumbar multifidus muscle five years after surgery for a lumbar intervertebral disc herniation. Spine 1993;18(5):568-74

361. Rasmussen H. Justification for intraveous magnesium therapy in acute myocardial infarction. Magnesium Res 1988;1:59-73

362. Reid D. Sports Injury Assessment and Rehabilitation. New York: Churchill Livingstone; 1992

363. Reis S et al. Low back pain: More than anatomy. J Fam Pract 1992;35(5):509-10

364. Ren K. The effects of a non-competitive NMDA receptor antagonist, MK-801, on behavioral hyperalgesia and dorsal horn neuronal activity in rats with unilateral inflammation. Pain 1991;50:331-44

365. Renaud S et al. Influence of long-term diet modification on platelet function and composition in Moselle farmers. Am J Clin Nutr 1986;43:136-50

366. Ridker P. Endogenous tissue-type plasminogen activator and risk of myocardial infarction. Lancet 1993;341:1165-68

367. Rishi M. Effects of reduced dietary magnesium on platelet production and function in hamsters. Lab Invest 1990;63(5):717-21

368. Roberts H, Lozier J. New perspectives on the coagulation cascade. Hosp Med 1992(Jan 15):97-112

369. Robson M. Eicosanoids, cytokines, and free radicals In Cohen, Diegelmann, Lindblad eds. Wound Healing: Biochemical and Clinical Aspects. Philadelphia: W.B. Saunders; 1992: p.292-304

370. Roitt I et al. Immunology (2nd ed). New York: Harper & Row; 1989

371. Rose D. Clinical Physiology of Acid-Base and Electrolyte Disorders (Third ed). New York: McGraw Hill; 1989: p.261-322

372. Rose S. Synaptic plasticity, learning and memory. In Baudry M et al. Synaptic Plasticity: Molecular, Cellular and Functional Aspects. Cambridge, MA: MIT Press. 1993: p.209-29

373. Ross E. The role of marine fish oils in the treatment of ulcerative colitis. Nutr Rev 1993;51(2):47-49

374. Ross R. The pathogenesis of atherosclerosis – An update. New Eng J Med 1986;314(8):488-99

375. Ross R. Atherogenesis. In Gallin I et al. Inflammation: Basic Principles and Clinical Correlates (2nd ed). New York: Raven Press; 1992: p.1051-59

376. Roy S, Irvin R. Sports Medicine: Prevention, Evaluation, Management, and Rehabilitation. Englewood Cliffs, NJ: Prentice-Hall; 1983: p.125-27

377. Ryan G. Inflammation. Kalamazoo, MI: The Upjohn Company; 1977

378. Saal J et al. High levels of inflammatory phopholipase A-2 activity in lumbar disc herniations. Spine 1990;15:674-78

379. Safayhi H et al. Boswellic acids: novel, specific, nonredox inhibitors of 5-lipoxygenase. J Pharmacol Exp Ther 1992;261-(3):1143-46

380. Salmon J, Terano T. Supplementation of the diet with eicosapentaenoic acid: a possible approach to the treatment of thrombosis and inflammation. Proc Nutr Soc 1985;44:385-89

381. Salonen J. Effects of antioxidant supplementation on platelet function: a randomized pair-matched, placebo-controlled, double-blind trial in men with low antioxidant status. Am J Clin Nutr 1991;53:1222-9

382. Salter R. Continuous Passive Motion. Baltimore: Williams & Wilkins; 1993

383. Saltman P. Oxidative stress: A radical view. Sem Hematol 1989;26(4):249-56

384. Sanders T et al. Studies of vegans: the fatty acid composition plasma choline phophoglycerides, erythrocytes, adipose tissue, and breast milk, and some indicators of susceptibility to ischemic heart disease in vegans and omnivore controls. Am J Clin Nutr 1978;31:805-13

385. Sanders T, Younger K. The effect of dietary supplements of n-3 polyunsaturated fatty acids on the fatty acid composition of platelets and plasma choline phophoglycerides. Brit J Nutr 1981;45:613-18

386. Sanders T. Dietary fat and platelet function. Clin Sci 1983;65:343-50

387. Sapolsky R. Stress, the Aging Brain, and the Mechanisms of Neuron Death. Cambridge, MA: MIT Press; 1992

387a. Sato Y et al. Reactions of cardiac postganglionic sympathetic neurons to movements of normal and inflamed joints. J Autonomic Nerv Sys 1985;12:1-13

388. Satoskar R et al. Evaluation of anti-inflammatory property of curcumin (diferuloyl methane) in patients with postoperative inflammation. Int J Clin Pharmacol ther Toxicol 1986;24(12):651-54

389. Saunders H. Physiotherapy for acute low back pain. In Kirkaldy-Willis W, Burton C. Managing Low Back Pain (3rd ed), New York: Churchill Livingstone; 1992: p.305-315

390. Say B. A panacea for all ills? Nurs Times 1991;87(15):5860

391. Schacter M. Kinins-A group of active peptides. Ann Rev Pharmacol 1964;34:60-61

392. Schaible H. Afferent and spinal mechanisms of joint pain. Pain 1993;55:5-54

393. Schechter M. Magnesium for acute MI: Although the mechanisms of its therapeutic effect are still being debated, the element seems likely to secure a place in the armamentarium against myocardial infarction. Emerg Med 1993(May):135-39

394. Schmidt K. Antioxidant vitamins and beta-carotene: effects on immunocompetence. Am J Clin Nutr 1991;53:383S-85S

395. Schmitt W. Prostaglandin E-1, E-2, and E-3 flow charts. Chapel Hill, NC, (919) 942-8516, 1986

396. Schneider C et al. Quercetin, a regulator of polymorphonuclear leukocyte functions. Adv Exp Med Biol 1979;121-:371-79

397. Schneider D et al. Fibrinolytic activity at rest and after cycle ergometry and treadmill running performed to volitional exhaustion in male triathletes. J Appl Sport Sci Res 1992;6(1):49-54

398. Schneider H. Nutrtional Suport of Medical Practice. New York: Harper and Row; 1977: p.103-106

399. Schneider M, Cohen J. Nimmo receptor tonus technique: A chiropractic approach to trigger point therapy. In Sweere J. Chiropractic Family Practice Manual. Gaithersburg, MD: Aspen Publishers; 1992: p.3.3:1-3.3:18

400. Schroeder H. Losses of vitamins and trace minerals resulting from processing and preservation of foods. Am J Clin Nutr 1971;24:562-73

401. Schwartz L.The Mast Cell. In Kelley W et al. eds. Textbook of Rheumatology (4th ed). Philadelphia: W. B. Saunders; 1993: p.304-18

402. Seaman D.,Annual ACA Council on Nutr Meeting, Orlando, FL, November/1992

403. Seaman D. Handbook for Chiropractic and Pain Control (2.2 ed). DRS SYSTEMS Inc. Hendersonville, NC; 1993

404. Sears B. Essential fatty acids and dietary endocrinology: A hypothesis for cardiovascular treatment. J Adv Med 1993;6(4):211-24

405. Sedgwick A. Initiation of the inflammatory response and its prevention. In Bonta, Bray, Parnham eds. Handbook of Inflammation, Vol 5. The Pharmacology of Inflammation. New York: Elsevier; 1985: p.227-47

406. Seelig M. Cardiovascular consequences of magnesium defiency and loss: Pathogenesis, prevalence and manifestations—Magnesium and chloride loss in refractory potassium repletion. Am J Card 1989;63:4G-21G

407. Seelig M. Consequences of magnesium deficiency on enhancement of stress reaction; Preventive and therapeutic implications (A Review). J Am Coll Nutr 1994;13(5):429-446

408. Sejersted O, Hargens A. Regional pressure and nutrition of skeletal muscle during isometric contraction. In Hargens A ed. Tissue Nutrition and Viability. New York: Springer-Verlag; 1986: p.263-83

409. Seplowitz A. Effects of lipoproteins on plasma viscosity. Atherosclerosis 1981;38:89-95

410. Shakib F. The role of IgG4 in food allergy. In Brostoff J, Challacombe S eds. Food Allergy and Intoloerance. Philadelphia: Bailliere Tindall; 1987: p.898-906

411. Sharma J. Involvement of the kinin-formation system in the physiopathology of rheumatoid inflammation. Agents Actions 1992;38(suppl/III):343-61

412. Sherman H.,The Science of Nutrition. New York: Columbia University Press; 1943

413. Shils M, Olsen J, Shike M. Modern Nutrition in Health and Disease (8th ed). Philadelphia: Lea & Febiger; 1994

414. Sierkerka J. Nutrition and biochemistry of the intervertebral dis. Chir Tech 1991;3(3):116-21

415. Siess W et al. Platelet-membrane fatty acids, platelet aggregation, and thromboxane formation during a mackerel diet. Lancet 1980;(Mar 1):441-44

416. Simmons D. Myofascial pain syndromes of the head, neck and low back. In Dubner R ed. Proceedings of the Vth World Congress on Pain. New York: Elsevier; 1988: p.186-200

417. Simopoulos A. Omega-3 fatty acids in health and disease and in growth and development. Am J Clin Nutr 1991;54:438-63

418. Sinat B. Variables affecting measurement of human red cell Na^+/K^+ ATPase activity: technical factors, feeding and aging. Am J Clin Nutr ????

419. Sinclair H. The relative importance of essential fatty acids of the linoleic and linolenic families: Studies with an eskimo diet. Prog Lipid Res 1981;20:897-99

420. Sinclair H. Essential fatty acids in perspective. Human Nutr: Clin Nutr 1984;38C:245-60

421. Sjostrom L. Morbitiy of severely obese subjects. Am J Clin Nutr 1992;55:508S-15S

422. Skover G. Cellular and biochemical dynamics of wound repair: Wound environment in collagen regeneration. Clin Pod Med Surg 1991;8(4):723-56

423. Slosberg M. Effects of altered articular afferent input on sensation, proprioception, muscle tone and sympathetic response. JMPT 1988; 11:400-8

424. Smith, L., Causes of delayed muscle soreness and the impact on athletic performance, J Appl Sport Rel Sci Res, 6(3):135-41, 1992

425. Smith N. Physical activity and dietary intakes. In White P, Mondeika T eds. Diet and Exercise: Synergism in Health and Disease. Chicago: American Medical Association; 1982: p.27-37

426. Smyth R. The systemic absorption of an orally administered proteolytic enzyme, bromelain. Am J Pharm 1961;8:294-98

427. Souba W, Wimore D. Diet and nutrition in the care of the patietn with surgery, trauma, and sepsis. In Shills M et al. Modern Nutrition in Health and Disease (8th ed). Philadelphia: W.B. Saunders; 1994: p.1207-40

427a. Sperling R. Dietary omega-3 fatty acids: Effects on lipid mediators of inflammation and rheumatoid arthritis. Rheum Dis Clin N Am 1991;17(2):373-89

428. Spiliolpoulou I. IgG and IgM concentration in the prolapsed human intervertebral disk and sciatica etiology. Spine 1994;19(12):1320-23

429. Srivastava K. Effects of aqueous extracts of onion, garlic and ginger on platelet aggregation and metabolism of arachidonic acid in the blood vascular system: In vitrol study. Prost Leuk Med 1984;13:22-35

430. Srivastava R. Effect of curcumin on platelet aggregation and vascular prostacyclin synthesis. Arzneim Forsch 1986;36(4):715-17

431. Srivastava K, Mustafa T. Ginger (Zingiber officinale) in rheumatism and musculoskeletal disorders. Med Hypoth 1992;39:342-48

432. Staal F. Glutathione deficiency and human immunodeficiency virus infection. Lancet 1992;339:883-87

433. Stewart J. Role for kinins in inflammation. In Henson P, Murphy R eds. Mediators of the Inflammatory Process. New York: Elsevier; 1989: p.189-217

434. Stewart J. Personal communication. 10/30/92

435. Stites D, Rodgers C. Clinical laboratory methods for detection of antigens and antibodies. Stites, D., Basic & Clinical Immunology (6th ed). Norwalk: Appleton & Lange; 1987: p.241-84

436. Subramanian N. Role of L-ascorbic acid on detoxifcation. Biochem Pharmacol 1973;22:1671-73

437. Suda H. Potentiative effects of a kininase II inhibitor (YS980) on carageenan-induced oedema in rat hind paw and roles of plasma kininogen. J Pharm Pharmacol 1982;34:60-61

438. Sudarsky L. Central mechanisms of fatigue. In Dawson D, Sabin T. eds. Chronic Fatigue Syndrome. Boston: Little, Brown , Co; 1993: p.109-29

439. Supplemental dietary potassium reduced the need for antihypertensive drug therapy. Nutr Rev 1992;50(5):144-45

440. Taber's Cyclopedic Medical Dictionary (16th ed). Philadelphia: F. A. Davis; 1989

441. Tate G et al. Suppression of acute and chronic inflammation by dietary gamma linolenic acid. J Rheumatol 1989;16:729-33

442. Taussig S. Bromelain: Its use in prevention and treatment of cardiovascular disease - present status. J Inter Assoc Prev Med 1979;6(1):139-51

443. Taussig S, Batkin S. Bromelain, the enzyme complex of pineapple (Ananas comosus) and its clinical application. An update. J Ethnopharmacol 1988;22:191-203

444. Tepperman J, Tepperman H. Metabolic and Endocrine Physiology (5th ed). Chicago: Year Book Medical Publishers; 1987: p.249-96

445. Terano T et al. Eicosapentanoic acid as a modulator of inflammation. Biochem Pharmacol 1986;35(5):779-85

446. Teylor T, Grover L. Forms of long-term potentiation induce by NMDA and non-NMDA receptor activation. In Baudry M et al. Synaptic Plasticity: Molecular, Cellular and Functional Aspects. Cambridge, MA: MIT Press; 1993: p.73-86

447. Thomas R. Monocytes and macrophages. In Kelley W et al. eds. Textbook of Rheumatology (4th ed). Philadelphia: W. B. Saunders; 1993: p.286-303

448. Tobian L. High potassium diets reduce stroke mortality and arterial and renal tubular lesions and sometimes even the blood pressure in hypertension. In Seldin D, Gievisch G eds. The Regulation of Potassium Balance. New York :Raven Press; 1989: p.347-68

449. Travell J, Simmons D. Myofascial Pain and Dysfunction: The Trigger Point Manual. Baltimore: Williams & Wilkins; 1983

450. Triano J. Interaction of spinal biomechanics and physiology. In Haldeman S ed. Principles and Practice of Chiropractic (2nd ed). Norwalk, CT: Appleton & Lange; 1992: p.225-57

451. Turek S. Orthopaedics: Principles and Practice (4th ed). Lippincott, Philadelphia; 1984

452. Turini M et al. Effects of fish-oil and vegetable-oil formula on aggregation and ethanolamine-containing lysophospholipid generation in activated human platelets and on leukotriene production in stimulated neutrophils, Am J Clin Nutr 1994;60:717-24

453. U.S. Dept Health & Human Services. The Surgeon General's Report on Nutrtion and Health: Summary and Recommendations, Government Printing Office; 1988

454. U.S. Government Printing Office. Dietary Goals for the United States, Select Committee on Nutrition and Human Needs - United States Senate. Washington, DC; 1977

455. Valone F. Platelets. In Kelley W et al. ed. Textbook of Rheumatology (4th ed). Philadelphia: W.B. Saunders; 1993: p.319-26

456. van den Berg W. Mechanisms of cartilage destruction in joint inflammation. Agents Actions 1993;39:49-60

457. van der Beek E et al. Thiamin, riboflavin, and vitamins B-6 and C: impact of combined restricted intake on functional performance in man. Am J Clin Nutr 1988;48:1451-62

458. Van Der Meulin, J. Present state of knowledge on processes of healing in collagen strutures. Int J Sports Med 1982;3(suppl 1):4-8

459. van Furth R. Development and distribution of mononuclear phagocytes. In Gallin, Goldstein, Snyderman eds. Inflammation: Basic Principles and Clinical Correlates (2nd ed). New York: Raven Press; 1992: p.325-39

460. Varma S. Scientific basis for medical therapy of cataracts by antioxidants. Am J Clin Nutr 1991;53:335S-45S

461. Vatassery G et al. Changes in vitamin E concentrations in human plasma and platelets with age. J Am Coll Nutr 1983;4:369-75

462. Vellini M et al. Possible involvement of eicosanoids in the pharmacological action of bromelain. Arzneim Rorsch 1986;3636:110-12

463. Venge P et al. Neutrophils and eosinophils. In Kelley W et al. eds. Textbook of Rheumatology (4th ed). Philadelphia: W. B. Saunders; 1993: p.269-85

464. Videman T. Experimental models of osteoarthritis: the role of immobilization. Clin Biomech 1987;2:223-29

465. Voelkel N. Role of platelet-derived growth factor and other growth factors in inflammation. In Henson P, Murphy R eds. Mediators of the Inflammatory Process. New York: Elsevier; 1989: p.269-99

466. Voet D, Voet J. Biochemistry. New York: John Wiley & Sons; 1990

467. von Schacky C et al. Long-term effects of dietary marine n-3 fatty acids upon plasma and cellular lipids, platelet function, and eicosanoid formation in humans. J clin Invest 1985;76:1626-31

468. Voorhees J. Leukotrienes and other lipoxygenase products in the pathogenesis and therapy of psoriasis and other dermatoses. Arch Dermatol 1983:119:541-47

469. Warso M. Lipid peroxidation in relation to prostacyclin and thromboxane physiology and pathophysiology. Brit Med Bull 1983;39(3):277-80

470. Wahl L. Inflammation. In Cohen, Diegelmann, Lindblad eds. Wound Healing: Biochemical and Clinical Aspects. Philadelphia: W.B. Saunders; 1992: p.40-62

471. Walker J et al.,Attenuation of contraction-induced skeletal muscle injury by bromelain. Med Sci Sport Exer 1992;24(1):20-25

472. Wallach J. Interpretation of Diagnostic Tests (4th ed). Boston: Little, Brown and Co; 1986: p.27

473. Weisburger J. Nutrition approach to cancer prevention with emphasis on vitamins, antioxidants, and carotenoids. Am J Clin Nutr 1991;53:226S-37S

474. Weiss L. The Cell. In Weiss L ed. Cell and Tissue Biology: A Textbook of Histology. Baltimore :Urban & Schwarzenberg; 1988: p.1-65

475. Weitzhandler M, Berfield M. Proteoglycan conjugates, In Cohen I et al. eds. Wound Healing: Biochemical & and Clinical Aspects. Philadelphia: W.B. Saunders; 1992: p.195-208

476. Werb Z. Phagocytic cells: Chemotaxis and effector function of macrophages and granulocytes. In Stites et al. eds. Basic and Clinical Immunology (6th ed). Norwalk :Appleton & Lange; 1987: p.96-113

477. Werb Z. Proteinases and matrix degradation. In Kelley W et al. eds. Textbook of Rheumatology (4th ed). Philadelphia: W. B. Saunders; 1993: p.248-68

478. West D et al. Angiogenesis induced by degradation products of hyaluronic acid. Science 1985;228:1324-26

479. Westphal S. Metabolic response to glucose ingested with various amounts of protein. Am J Clin Nutr 1990:52:267-72

480. Whalen G, Zetter B. Angiogenesis. In Cohen I et al. Wound Healing: Biochemical and Clinical Aspects. Philadelphia: W.B. Saunders; 1992: p.77-95

481. National Research Council, Recommended Dietary Allowances (10th ed.). Washington, D.C.: National Acadamy Press; 1989

482. Wiggins D. Intermediate Metabolism. Milwaukee, WI: P-L Biochemicals; 1982

483. Williams M. Internal exchanges of potassium. In Seldin D, Giebisch G eds. The Regulation of Potassium Balance. New York: Raven Press; 1989: p.3-29

484. Williams R et al. Induced thiamine (vitamin B-1) deficiency in man. Arch Int Med 1943;71:38-53

485. Willis A. Nutritional and pharmacological factors in eicosanoid biology. Nutr Rev 1981;39(8):289-301

486. Windham Guidelines - Practice Guidelines for Straight Chiropractic, World Chiropractic Alliance, Chandler, AZ, 1993

487. Woolf C. Evidence for a central component of post-injury pain hypersensitivity. Nature 1983;306:686-88

488. Woolf C. The dorsal horn: state-dependent sensory processing and the generation of pain. In Wall P, Melzack R eds. Testbook of Pain (3rd ed). New York: Churchill Livingstone; 1994: p.101-12

489. Wright S. Receptors for complement and the biology of phagocytosis. In Gallin, Goldstein, Snyderman eds. Inflammation: Basic Principles and Clinical Correlates (2nd ed). New York: Raven Press; 1992: p.477-95

490. Wyke B. The neurological basis of thoracic spinal pain. Rheum Phys Med 1970;10(7):356-67

491. Wyke B. Neurological aspects of pain therapy. In The Therapy of Pain. Swerdlow M ed. J.B. Philadelphia: Lippincott; 1980: p.1-30

492. Wyke B. Articular neurology and manipulative therapy. In Glasgow E et al. Aspects of Manipulative Therapy. New York: Churchill Livingstone; 1985: p.72-77

493. Wyke B. The neurology of low back pain. In Jayson M ed. The Lumbar Spine and Back Pain (3rd ed). Churchill Livingstone; 1987: p.56-99

494. Wyke B. Articular Neurology and the Neurology of Pain. Postgraduate Seminar at New York Chiropractic College, 6/4-5/88

495. Yaksh T, Malmberg A. Central pharmacology of nociceptive transmission. In Wall P, Melzack R ed. Testbook of Pain (3rd ed). New York: Churchill Livingstone; 1994: p.165-90

496. Yoshimoto T. Flavonoids: Potent inhibitors of arachidonate 5-lipoxygenase. Biochem Biophys Res Commun 1983;16:612-18

497. Young C. Chymoral-100 and swelling—Fact or fiction. J Am Pod Assoc 1979;69(7):421-24

498. Yu B. Free Radicals in Aging. Boca Raton, FL: CRC Press; 1993

499. Yudkin J. Evolutionary and historical changes in dietary carbohydrates. Am J clin Nutr 1967;20(2):108-15

500. Yudkin J et al. Dietary sucrose affects plasma HDL cholesterol concentration in young men. Ann Nutr Metab 1986;30:261-66

501. Yusuf S. Intravenous magnesium in acute myocardial infarction: An effect, safe, simple and inexpensive intervention. 1993;87(6):2043-46

502. Zanelli G. Proteolytic enzymes in the management of some morbid forms of angiological interest. Minerva Cardioangioloica 1974;22:379-82

503. Zeman F. Clinical Nutrition and Dietetics (2nd ed). New York: MacMillan Pub; 1993: p.6-15

504. Zimmerman M. Physiological mechanisms of pain of the musculoskeletal system. In Emre M, Mathies H eds. Muscle Spasms and Pain. Park Ridge, NJ: Parthenon Pub; 1988: p.7-17

505. Zimmerman G. Platlete-activating factor: A fluid-phase and cell-associated mediator of inflammation. In Gallin, Goldstein, Snyderman eds. Inflammation: Basic Principles and Clinical Correlates (2nd ed). New York: Raven Press; 1992: p.149-76

506. Zurier R, Ballas M. Prostaglandin E-1 (PGE-1) suppresion of adjuvant arthritis. Arth Rheum 1973;16(2):251-58

507. Zvaifler N. New perspectives on the pathogenesis of rheumatoid arthritis. Am J Med 1988;85(suppl 4A):12-17

508. Light A. The initial processing of pain and its descending control: Spinal and trigeminal systems. New York: Karger; 1992

509. Behrens F. Alteration of rabbit articular cartilage by intr-articular injection of glucocorticoids. J Bone Joint Surg (Am) 1975;57:70

510. Bentley G. Disorganization of the knees following intra-articular hydrocortisone injections. J Bone Joint Surg (Br) 1969;51:498-504

511. Borenstein D. Medical therapy of low back pain. Drug Therapy 1992;22(10):93-102.

512. Fisher D. Corticosteroid-induced avascular necrosis. J Bone Joint Surg (Am) 1971;53:859

513. Gibson G. Colitis induced by nonsteroidal anti-inflammatory drugs: report of four cases and review of the literature. Arch Int Med 1992;152:625-32

514. Gilman A, et.al. The Pharmacologic Basis of Disease (7th ed). New York: MacMillan Pub. Co; 1985

515. Goldfien A. Adrenocorticosteroids & adrenocortical antagonists. In Katzung B, editor.Basic and clinical pharmacology (3rd ed), Lange & Appleton, Norwalk, CT, 1987 p.449-60

516. Goldyne M. Prostaglandins and other eicosanoids. In Katzung B, editor. Basic and clinical pharmacology (3rd ed). Norwalk CT: Lange & Appleton; 1987: p.211-21

517. Gray R. Intra-articular corticosteroids: an updated assessment. J Orthop Relat Res 1983;177:235-63

518. Hench P. Effects of cortisone acetate and pituitary ACTH on rheumatoid arthritis, rheumatic fever and certain other conditions. Arch Int Med 1950;85:545-66

519. Kapetanos G. The effect of the local corticosteroids on the healing and biomechanical properties of the partially injured tendon. Clin Orthop Relat Res 1982;162:170-9

520. Malmberg A. Hyperalgesia mediated by spinal glutamate or substance P receptor blocked by spinal cyclo-oxygenase inhibition. Science 1992:257:1276-79

521. Manning M. Aspirin sensitivity. Postgrad Med 1991:90(5):227-33

522. Med Adv News. Arthritis unyielding to drugs. May/1991; p.26-7

523. McEvoy G. AHFS Drug Information. Bethesda, MD: American Society of Hospital Pharmacists, Inc. 1989: p.1662-85

524. Miller R. Skeletal muscle relaxants. In Katzung B, editor. Basic and clinical pharmacology (3rd ed). Norwalk, CT: Lange & Appleton; 1987: p.295-305

525. Newman N. Acetabular bone destruction related to non-steroidal anti-inflammatory drugs. Lancet 1985; (Jul 6):11-3

526. Richter J. Gastroesophageal reflux: Diagnosis and management. Hosp Practice, 1992; (Jan 15):59-66

527. Roubenoff R. Catabolic effects of high-dose corticosteroids persist despite therapeutic benefit in rheumatoid arthritis. Am J Clin Nutr 1990;52:1113-7

528. Shearn M. Nonsteroidal anti-inflammatory agents; nonopiate analgesics; drugs used in gout. In Katzung B, editor. Basic and clinical pharmacology (3rd ed). Norwalk, CT: Appleton & Lange. 1987: p.396-413

529. Silverman S. Corticosteroid-induced osteoporosis: assessment, prevention, and treatment," J Musculoskeletal Med 1990;7(7):14-27

530. Sweetnam R. Editorial and annotations, corticosteroid arthrompathy and tendon rupture. J Bone Joint Surg (Br) 1969;51:397

531. Lokken P, Skoglund L. Anti-inflammatory efficacy of treatments with aspirin and aceaminophen. PAIN 1995;60(2):231-2

532. Abbas AK, Lichtman AH, Pober JS. Cellular and molecular immunology. 3rd ed. Philadelphia: WB Saunders; 1997

533. Abernethy DR, Greenblatt DJ, Divoll M, Shader RI. Enhanced glucuronide conjugation of drugs in obesity: studies of lorazepam, oxazepam, and acetaminophen. J Lab Clin Med 1983;101:83-0

534. Abraham GE, Grewal H. A total dietary program emphasizing magnesium instead of calcium: effect on the mineral density of calcaneous bone in postmenopausal women on hormonal therapy. J Reproductive Med 1990;35:503-507

535. Adler AJ, Holub BJ. Effect of garlic and fish-oil supplementation on serum lipid and lipoprotein concentrations in hypercholesterolemic men. Am J Clin Nutr 1997; 65:445-50

536. Ali M, Thomson M. Consumption of a garlic clove a day could be benficial in preventing thrombosis. Prost Leuk Ess Fatty Acids 1995; 53:211-12

537. Altura BT Brust M, Bloom S. Magnesium dietary intake modulates blood lipid levels and atherogenesis. Proc Natl Acad Sci 1990;87:1840-44

538. American Cancer Society 1996 Advisory Committee on Diet, Nutrition, and Cancer Prevention. Nestle M, Bal D, Birt D et al. Guidelines on diet, nutrition, and cancer prevention: Reducing the risk of cancer with healthy food choices and physical activity. CA–A Cancer J Clinicians 1996;46:325-41

539. Anderson JW, Zettwoch N, Feldman T et al. Cholesterol-lowering effects of psyllium hydrophilic mucilloid for hypercholesterolemic men. Arch Int Med 1988;148:292-96

540. Anderson KE, Kappas A. Dietary regulation of cytochrome P-450. Annu Rev Nutr 1991;11:141-67

541. Anderson RA. Chromium metabolism and its role in disease processes in man. Clin Physiol Biochem 1986;4:31-41

542. Anderson RA. Nutritional factors influencing the glucose/insulin system: chromium. J Am Coll Nutr 1997; 16:404-11

543. Appendix, Table A-24A. In Shils ME, Olson JA, Shike M. eds. Modern nutrition in health and disease. 8th ed. Philadelphia: WB Saunders; 1994: p.A-135

544. Appendix, Table A-34. In Shils ME, Olson JA, Shike M. eds. Modern nutrition in health and disease. 8th ed. Philadelphia: WB Saunders; 1994: p.A-171

545. Armstrong AM, Chestnutt JE, Gormley MJ, Young IS. The effect of dietary treatment on lipid peroxidation and antioxidant status in newly diagnosed noninsulin dependent diabetes. Fre Rad Biol Med 1996; 21:719-26

546. Arnason JA, Gudjonsson H, Freysdottir J, Jonsdottir I, Valdimarsson H. Do adults with high gliadin antibody concentrations have subclinical gluten intolerance? Gut 1992; 33:194-97

547. Atalay M, laaksonen DE, Niskanen L, Uusitupa M, Hanninen O, Sen CK. Altered antioxidant enzyme defences in insulin-dependent diabetic men with increased resting and exercise-induced oxidative stress. Act Physiol Scand 1997;161(2):195-201

548. Aw TY, Jones DP. Nutrient supply and mitochondrial function. Ann Rev Nutr 1989;9:229-51

549. Barri YM, Wingo CS. The effects of potassium depletion and supplementation on blood pressure: a clinical review. Am J Med Sci 1997; 31:37-40

550. Bartoszyk GD, Wild A. Antinociceptive effects of pyridoxine, thiamine, and cyanocobalamin in rats. Ann N Y Acad Sci 1990; 585:473-76

551. Bauer JD. Clinical laboratory methods. 9th ed. St. Louis: Mosby; 1982: p.542-543

552. Beecher GR. Nutrient content of tomatoes and tomato products. Proc Soc Exp Biol med 1998;21:98-100

553. Bell RR, Spencer MJ, Sheriff JL. Voluntary exercise and monounsaturated canola oil reduce fat gain in mice fed diets high in fat. J Nutr 199;127:2006-10

554. Bergstrom E, Hernell O, Persson LA, Vessby B. Insulin resistance syndrome in adolescents. Metabolism 1996;45(7):908-14

555. Bernhardt R. Cytochrome P450: structure, function , and generation of reactive oxygen species. Rev Physiol Biochem Pharmacol 1996;127:137-221

556. Berry E. Dietary fatty acids in the management of diabetes mellitus. Am J Clin Nutr 1997; 66(suppl):991S-97S

557. Bezard J, Blond JP, Bernard A, Clouet P (1994). The metabolism and availability of essential fatty acids in animal and human tissues. Reprod. Nutr. Dev. 34(6): 539-568.

558. Bingham SA, Cassidy A, Cole TJ et al. Validation of weighed records and other methods of dietary assessment using the 24 h urine nitrogen technique and other biological markers. Brit J Nutr 1995;75:531-50

559. Bland JS, Bralley JA. Nutritional upregulation of hepatic detoxication enzymes. J Appl Nutr 1992;44:243-56

560. Block G, Patterson B, Subar A. Fruit, vegetables, and cancer prevention: a review of the epidemiological evidence. Nutr Canc 1992;18:1-29

561. Bolufer P, Gandia A, Rodriguez A, Antonio P. Salivary corticosteroids in the study of adrenal function. Clin Chim Acta 1989; 183:217-26

562. Bordia T, Mohammed N, Thomson M, Ali M. An evaulation of garlic and onion as antithrombotic agents. Prost Leuk Ess Fatty Acids 1996; 54(3):183-86

563. Borkman ML, Storlien LH, Pan DA, Jenkins, AB, Chisholm DJ, Campbell LV. The relation between insulin sensitivity and the fatty-acid composition of skeletal-muslce phospholipids. N Eng J Med 1993;328:238-44

564. Bradley H, Wating RH, Emery P, Arthur V. Metabolism of low-dose paracetamol in patients with rheumatoid arthritis. Xenobiotica 1991;21(5):689-93

565. Brenner RR. Nutritional and hormonal factors influencing desaturation of essential fatty acids. Prog Lip Res 1981; 20:41-47

566. Brockmoller J, Roots I. Assessment of liver metabolic function: clinical implications. Clin Pharmacokinet 1994;27:216-48

567. Brostoff J, Challacombe SJ. eds. Food allergy and intolerance. Philadelphia: Bailliere Tindall; 1987

568. Broughton DL, Taylor R. Review: Deterioration of glucose tolerance with age: The role of insulin resistance. Age Aging 1991;20:221-25

569. Buffington CK, Pourmotabbed G, Kitabchi AE. Case report: amelioration of insulin resistance in diabetes with dehydroepiandrosterone. Am J Med Sci 1993;306:320-24

570. Burt AM. Textbook of neuroanatomy. Philadelphia: WB Saunders; 1993

571. Caballero B. Vitamin E improves the action of insulin. Nutr Rev 1993;51:339-40

572. Calder PC. n-3 polyunsaturated fatty acids and cytokine production in health and disease. Ann Nutr Metab 1997;41(4):203-34

573. Calder PC. Dietary fatty acids and the immune system. Nutr Rev 1998; (II):S70-S83

574. Campan P, Planchard PO, Duran D. Polyunsaturated n-3 fatty acids in the treatment of experimental human gingivitis. Bull Group Int Rech Sci Stomatol Odontol 1996; 29(1-2):25-31

575. Campan P, Planchard PO, Duran D. Pilot study on n-3 polyunsaturated fatty acids in the treatment of experimental human gingivitis. J Clin Periodontol 1997; 24(12):907-13

576. Catapano AL. Antioxidant effect of flavonoids. Angiology 1997;48:39-44

577. Chandra RK. Food intolerance. New York: Elsevier; 1984

578. Chen L, Mohr SN, Yang CS. Decrease of plasma and urinary oxidative metaboites of acetaminophen after consumption of watercress by human volunteers. Clin Pharmacol Ther 1996;60:651-60

579. Clinton SK. Lycopene: chemistry, biology, and implications for human health and disease. Nutr Rev 1998; 56:35-51

580. Coleman E. Debunking the "eicotec" myth. Sports Med Dig 1993;15:6-7

581. Coleman EJ. The biozone nutrition system: a dietary panacea? Int J Sport Nutr 1996; 6:69-71

582. Coleman EJ. Carbohydrate unloading. Phys Sportsmed 1998;25:97-98

583. Coleman EJ. Carbohdrate—The master fuel. In: Berning JR, Steen SN. Eds. Nutrition for sport and exercise. Gaithersburg: Aspen Publishers; 1998: p.21-44

584. Conner E, Grisham M. Inflammation, free radicals, and antioxidants. Nutrition 1996; 12:274-77

585. Connon JJ. Celiac disease. In Shils ME, Olson JA, Shike M. eds. Modern nutrition in health and disease. 8ᵗʰ ed. Philadelphia: WB Saunders; 1994: p.1060-1065

586. Connor S, Connor W. Are fish oils beneficial in the prevention and treatment of coronary artery disease? Am J Clin Nutr 1997; 66(suppl):1020S-31S

587. Cononie CC, Goldberg AP, Rogus E, Hagberg JM. Seven consecutive days of exercise lowers plasma insulin responses to an oral glucose challenge in sedentary elderly. J Am Geriatr Soc 1994;42: 394-98

588. Corcoran GB, Racz WJ, Smith CV, Mitchell JR. Effects of N-acetylcysteine on acetaminophen covalent binding and hepatic necrosis in mice. J Pharmacol Experimental Therapeut 1985;232(3):864-72

589. Coulston AM, Liu GC, Reaven GM. Plasma glucose, insulin and lipid responses to high-carbohydrate low-fat diets in normal subjects. Metabolism 1983; 32:5256

590. Craig W. Phytochemicals: Guardians of our health. J Am Diet Assoc 1997;97(10 suppl 2):S199-S204

591. da Camara CC, Dowless GV. Glucosamine sulfate for osteoarthritis. Ann Pharmacother 1998;32(5):580-87

592. Das U. Benefical effect of EPA and DHA in the management of systemic lupus erythematosus and its relationship to the cytokine network. Prost Leuk Ess Fat Acids 1994; 51:207-13

593. Davidson MH, Maki KS, Kong JC et al. Long-term effects of consuming foods containing psyllium seed husk on serum lipids in subjects with hypercholesterolemia. Am J Clin Nutr 1998;67:367-6

594. De Castro J. Methodology, correlational analysis, and interpretation of diet diary records of the food and fluid intake of free-living humans. Appetite 1994;23:179-92

595. Decker EA. The role of phenolics, conjugated linoleic acid, carnosine, and pyrroloquinoline quinone as nonessential dietary antioxidants. Nutr Rev 1995; 53(3):49-58

596. de Feo P, Perriello G, Torlone E et al. Contribution of cortisol to glucose counterregulation in humans. Am J Physiol 1989;257:E35-E42

597. de Groot H, Rauen U. Tissue injury by reactive oxygen species and the protective effects of flavonoids. Fundam Clin Pharmacol 1998; 12(3):249-55

598. Dekkers JC, van Doornen LJ, Kemper HC. The roel of antioxidant vitamins and enzymes in the prevention of exercise-induced muscle damage. Sports Med 1996;21(3):213-38

599. de Lorgeril M, Renaud S, Mamelle N et al. Meditarranean alpha-linolenic acid-rich diet in secondary prevention of coronary artery disease. Lancet 1994;343:1454-59

600. de Lorgeril M, Salen P, Martin JL, Monjaud I, Boucher P, Mamelle N. Mediteranean dietary pattern in a randomized trial: Prolonged survival and possible reduced cancer rate. Arch Int Med 1998; 158:1181-87

601. de Lorgeril M. Mediterranean diet in the prevention of coronary artery disease. Nutrition 1998;14(1):55-57

602. Diagnos-Techs, A clinical and research laboratory. Kent, Washington. Unpublished results.

603. Diagnos-Techs, A clinical and research laboratory. Kent, Washington. Application guide

604. Diaz M, Frei B, Vita J, Keaney J. Antioxidants and atherosclerotic heart disease. New Eng J Med 1997; 337(6):408-16

605. Dolara P, Ludovici M, Salvadori M. Urinary 6-betaOH-cortisol and paracetamol metabolites as a probe for assessing oxidation and conjugation of chemicals. Pharmacol Res Comm 1987;19(4):261-73

606. Dutta-Roy AK. Insulin mediated processes in platelets, erythrocytes and monocytes/macrophages: effects of essential fatty acid metabolism. Pros Leuk Ess Fatty Acids 1994;51:385-99

607. Dvorak J, Dvorak V. Manual medicine: Diagnostics. New York: Thieme Medical Publishers; 1990

608. Eaton SB, Eaton SB, Konner MJ, Shostak M. An evolutionary perspective enhances understanding of nutritional requirements. J Nutr 1996; 126:1732-40

609. Elin R. Magnesium in health and disease. Disease-a-Month 1988(April):163-219

610. Eisinger J, Gandolfo C, Zakarian H, Ayavou T. Reactive oxygen species, antioxidant status and fibromyalgia. J Musculoskeletal Pain 1997; 5(4):5-15

611. Eliasson M, Roder M, Dinesen B, Evrin P, Lindahl B. Proinsulin, intact insulin, and fibrinolytic variables and fibrinogen in healthy subjects. Diabetes Care 1997;20(8):1252-55

612. Facchinetti F, Sances G, Borella P, Genazzani AR, Nappi G. Magnesium prophylaxis of menstrual migraine: effects on intracellular magnesium. Headache 1991;31:298-301

613. Feldman E. Nutrition and diet in the management of hyperlipidemia and atherosclerosis. In: Shils ME, Olson JA, Shike M. eds. Modern nutrition in health and disease. 8th ed. Philadelphia: WB Saunders; 1994: p.1298-1316

614. Fernandes G, Venkatraman J. Role of omega-3 fatty acids in health and disease. Nutr Res 1993; 13(suppl 1):S19-S45

615. Fickova M, Hubert P, Klimes I et al. Dietary fish oil and olive oil improve the liver insulin receptor tyrosine kinase activity in high sucrose fed rats. Endocr Regul 1994; 28:187-97

616. Flagg E, Coates R, Greenburg R. Epidemiologic studies of antioxidants and cancer in humans. J Am Col Nutr 1995; 14:419-27

617. Flynn MA, Nolph GB, Flynn TC, Kahrs R, Krause G. Efect of dietary egg on human serum cholesterol and triglycerides. Am J Clin Nutr 1979;32:1051-57

618. Folkers K, Langsjoen P, Willis R, Richardson P, Xia LJ, Ye CQ, et al. Lovastatin decreases coenzyme Q levels in humans. Proc Natl Acad Sci USA 1990;87(22):8931-34

619. Folkers K, Wolaniuk J, Simonsen R, Morishita M, Vadhanavikit S. Biochemical rationale and the cardiac response of patients with muscle disease to therapy with coenzyme Q10. Proc Natl Acad Sci USA 1985;82(13):4513-16

620. Folkers K, Wolaniuk A. Research on coenzyme Q10 in clinical medicine and in immunomodulation. Drugs Exp Clin Res 1985;11(8):539-45

621. Forbes GB. Potassium: the story of an element. Pers Biol Med 1995; 38:554-66

622. Foster-Powell K, Miller JB. International tables of glycemic index. Am J Clin Nutr 1995; 62:871S-93S

623. Garg A, Grundy SM. Should NIDDM patients be on high-carbohydrate, low fat diets? Negative. Hosp Pract 1992;27(suppl 1):11-14

624. Garg A, Bantle JP, Henry RR et al. Effects of varying carbohydrate content of diet in patients with non-insulin dependent diabetes mellitus. JAMA 1994; 271(18):1421-28

625. Garg A. High-monounsaturated-fat diets for patients with diabetes mellitus: a meta-analysis. Am J Clin Nutr 1998;67(suppl):57S-82S

626. Gartner C, Stahl W, Sies H. Lycopene is more bioavailable from tomato paste than from fresh tomatoes. Am J Clin Nutr 1997; 6:116-22

627. Gates D. The body ecology diet. Atlanta: B.E.D. Publishing; 1996

628. Gaziano JM. Antioxidants in cardiovascular disease: randomized trials. Nutrition. 1996; 12:583-88

629. Gerster H. The potential role of lycopene for human health. J Am Coll Nutr 1997;16:109-26

630. Ghirlanda G, Oradei A, Manto A, Lippa S, Uccioli L, Caputo S, et al. Evidence of plasma CoQ10-lowering effect by HMG-CoA reductase inhibitors: a double-blind, placebo-controlled study. J Clin Pharmacol 1993;33(3):226-29

631. Golay A, Eigenheer C, Morel Y, Kujawaski P, Lehmann T, de Tonnàc N. Weight-loss with low or high-carbohydrate diet? In t J Obesity 1996;20:1067-72

632. Gottlieb MS. Conservative management of spinal osteoarthritis with glucosamine sulfate and chiropractic treatment. J Manipulative Physiol Ther 1997;20(6):400-414

633. Great Smokies Medical Laboratory. Application guide: Detoxification profile. 11 pages. www.greatsmokieslab.com

634. Great Smokies Medical Laboratory. Patient information: Detoxification profile. 2 pages. www.greatsmokieslab.com

635. Grey N, Kipnis DM. Effect of diet composition on the hyperinsulinemia of obesity. N Eng J Med 1971;285:827-31

636. Grimble RF. Nutritional modulation of cytokine biology. Nutrition 1998;14:634-40

637. Grimble RF. Modulation of inflammatory aspects of immune function by nutrients. Nutrition Research 1998;18(7):1297-1317

638. Groop L, Forsblom C, Lehtovirta M. Characterization of the prediabetic state. Am J Hypertension 1997; 10:172S-80S

639. Guechot J. Lepine JP, Cohen C, Fiet J, Lemperiere T, Dreux.. Simple laboratory test of neuroendocrine disturbance in depression: 11 PM saliva cortisol. Neuropsychobiology 1987; 18:1-4

640. Guengerich FP. Effects of nutritive factors on metabolic processes involving bioactivation and detoxication of chemicals. Ann Rev Nutr 1984;4:207-31

641. Guengerich FP. Influence of nutrients and other dietary materials on cytochrome P-450 enzymes. Am J Clin Nutr 1995;61(suppl):651S-8S

642. Guengerich FP. Comparisons of catalytic selectivity of cytochrome P450 subfamily enzymes from different species. Chem Biol Interact 1997;106(3):161-82

643. Guengerich FP. Role of cytochrome P450 enzymes in drug-drug interactions. Adv Pharmacol 1997;43:7-35

644. Guyenet PG. Role of the ventral medulla oblongata in blood pressure regulation. In Loewy AD, Spyer KM. eds. Central Regulation of Autonomic Functions. New York: Oxford Univ Press; 1990: p.145-167

645. Haber B. The Mediterranean diet: a view from history. Am J Clin Nutr 199;66(suppl):1053S-57S

646. Haenni A, Ohrvall M, Lithell H. Atherogenic lipid fractions are related to ionized magnesium status. Am J Clin Nutr 1998;67:202-207

647. Halliwell B. Free radicals, antioxidants, and human disease: curiosity, cause, or consequence? Lancet 1994; 344:72124

648. Halliwell B, Evans P, Kaur H, Aruoma O. Free radicals, tissue injury, and human disease: A potential of therapeutic use of antioxidants? In: Kinney J, Tucker H. eds. Organ Metabolism and Nutrition: Ideas for Future Critical Care. New York: Raven Press, 1994:425-45

649. Halliwell B. Antioxidants in human health and disease. Ann Rev Nutr 1996; 16:33-50

650. Hannington-Kiff JG. Sympathetic nerve blocks in painful limb disorders. In Wall PD, Melzack R. eds. Testbook of pain. 3rd ed. New York: Churchill Livingtsone; 1994: p.1035-1052

651. Harakeh S, Jariwalla RJ. Ascorbate effect on cytokine stimulation of HIV production. Nutrition 1995;11:684-88

652. Harman SK, Parnell WR. The nutritional health of New Zealand vegetarian and non-vegetarian Seventh-day Adventists: selected vitamin, mineral and lipid levels. N Z Med J 1998; 111:91-94

653. Harrats D et al. Citrus fruit supplementation reduces lipoprotein oxidation in young men ingesting a diet high in saturated fat: presumptie evidence for an interaction between vitamins C and E in vivo. Am J Clin Nutr 1998; 67:240-45

654. Heafield MT, Fearn S, Steventon GB, Waring RH, Williams AC, Sturman SG. Plasma cysteine and sulphate levels in patients with motor neurone, Parkinson's and Alzheimer's disease. Neuroscience Letters 1990;110:216-20

655. Heller PH, Green PG, Tanner KD, Miao FJ, Levine JD. Peripheral neural contributions to inflammation. In: Fields HL, Liebeskind JC. Eds. Pharmacological approaches to the treatment of chronic pain: new concepts and critical issues. Progress in pain research and management. Vol 1. Seattle: IASP Press; 1994: p.31-42

656. Hertog MG, Kromhout D, Aravanis C et al. Flavonoid intake and long-term risk of cornary heart disease an cancer in the seven countries study. Arch Int Med 1995;155:381-86

657. Hibbeln JR, Salem N. Dietary polyunsaturated fatty acids and depression: when cholesterol does not satisfy. Am J Clin Nutr 1995;62:1-9

658. Hogan WJ, Kaplan R. The therapeutic effect of magnesium orotate in serum lipid reduction. J Manipulative Physiol Ther 1978;1:27-31

659. Hu FB, Stampfer MJ, Manson JE, Rimm E, Colditz GA, Rosner BA, et al. Dietary fat intake and the risk of coronary heart disease in women. N Engl J Med 1997;337:1491-9

660. Hunt T, Dunphy J.eds. Fundamentals of wound management. Norwalk (CT): Appleton & Lange; 1979: p.36

661. Hunter JO. Food allergy-or enterometabolic disorder? Lancet 1991;338:495-6

662. Ioannides C, Parke DV. The cytochromes P-448—A unique family of enzymes involved in chemical toxicity and carcinogenesis. Biochem Pharmacol 1987;36(24):4197-4207

663. Ioannides C, Parke DV. Induction of cytochrome P-4501 as an indicator of potential chemical carcinogenesis. Drug Metab Rev 1993; 25(4):485-501

664. James RC, Harbison RD, Roberts SM. Phenylpropanolamine potentiation of acetaminophen-induced hepatotoxicity: evidence for a glutathione-dependent mechanism. Toxicol Appl Pharmacol 1993;118:159-68

665. Janig W. the puzzle of "relfex sympathetic dystrophy": Mechanisms, hypotheses, open questions. In: Janig W, Stanton-Hicks M. eds. Reflex sympathetic dystrophy: A reappraisal. Progress in pain research and management. Vol 6. Seattle: IASP Press; 1996: p.1-24

666. Jansson B. Seneca County, New York: an area with low cancer mortality rates. Cancer 1981; 48:2542-46

667. Jansson B, Jankovic J. Low cancer rates among patients with Parkinson's disease. Ann Neurol 1985; 17:505-509

668. Jansson B. Geographic mappings of colorectal cancer rates: a retrospect of studies, 1974-1984. Cancer Detect Prev 1985; 8:341-48

669. Jansson B. Geographic cancer risk and intracellular potassium/sodium ratios. Cancer Detect Prev 1986; 9:171-94

670. Jansson B. Dietary, total body, and intracellular potassium-to-sodium ratios and their influence on cancer. Cancer Detect Prev 1990;14:563-65

671. Jansson B. Potassium, sodium, and cancer: a review. J Environ Pathol Toxicol Oncol 1996; 15(2-4):65-73

672. Jenkins DJA, Kendall CWC, Ransom TPP. Dietary fiber, the evolution of the human diet and coronary artery disease. Nutr Res 1998; 18:633-52

673. Jeppesen J, Schaaf P, Jones C et al. Effects of low-fat, high-carbohydrate diets on risk factors for ischemic heart disease in postmenapausal women. Am J Clin Nutr 1997; 65:1027-33

674. Jost G, Wahllander A, von Mandach U, Preisig R. Overnight salivary caffeine clearance: a liver function test suitable for routine use. Hepatology 1987;7(2):338-44

675. Jurna I, Carlson KH, Bonke D, Fu QG, Zimmerman M. Suppression of thalamic and spinal nociceptive neuronal responses by pyridoxine, thiamine, and cyanocobalamin. Ann N Y Acad Sci 1990; 585:492-95

676. Kahn J, Rubinow DR, Davis CL, Kling M, Post RM. Salivary cortisol: A practical method for evaluation of adrenal function. Biol Psychiatry 1988; 23:335-49

677. Kalmijn S, Launer LJ, Ott A, Witteman JC, Hofman A, Breteler MMB. Dietary fat intake and the risk of incident dementia in the Rotterdam study. Ann Neurol 1997;42:776-82

678. Kamikawa T, Kobayashi A, Yamashita T, Hayashi H, Yamazaki N. Effects of Coenzyme Q10 on exercise tolerance in chronic stable angina pectoris. Am J Cardiol 1985;56:247-51

679. Kanter M. Free radicals, exercise, and antioxidant supplementation. Proc Nutr Soc 1998;57:9-13

680. Karlowsky JA, Zhanel GG, Klym KA, Hoban DJ, Kabani AM. Candidemia in a Canadian tertiary car hospital from 196 to 1996. Diagn Microbiol Infect Dis 1997;29(1):5-9

681. Katan M, Zock PL, Mensink RP. Trans fatty acids and their effects on lipoprotein in humans. Annu Rev Nutr 1995;15:473-93

682. Katsouyanni K, Skalkidis Y, Petridou E, Polychronopoulou-Trichopoulou, Willet W, Trichopoulos D. Diet and peripheral arterial occlusive disease: The role of poly-, mono-, and saturated fatty acids. Am J Epidemiol 1991;133:24-31

683. Kelly GS. The role of glucosamine sulfate and chondroitin sulfates in the treatment of degenerative joint disease. Altern Med Rev 1998;3(1):27-39

684. Keltikangas-Jarvinen L, Ravaja N, Raikkonen K, Lyytinen H. Insulin resistance syndrome and autonomically mediated physiological responses to experimentally induced mental stress in adolescent boys. Metabolism 1996;45: 614-21

685. Kennedy E, Shaw A, Davis C. Essential fatty acids and USDA's food guide pyramid. Letter to the editor-reply to Siguel and Lerman. Am J Clin Nutr 1995; 62:645-46

686. Kholsa P, Hayes KC. Dietary trans-monounsaturated fatty acids negatively impact plasma lipids in humans: Critical review of the evidence. J Am Coll Nutr 196;15:325-39

687. Kimura Y, Murase M, Nagata Y. Change in glucose homeostasis in rats by long-term magnesium-deficient diet. J Nutr Sci Vitaminol 1996;42:407-22

688. Knapp H. Omega-3 fatty acids in respiratory diseases: a review. J Am Coll Nutr 1995;14(10):18-23

689. Knoke M. Fungi in the oro-intestinal tract and their scientifically founded status. Z Artztl Fortbild Qualitatssich 1998;92(3):157-62 Abstract-(German)

690. Kohlmeier L, Simonses N, van 't Veer P et al. Adipose tissue trans fatty acids and breast cancer in the European community multicenter study on antioxidants, myocardial infarctions, and breast cancer. Can Epidemiol Biomarkers Prev 1997;6(9):705-10

691. Kozlovsky AS, Moser PB, Reiser S, Anderson RA. Effects of diets high in simple sugars on urinary chromium losses. 1986;35:515-18

692. Kremer J. Clinical studies of omega-3 fatty acid supplementation in patients who have rheumatoid arthritis. Rheum Dis Clin N Am 1991;17(2):391-402

693. Kremer JM, Lawrence DA, Petrillo GF et al. Effects of fish oil on rheumatoid arthritis after stopping nonsteroidal antiinflammatory drugs. Arthr Rheum 1995;38:1107-1114

694. Kritchevsky D, Tepper SA, Klurfeld DM, Vessilinovitch D, Wissler RW. Experimental atherosclerosis in rabbits fed cholesterol-free diets. Part 12. Comparison of peanut and olive oils. Atherosclerosis 1984; 50:253-59

695. Kroker GF. Chronic candidiasis and allergy. In: Brostoff J, Challacombe SJ. eds. Food allergy and intolerance. Philadelphia: Bailliere Tindall; 1987: p. 850-872

696. Langsjoen PH, Folkers K, Lyson K, Muratsu K, Lyson T, Langsjoen P. Effective and safe therapy with coenzyme Q10 for cardiomyopathy. Klin Wochenscher 1988;66(13):583-90

697. Laudat MH, Cerdas S, Fournier D, Guiban D, Guilhaume B, Luton JP. Salivary cortisol measurement: a practical approach to assess pituitary-adrenal function. J Clin Endocrinol Metab 1988;66:343-48

698. Lauler DP. Introduction: magnesium—coming of age. Am J Cardiol 1989;63:1G-3G

699. Lee RD, Nieman DC, Rainwater M. Comparison of eight microcomputer dietary analysis programs with the USDA Nutrient Data Base for Standard Reference. J Am Diet Assoc 1995;95(8):858-67

700. Leslie K. Undesirable inflammatory responses. In: Thornborough J. ed. Inflammation I. PreTest Key Concepts Series. Volume 3. New York: McGraw-Hill, 1995: p.121-76

701. Levine J, Dardick SJ, Roizen MS, Helms MS, Basbaum AI. Contribution of sensory afferents and sympathetic efferents to joint injury in experimental arthritis. J Neurosci 1986; 6:3423-29

702. Levy G. Pharmacokinetics of salicylate elimination in man. J Pharmaceut Sci 1965;54(7):959-67

703. Levy G. Sulfate conjugation in drug metabolism: role of inorganic sulfate. Federation Proc 1986;45:2235-40

704. Lewis DF, Ioannides C, Parke DV. Molecular dimensions of the substrate binding site of cytochrome P-448. Biochem Pharmacol 1986; 35(13):2179-85

705. Lin MC, Wang EJ, Patten C, Lee MJ, Xiao F, Reuhl KR, et al. Protective effect of diallyl sulfone against acetaminophen-induced hepatotoxicity in mice. J Biochem Toxicol 1996;11(1):11-20

706. Lindahl M, Tagesson C. Flavonoids as phospholipase A2 inhibitors: importance of their structure for selective inhibition of group II phopholipase A2. Inflammation 1997;21:34-56

707. Lindberg JS, Zobitz MM, Poindexter JR, Pack CYC. Magnesium bioavailability from magnesium citrate and magnesium oxide. J Am Coll Nutr 1990;9:48-55

708. Lindh E, Ljunghall S, Larsson K, Lavo B. Screening for antibodies against gliadin patients with osteoporosis. J Internal Med 1992; 231:403-406

709. Lipworth L, Martin ME, Angell J, Hsieh AJ, Trichopoulos D. Olive oil and human cancer: an assessment of the evidence. Prev Med 1997; 26:181-90

710. Luster AD. Chemokines – chemotactic cytokines that mediate inflammation. N Eng J Med 1998;338(7):436-45

711. Machiex JJ, Fleuriet A, Billot J. Fruit phenolics. Boca Raton: CRC Press; 1990; p.272-73

712. Mader R, Deutsch H, Siebert GK, Gerbershagen HU, Gruhn E, Behl M, et al. Vitamin status on inpatients with chronic cephalgia and dysfunction pain syndrome and effects of a vitamin supplementation. Internat J Vita Nutr Res 1988;58:436-41

713. Maffetone P. Complementary sports medicine. Champaign (IL): Human Kinetics; (in press for 1999)

714. Mascolo N, Pinto A, Capasso F. Flavonoids, leucocyte migration and eicosanoids. J Pharm Pharmacol 1988;40:293-95

715. Mataix J, Quiles JL, Huertas JR, Battino M, Manas M. Tissue specific interactions of exercise, dietary fatty acids, and vitamin E in lipid peroxidation. Free Radical Biol Med 1998; 24(4):511-21

716. Mataix J, Manas M, Quiles J, Battino M et al. Coenzyme Q content depends on oxidative stress and dietary fat unsaturation. Mol Aspects Med 1997; 18(suppl):S129-35

717. Maxwell SR. Prospects for the use of antioxidant therapies. Drugs 1995; 49(3):345-61

718. McCabe RD, Bakarich MA, Srivistava K, Young DB. Potassium inhibits free radical formation. Hypertension 1994; 24:77-82

719. McCarty MF. The neglect of glucosamine as a treatment for osteoarthritis—a personal perspective. Med Hypoth 1994;42:323-27

720. McCarty MF. Magnesium taurate and fish oil for the prevention of migraine. Med Hypoth 1996;47:461-66

721. McCollister RJ, Flink EB, Lewis MD. Urinary excretion of magnesium in man following ingestion of ethanol. Am J Clin Med 1963;12:415-20

722. McGanity W, Dawson EB, Fogleman A. Nutrition in pregnancy and lactation. In: Shils M, ME, Olson JA, Shike M. eds. Modern Nutrition in Health and Disease. 8th ed. Philadelphia: WB Saunders; 1994: p.705-27

723. McGarry JD. Glucose—fatty acid interactions in health and disease. Am J Clin Nutr 1998;67(suppl):500S-504S

724. McMillan SA, Watson RP, McCrum EE, Evans AE. Factors associated with serum antibodies to reticulin, endomysium, and gliadin in an adult population. Gut 1996;39:43-47

725. Meneely GR, Battarbee HD. Sodium and potassium. Nutr Rev 1976; 34(8):225-35

726. MetaMetrix Medical Research Laboratory. Norcross, Georgia

727. Meydani M, Evans WJ. Free radicals, exercise, and aging. In: Yu,,BP. ed. Free radicals in aging. Boca Raton: DRD Press, 1993: p.183-204

728. Meydani M. Nutrition, immune cells, and atherosclerosis. Nutr Rev 1998; 56:S177-82

729. Meydani S. Effect of (n-3) polyunsaturated fatty acids on cytokine production and their biologic function. Nutrition 1996; 12:S8-S14

730. Moan A, Eide IK, Kjeldsen SE. Metabolic and adrenergic characteristics of young men with insulin resistance. Blood Press. 1996;5(Suppl 1):30-37

731. Morgan SA, O'Dea K, Sinclair AJ. A low-fat diet supplemented with monounsaturated fat results in less HDL-C lowering than a very-low-fat diet. J Am Diet Assoc 1997; 97:151-56

732. Mosca L, Rubenfire M, Mandel C, et al. Antioxidant nutrient supplementation reduces the susceptibility of low density lipoprotein to oxidation in patients with coronary artery disease. J Am Coll Cardiol 1997; 30(2):392-99

733. Muhlbauer B, Schwenk M, Coram WM et al. Magnesium-L-aspartate-HCL and magnesium-oxide: bioavailability in healthy volunteers. Eur J Clin Pharmacol 1991;40:43-3

734. Mutschler E, Derendorf H, Schager-Korting M, Elrod K, Estes KS. Drug actions. Boca Raton: CRC Press; 1995

735. Navarro MD, Periago JL, Pita ML, Hortelano P. The n-3 polyunsaturated fatty acid levels in rat tissue lipids increase in response to dietary olive oil relative to sunflower oil. Lipids 1994; 29(12):845-49

736. Nebert DW, McKinnon RA. Cytochrome P450: evolution and functional diversity. Prog Liver Dis 1994;12:63-97

737. Nettleton J. Omega-3 fatty acids and health. New York: Chapman & Hall; 1995. p.67-73

738. Newmark HL. Squalene, olive oil, and cancer risk: a review and hypothesis. Cancer Epidemiol Biomarkers Prev 1997; 6(12):1101-03

739. Nutrition Reviews editorial. Vitamin P and increased capillary fragility. Nutr Rev 1942;2:309-10

740. Nutrition Reviews. Brief critical review. Is fibromyalgia caused by a glycolysis impairment? Nutr Rev 1994;52:248-50

741. Ophir O et al. Low blood pressure in vegetarians: the possible role of potassium. Am J Clin Nutr 1983; 37:755-62

742. Orekhov AN, Grunwald J. Effects of garlic on atherosclerosis. Nutrition 1997;13:656-63

743. Orlov MV, Brodsky MA, douban S. A review of magnesium, acute myocardial infarction and arrhythmia. J Am Coll Nutr 1994;13:127-32

744. Packer L. Oxidants, antioxidant nutrients and the athlete. J Sports Sci 1997;15(3):353-63

745. Paolisso G, Sgambato S, Gambardell A et al. Daily magnesium supplements improve glucose handling in elderly subjects. 1992;55:1161-67

746. Parke DV, Ioannides C, Lewis DF. Metabolic activation of carcinogens and toxic chemicals. Hum Toxicol 1988; 7(5):397-404

747. Parker DR, Weiss ST, Troisi R, Cassano PA, Vokonas PS, Landesberg L. Relationship of dietary saturated fatty acids and body habitus to serum insulin concentrations: the normative aging study. Am J Clin Nutr 1993; 58:129-36

748. Parker LN, Levin ER, Lifrak ET. Evidence for adrenocortical adaptation to severe illness. J Clin Endocrinol Metab 1985;60:947-52

749. Parkinson D. Adrenergic receptors in the autonomic nervous system. In Loewy AD, Spyer KM. eds. Central Regulation of Autonomic Functions. New York: Oxford Univ Press; 1990: p.17-27

750. Patel DK, Ogunbona A, Notarianni, Bennett PN. Depletion of plasma glycine and effect of glycine by mouth on salicylate metabolism during aspirin overdose. Human Exp Toxicol 1990;9:389-95

751. Patel M, Tang BK, Kalow W. Variability of acetaminophen metabolism in caucasians and orientals. Pharmacogenetics 1992;2:38-45

752. Patel M, Tang BK, Grant DM, Kalow W. Interindividual variability in the glucuronidation of (S) oxazepam contrasted with that of (R) oxazepam. Pharmacogenetics 1995;5:287-97

753. Peet M et al. Essential fatty acid deficiency in erythrocyte membranes from chronic schizophrenic patients, and the clinical effects of dietary supplementation. Prost Leuk Ess Fat Acids 1996;55(1&2):71-75

754. Peet M, Murphy B, Shay J, Horrobin D. Depletion of omega-3 fatty acid levels in red blood cell membranes of depressive patients. Biol Psychiatry 1998;43:315-19

755. Pelletier X, Thouvenot P, Belbraouet S et al. Efect of egg consumption in healthy volunteers: influence of yolk, white or whole-egg on gastric emptying and on glycemic and hormonal responses. Nutr Metab 1996; 40:109-15

756. Percival M. Nutritional support for detoxification. Clin Nutr Insights. Advanced Nutrition Publications; 1998

757. Perseghin G, Ghosh S, Gerow K, Shulman GI. Metabolic defects in lean nondiabetic offspring of NIDDM parents: a cross sectional study. Diabets 1997;46:1001-1009

758. Peterson DB. Long-chain fatty acids and cardiovascular disease risk in non-insulin-dependent-diabetes. Nutrition 1998; 316-18

759. Petroni A, Blasevich M, Salami M, Papini N, Montedoro GF, Galli C. Inhibition of platelet aggregation and eicosanoid production by phenolic components of olive oil. Thromb Res 1995; 78(2):151-60

760. Pierno S, DeLuca A, Tricarico D, Roselli A, Natuzzi F, Ferrannini E, et al. Potential risk of myopathy by HMG-CoA reductase inhibitors: a comparison of pravastatin and simvastatin effects on membrane electrical properties of rat skeletal muscle fibers. J Pharmacol Exp Ther 1995;25(3):1490-96

761. Plotnick GD, Corretti MS, Bogel RA. Efect of antioxidant vitamins on the transient impairment of endothelium-dependent brachial artery vasoactivity following a single high-fat meal. JAMA 1997; 28:1682-86

762. Pressman AH. Metabolic toxicity and neuromuscular pain, joint disorders, and fibromyalgia. ACA J Chiro 1993; (Sept):77-78

763. Preuss H. Effects of glucose/insulin perturbations on aging and chronic disorders of aging: the evidence. J Am Coll Nutr 1997;16(5):397-403

764. Raitakaari OT, Porkka KV, Ronnemaa T et al. The role of insulin of serum lipids and blood pressure in children and adolescents. The cardiovascular risk in young Finns study. Diabetologia 1995;38:1042-50

765. Ramadan NM, Halvorson H, Vande-Linde A, Levine SR, Helpern JA, Welch KMA. Low brain magnesium in migraine. Headache 1989; 29:590-93

766. Rang HP, Perkins MN. The role of B1 and B2 bradykinin receptors in inflammatory pain. In : Borsook D. ed. Molecular neurobiology of pain. Seattle: IASP Press; 1997: p.221-23

767. Reaven GM. Role of insulin resistance in human disease. Diabetes 1988; 37:1595-1607

768. Reaven GM. Pathophysiology of insulin resistance in human disease. Physiol Rev;1995; 75:473-86

769. Reaven GM. Do high carbohydrate diets prevent the development or attenuate the manifestations (or both) of syndrome X? A viewpoint strongly against. Curr Opin Lipid 1997; 8:23-27

770. Renaud SC. Dietary management of cardiovascular diseases. Prost Leuk Essent Fatty Acids 1997;(57):423-27

771. Renner E, Wietholtz H, Huguenin P, Arnaud MJ, Preisig R. Caffeine: a model compound for measuring liver function. Hepatology 1984;4(1):38-46

772. Riales R, Albrink M. Effect of chromium chloride supplementation on glucose tolerance and serum lipids including high-density lipoprotein of adult men. Am J Clin Nutr 1981;34:2670-78

773. Ridker PM, Cushman M, Stampfer MJ, Tracy RP, Hennekens CH. Inflammation aspirin and the risk of cardiovascular disease in apparently healthy men. New Eng J Med 1997;336:973-79

774. Robbins RC. Flavones in citrus exhibit antiadhesive action on platelets. Internat J Vit Nutr Res 1988;58:418-22

775. Roberts S, Eisenstein SM, Megae J, Evans EH, Ashton IK. Mechanoreceptors in intervertebral discs. Spine 1995;20:2645-51

776. Robinson D, Mirovsky Y, Halperin N, Evron Z, Nevo Z. Changes in proteoglycans of intervertebral disc in diabetic patients. Spine 1998; 23(8):849-56

777. Rogers M, King DS, Hagberg JM, Ehsani AA, Holloszy JO. Effect of 10 days of physical inactivity on glucose tolerance in masters athletes. J Appl Physiol 1990;68:1833-37

778. Rose D. Dietary fatty acids and cancer. Am J Clin Nutr 1997; 66(suppl):998S-1003S

779. Rosolova H, Mayer O Jr, Reaven G. Effect of variations in plasma magnesium concentration on resistance to insulin-mediated glucose disposal in nondiabetic subjects. J Clin Endocrinol Metab 1997;82:3783-85.

780. Ross R. The pathogenesis of atherosclerosis: a perspective for the 1990s. Nature 1993;362:801-809

781. Rude RK. Physiology of magnesium metabolism and the important role of magnesium in potassium deficiency. Am J Cardiol 1989;63:31G-34G

782. Rude RK. Magnesium deficiency: a cause of heterogenous disease in humans. J Bone Min Res 1998; 13:749-58

783. Ruderman NB, Schneider SH, Berchtold P. The "metabolically-obese," normal-weight individual. Am J Clin Nutr 1981;34:1617-621

784. Rudin D. The major psychoses and neuroses as omega-3 essential fatty acid deficiency syndrome: substrate pellagra. Med Hypoth 1981; 16(9):837-50

785. Rudin D. The dominant diseases of modernized societies as omega-3 fatty essential fatty acid deficiency syndrome: Substrate beriberi. Med Hypoth 1982;8:17-47

786. Ruiz-Gutierrez V, Morgado N, Prada JL, Perz-Jimenez F, Muriana FJ. Composition of human VLDL triacylglycerols after ingestion of olive oil and high oleic safflower oil. J Nutr 1998; 128(3):570-76

787. Salmeron J, Ascherio A, Blum EB et al. Dietary fiber, glycemic load, and risk of NIDDM in men. Diab Care 1997; 20:545-550

788. Salomaa V, Salminen I, Rasi V, Vahtera E, Aro A, Myllyla G. Association of the fatty acid composition of serum phospholipids with hemostatic factors. Aterioscler Thromb Vas Biol 1997;17:809-13

789. Sampugna J, Teter BB. Trans fatty acid content should be included on food labels. J Am Coll Nutr 1996; 15:321-322

790. Schoenthaler S. Malnutrition and maladaptive behavior: Two correlational anlayses and a double-blind placebo-controlled challenges in five states. In: Essman W. ed. Nutrients and brain function. New York: Karger, 1987: p.198-218

791. Schwieger G, Karl H, Schonhaber E. Relapse prevention of painful vertebral syndromes in follow-up treatment with combination of vitamins B1, B6, and B12. Ann N Y Acad Sci 1990; 585:540-42

792. Scott RD. The clinical importance of magnesium. Scot Med J 1976;21:9-10

793. Seaman DR. Letter to editor. Spine 1996;21:1609-10

794. Seaman DR. Proprioceptor: an obsolete, inaccurate word. J Manipulative Physiol Ther 1997;20:279-84

795. Seaman DR. Joint Complex Dysfunction, a novel term to replace subluxation/subluxation complex: Etiological and treatment considerations. J Manipulative Physiol Ther 1997;20:634-44

796. Seaman DR, Wintestein JF. Dysafferentation: a novel term to describe the neuropathophysiological effects of joint complex dysfunction. A look at likely mechanisms of symptom generation. J Manipulative Physiol Ther 1998; 21:267-80

797. Seaman DR, Cleveland CS. Spinal pain syndromes: nociceptive, neuropathic, and psychologic mechanisms. J Manipulative Physiol Ther (in press)

798. Seaman DR. How can you and your patients profit from nutrition? Chiro Econ 1998; (Mar/April):72-77,91-92

799. Sears B. The Zone. New York: Harper Collins, 1995

800. Sears B. Essential fatty acids, eicosanoids, and cancer. In Quillin P, Williams R. eds. Adjuvant nutrition in cancer treatment. Arlington Heights (IL): Cancer Treatment Research Foundation; 1993:267-82

801. Seidell JC. Dietary fat and obesity: an epidemiologic perspective. Am J Clin Nutr 1998;67:3 (suppl):546S-550S

802. Sen CK. Oxidants and antioxidants in exercise. J Appl Physiol 1995; 79(3):675-86

803. Shaw A, Fulton L, Davis C, Hogbin M. Using the food guide pyramid: a resource for nutrition educators. US Department of Agriculture. Food, Nutrition, and Consumer Services. Center for Nutrition Policy and Promotion. Downloaded from the website of the USDA. (www.nal.usda.gov/fnic/Fpyr/pyramid.html)

804. Sheehan J. Importance of magnesium chloride repletion after myocardial infarction. Am J Cardiol 1989;63:35G-38G

805. Shils ME. Magnesium. In Shils ME, Olson JA, Shike M. eds. Modern nutrition in health and disease. 8th ed. Philadelphia: WB Saunders, 1994: p.164-84

806. Shimada T, El-Bayoumy K, Upadhyaya P, Sutter TR, Guengerich FP, Yamazaki H. Inhibition of human cytochrome P450-catalyzed oxidation of xenobiotics and procarcinogens by synthetic organoselenium compounds. Cancer Res 1997;57(21):4757-64

807. Siguel EN, Lerman RH. Role of essential fatty acids: dangers in the US Department of Agriculture dietary recommendations ("pyramid") and low-fat diets. Letter to the editor. Am J Clin Nutr 1994; 60:973-74

808. Siguel EN, Lerman RH. Letter to the editor-Reply to Kennedy et al. Am J Clin Nutr 1995; 62:646-47

809. Simopoulos AP. Fatty acid composition of skeletal muscle membrane phosopholipids, insulin resistance and obesity. Nutr Today 1994; 29:12-16

810. Simopoulos AP. The role of fatty acids in gene expression: health implications. Ann Nutr Metab 1996;40:303-11

811. Simopoulos AP. Robinson J. The Omega Plan. New York: HarperCollins; 1998: p.25

812. Singh RB, Gupta UC, Mittal N, Niaz MA, Ghosh S, Rastogi V. Epidemiologic study of trace elements and magnesium on risk of coronary artery disese in rural and urban Indian populations. J Am Coll Nutr 1997; 16:62-67

813. Smilkstein MJ, Douglas DR, Daya MR. Acetaminophen poisoning and liver function [letter]. N Engl J Med 1994; Nov 10:1310-11

814. Smilkstein MJ, Knapp GL, Kulig KW, Rumack BH. Efficacy of oral N-acetylcysteine in the treatment of acetaminophen overdose. Analysis of national multicenter study (1976 to 1985). N Engl J Med 1988;319(24):1557-62

815. Sorkin LS, Xiao WH, Wagner R, Myers RR. Tumour necrosis factor-alpha induces ectopic activity in nociceptive primary afferent fibres. Neuroscience 1997;81(1):255-62

816. Steinmetz K, Potter J. Vegetables, fruit, and cancer prevention: A review. J AM Diet Assoc 1996;96:1027-39

817. Stenson WF, Cort D, Beeken W et al. Dietary supplementation with fish oil in ulcerative colitis. Ann Int Med 1992; 116:609-13

818. Steventon GB, Heafield MTE, Waring RH, Williams AS, Sturman S, Green M. Metabolism of low-dose paracetamol in patients with chronic neurological disease. Xenobiotica 1990;20(1):117-22

819. Steventon GB, Heafield MT, Waring RH, Williams AC. Xenobiotic metabolism in Parkinson's disease. Neurology 1989;39:883-7

820. Stoll BA. Macronutrient supplements may reduce breast cancer risk: how, when, which? Eur J Clin Nutr 1997;51:573-77

821. Stoll BA. Essential fatty acids, insulin resistance, and breast cancer risk. Nutr Cancer 1998; 31:2-7

822. Stone J, Doube A, Dudson D, Wallace J. Inadequate calcium, folic acid, vitamin E, zinc, and selenium intake in rheumatoid arthritis patients: results of a dietary survey. Semin Arthritis Rheum 1997;27(3):180-85

823. Storlien LH, Kriketos AD, Calvert GD, Baur LA, Jenkins AB. Fatty acids, triglycerides and syndromes of insulin resistance. Prost Leuk Ess Fatty Acids 1997;57:379-85

824. Sugawa M et al. Oxidized low density lipoprotein caused by CNS neuron cell death. Brain Res 1997; 61:165-72

825. Sugita M, Aikawa H, Suzuki K, Yamasaki T, Minowa H, Etoh R, et al. Urinary hippuric acid excretion in everyday life. Tokai J Exp Clin Med 1988;13(4):185-90

826. Suter PM. Potassium and hypertension. Nutr Rev 1998; 56(5):151-53

827. Talent JM, Gracy RW. Pilot study of oral polymeric N-acetyl-D-glucosamine as a potential treatment for patients with osteoarthritis. Clin Ther 1996;18(6):1184-90

828. Thomas GD, Hansen J, Victor RG. ATP-sensitive potassium channels mediate contraction-induced attenuation of sympathetic vaoconstriction in rat skeletal muscle. J Clin Invest 1997;99(1):2602-09

829. Thomas GD, Victor RG. Nitric oxide mediates contraction-induced attentuation of sympathetic vasoconstriction in rat skeletal muscle. J Physiol (lond): 1998;506(Pt 3):817-826

830. Thomas P. ed. Weighing the options: Criteria for evaluating weight-management programs. Washington: Academic Press, 1995:186

831. Timbrell JA. Principles of biochemical toxicology. 2nd ed. London: Taylor & Francis; 1991

832. Torjesen PA, Birkeland KI, Anderssen SA et al. Lifestyle changes may reverse development of the insulin resistance syndrome. Diab Care 1997;20:2631

833. Towle HC, Kaytor EN, Shih H. Regulation of the expression of lipogenic enzyme genes by carbohydrate. Ann Rev Nutr 1997;17:405-33

834. Trichopoulou A, Katsouyanni K, Stuver S et al. Consumption of oilive oil and specific food groups in relation to breast cancer risk in Greece. J Natl Cancer Inst 1995;7:110-16

835. Tsuyusaki T, Noro C, Kikawada R. Mechanocardiography of ischemic or hypertensive heart failure. In: Yamamura Y, Folkers K, Ito Y. eds. Biomedical and clinical aspects of coenzyme Q. Vol 2. New York: Elsevier; 1980: p.273-88

836. van de Vijver LPL, Kardinaal AFM, Grobbee DC, Princen HMG, van Poppel G. Lipoprotein oxidation, antioxidants and cardiovascular risk: epidemiologic evidence. Prost Leuk Essen Fat Acids 1997; 57(4&5):479-87

837. van der Beek EJ, van Dokkum W, Wedel M, Schrijver J, van den Gerg H. thiamin, riboflavin and vitamin B6: impact of restricted intake on physical performance in man. J Am Coll Nutr 1994;13:629-40

838. Varma RS. Dietary bioflavonoids, chalcones, and related alkenones in prevention and treatment of cancer. Nutrition 1996;12(9):643-45

839. Vining R, McGinley R. The measurement of hormones in saliva: Possibilities and pitfalls. J Steroid Biochem 1987; 27(1-3):81-94

840. Vinson JA, Dabbagh YA. Tea phenols: antioxidant effectiveness of teas, tea components, tea fractions and their binding with lipoproteins. Nutr Res 1998;18:1067-75

841. Visioli F, Bellomo G, Mantedoro G, Galli C. Low density lipoprotein oxidation is inhibited in vitro by olive oil constituents. Atherosclerosis 1995; 117:25-32

842. Visioli F, Galli C. The effect of minor constituents of olive oil on cardiovascular disease: new findings. Nutr Rev 1998;56:142-47

843. Vorster HV, Benade AJ, Barnard HC et al. Egg intake does not change plasma lipoprotein and coagulation profiles. Am J Clin Nutr 1992; 55:400-410

844. Walker KZ, O'Dea K, Johnson L et al. Body fat distribution and non-insulin-dependent diabetes: comparison of a fiber-rich, high-carbohydrate, low-fat (23%) diet and a 35% fat diet high in monounsaturated fat. Am J Clin Nutr 1996;63:254-60

845. Walker R. Salivary cortisol determinations in the assessment of adrenal activity. Front Oral Physiol 1984; 5:33-50

846. Wall SD, Jones B. Gastrointestinal tract in the immunocompromised host: opportunistic infections and other complications. Radiology 1992;185:32-35

847. Watson RG, McMillan SA, Dickey W, Biggart JD, Porter KG. Detection of undiagnosed coeliac disease with atypical features using antireticulin and antigliandin antibodies. Q J Med 1992; 84(305):713-18

848. Weiss EL. Connective tissue in wound healing. McCulloch JM, Kloth LC, Feedar JA. Wound healing: Alternatives in management. 2nd ed. Philadelphia: FA Davis; 1995: p.16-31

849. Wells AS, Read NW, Langharne JDE, Ahluwalia NS. Brit J Nutr 1998;79:23-30

850. Wester PO, Dyckner T. The importance of the magnesium ion. Magnesium deficiency-symptomatology and occurrence. Acta Med Scand (Suppl)1982;661:3-4

851. Willet WC. Is dietary fat a major determinant of body fat. Am J Clin Nutr 1998;67(suppl):556S-62S

852. Wiseman SA, Mathot JN, de Fouw NJ, Tijburg LB. Dietary non-tocopherol antioxidants present in extra virgin olive oil increase the resistance of low density lipoproteins to oxidation in rabbits. Atherosclerosis 1996; 120(1-2):15-23

853. Wolever TM, Katzman-Relle L, Jenkins AL, Vuksan V, Josse RG, Jenkins DJ. Glycaemic index of 102 complex carbohydrate foods in patients with diabetes. Nutr Res 1994; 14:651-69

854. Wolever TM. The glycemic index: flogging a dead horse? Diab Care 1997;20:452-56

855. Wolk A, Bergstrom R, Hunter D et al. A prospective study of association of monounsaturated fat and other types of fat with risk of breast cancer. Arch Int Med 1998;158:41-45

856. Xiao W, Wagner R, Myers RR, Sorkin LS. Tumor necrosis factor alpha applied to the sciatic nerve trunk elicits background firing in nociceptive primary afferents. In: Jensen TS, Turner JA, Wiesenfeld-Hallin Z. eds. Proceedings 8th World Congress on Pain. Progess Pain Research Management, Vol 8. Seattle: IASP Press; 1997:293-302

857. Yam D, Eliraz A, Bery EM. Diet and disease—The Israeli paradox: possible dangers of a high omega-6 polyunsaturated fatty acid diet. Isr J Med Sci 1996;32:1134-1143

858. Yang CS, Yoo JSH. Nutrition and hepatic xenobiotic metabolism. In: Rowland IR. ed.. Nutrition, toxicity and cancer. Boca Raton: CRC Press; 1991:p.53-91

859. Yaqoob P, Knapper JA, Webb DH, Williams CM, Newsholme EA, Calder PC. Effect of olive oil on immune function in middle-aged men. Am J Clin Nutr 1998;67:129-35

860. Yasuma T, Arai K, Suzuki F. Age-related phenomena in the lumbar intervertebral discs: Lipofuscin and amyloid deposition. Spine 1992;17(10):1194-98

861. Young DB, Huabao L. McCabe RD. Potassium's cardiovascular protective mechanisms. Am J Physiol 1995; 268:R825-37

862. Zehender M, Meinertz T, Faber T. Antiarrhythmic effects of increasing the daily intake of magnesium and potassium in patients with frequent ventricular arhythmias. J Am Coll Cardiol 1997;29:1028-34

863. Zhang H, Osada K, Maebashi M, Ito M, Komai M, Furukawa Y. A high biotin diet improves the impaired glucose tolerance of long-term spontaneously hyperglycemic rats with non-insulin-dependent diabetes mellitus. J Nutr Sci Vitaminol 1996;42:517-26

864. Zhang H, Osada K, Sone H, Furukawa Y. Biotin administration improves impaired glucose tolerance of streptozotocin-induced diabetic wistar rats. J Nutr Sci Vitaminol 1997;43:271-80

865. Zimmerman M, Bartoszyk GD, Bonke D, Jurna I, Wild A. Antinociceptive properties of pyridoxine: neurophysiological and behavioral findings. Ann NY Acad Science 1990;585:219-30

866. Zimmet PZ, Collins VR, Dowse GK, Knight LT. Hyperinsulinaemia in youth is a predictor of Type 2 (non-insulin-dependant) diabetes mellitus. Diabetologia 1992;35:534-41

Appendix A

NUTRITION EDUCATION FOR PATIENTS

#1 – NUTRITION AND PAIN CONTROL

Express to your audience that today/tonight they are going to learn about health and nutrition, and how poor dietary habits can promote pain syndromes and joint restriction. Explain that chiropractors adjust joints that are stiff and restricted from moving normally, and that the adjustment restores motion to restricted joints which improves biomechanical and neurological function. This presentation, entitled Nutrition and Pain Control, will demonstrate how proper nutrition promotes a healthy body chemistry that can, in turn, help

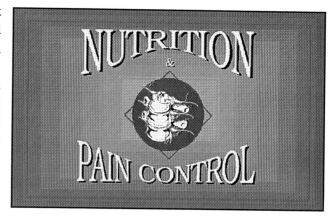

to biochemically eliminate pain and joint complex dysfunction. State that it is true that what we eat can influence pain and joint function.

Have your audience take note of the picture of the spinal cord on this slide and state that the information contained in this presentation is based upon well known principles of neurology and biochemistry, which will be translated into laymen's terms for easy understanding.

Go to the next slide.

NOTES:

#2 – OHH THE PAIN

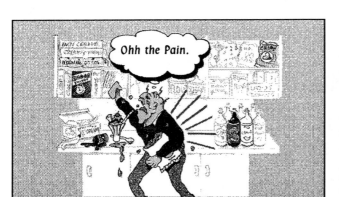

Ask your audience, how many of us here today/tonight believe that what we eat directly relates to the aches/pain we experience? Regardless of how many people agree or disagree, skepticism about this topic abounds in most peoples minds. Most people simply do not believe that there is a relationship between what we eat and the experience of pain. Thus, people do not want to believe what they see in slide #2. The basic problem is that people do not want to give up munching on all the goodies that are stockpiled in the cupboard.

Tell your audience that by the end of this presentation, they will see very clearly how proper nutrition can help reduce pain and joint restriction. Everyone should listen closely and take the information to heart because eating properly can help reduce the need to be adjusted which can save [patients] a lot of money.

Go to the next slide.

♦ For the Doctor ♦

I myself have been told by numerous DCs, MDs, PhDs and laymen that such a relationship does not exist. The point is that we should be prepared for such skepticism from the people in our audiences, especially if we address groups with backgrounds in science.

We as presenters of this information should appreciate that nutrition is the last mode of therapy that most people would associate with the treatment of pain. This is very reasonable because there is not a great deal of research that directly discusses the topic of nutrition and pain control, much less, the topic of nutrition and joiny complex dysfunction. However, there are countless articles which discuss the biochemistry of pain/pain control, and there are countless articles which discuss the relationship between nutrition and biochemistry. By linking the data from each specialty, we can examine the nutritional biochemistry of pain control, which can be extrapolated to help define the nutritional biochemistry of the joint complex dysfunction. This is very important, because ultimately we are not only making nutritional recommendations to fight pain. Rather, I believe that we should provide nutritional recommendations to help our patients pursue health, and also for the purpose of biochemically reducing joint complex dysfunction.

NOTES:

#3 – YOU ARE WHAT YOU EAT

Ask your audience- How many of us here today/tonight have heard the following statement: "You are what you eat." Wait for their response and state, "unfortunately most people do not take this fundamental truth to heart." Ask your audience if they believe this statement is true. Continue and ask for a show of hands to see how many consider this biological fact as they eat their meals. Regardless of your audience's response, the truth is that very few, at best, consider that "they are what they eat."

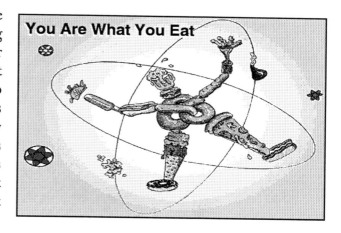

We need to consider the degree to which ignoring this fact can detrimentally influence a normal healthy existence. <u>The Surgeon General's Report on Nutrition and Health</u>, which was published in 1988, states that heart disease, cancer and strokes are the three leading causes of death in America, totaling close 75% of all deaths. We are also told that these are diet-related diseases. The Report concludes, "one personal choice seems to influence long-term health prospects more than any other: what we eat"[1].

The only problem with this information is that we, in today's day and age, rarely if ever seriously think about how our current habits, such as eating, affect our long term well-being. We also tend to have a false sense of invulnerability and therefore, do not pay attention to nutritional recommendations. Concerning this issue, a <u>New York Times</u> article discussed the results of a poll which questioned dietary habits. "Among the most startling findings is that people age 18 to 29 – the generation that grew up amid a flood of nutrition research – have poorer eating habits than their elders"[2]. The truth is that, on a national level, our intake of health-promoting foods such as fresh fruits, vegetables and whole grains is grossly inadequate[3]. This is very sad. Consider how we act when friends or family members become ill. We run to the doctor for a cure, and often go as far as to blame doctors for not having adequate therapies. This is very unfair. We must realize that because most diseases can be prevented by adopting a healthy life-style, most of our so-called health problems are self-inflicted.

A lot of people cannot take such a pointed explanation. Thus, in a humorous manner, we must appeal to our audience's ability to reason and think logically. Tell your audience to look at the Pretzel Man. Explain that, in reality, if you eat only pretzels for a year, you won't really turn into a pretzel, or a can of beer, or a hot dog. However, pretzels, beer and hot dogs are deficient in a variety of nutrients which are required for the maintenance of healthy tissues. Thus, normal tissue repair can be hampered and the result is unhealthy cells/tissues/organs, and such is the case of the man in the next slide...

Go to the next slide.

1.   <u>The Surgeon General's Report on Nutrition and Health</u>, U.S. Dept. Health & Human Services, U.S. Government Printing Office, Wash., DC., 1988
2.   Burros, M., *"What Americans Really Eat: Nutrition Can Wait,"* p.C1 & C6, <u>The New York Times</u>, 1/6/88
3.   Block, G., *"Dietary guidelines and the results of food consumption surveys,"* <u>Am J Clin Nutr</u> 53:356S-57S, 1991

#4 – THE UNHEALTHY MAN

This slide clearly depicts the average American...a sedentary pill-popping junkfood-junkie. Compare this individual with...

Go to the next slide.

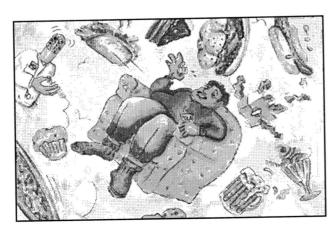

♦ *For the Doctor* ♦

The gentleman in this slide can be characterized as obese. Obesity is defined as body weight 20% or more above desirable levels in women and 25% or more above desirable levels in men[1]. In 1980 there were approximately 34 million obese adults in the United States[2]. Realize that this number does not include the millions of children who are obese or the countless adults who are moderately overweight.

The overweight condition has an enormous economic impact on our society. Obesity is associated with increased risk of non-insulin-dependent diabetes mellitus, hypertension, cardiovascular disease, gallbladder disease and cholecystectomy, and colon and postmenopausal breast cancer. A conservative estimate of the economic costs of obesity was $39.3 billion, for the year of 1986 [2].

Consider the following quote: "Visceral obesity constitutes one subgroup at high risk. It seems possible to link diabetes, hypertriglyceridemia, *reduced fibrinolysis*, and hypertension to elevated portal free fatty acid concentrations because of an increased visceral adipose tissue depot[3]." Notice that *reduced fibrinolysis* has been italicized. This is very important information because an emerging body of research suggests that a metabolic defect in fibrinolytic activity is associated with the development of chronic pain syndromes[4,5]. See Chapter 8 for more information concerning this topic.

Regarding the treatment of obesity, it seems that Richard Simmons' approach is the most successful. He has people make healthy meal choices and exercise regularly.

In my experience, I have found that fat/weight loss is a natural by-product of a diet rich in vegetables and fruits. In my opinion, the best way to manage an overweight/obese patient is to make sure that they eat large quantities of vegetables and fruits, and exercise everyday.

Go to the next slide

1.   Zeman, F., <u>Clinical Nutrition and Dietetics</u> (2nd ed), p.479, MacMillan Pub, New York, 1991
2.   Colditz, G., *"Economic costs of obesity,"* <u>Am J Clin Nutr</u> 55:503S-7S, 1992
3.   Sjostrom, L., *"Morbidity of severely obese subjects,"* <u>Am J Clin Nutr</u> 55:508S-15S, 1992
4.   Jayson, M., *"Chronic inflammation and fibrosis in back pain syndromes,"* p.411-18, in Jayson, M., editor, <u>The Lumbar Spine and Back Pain</u> (3rd ed), Churchill Livingstone, New York, 1987
5.   Haaland, A., *"Fibrinolytic activity as a predictor of the outcome of prolapsed intervertebral lumbar disc surgery with reference to background variables: Results of a prospective cohort study,"* <u>Spine</u> 17(9):122-27, 1992

NOTES:

#5 – THE HEALTHY MAN

Ask you audience: Do you think the sedentary pill-popping junkfood-junkie or the man in this slide would be more likely to have aches, pains and other health problems? Wait for their response. Most will state that the man on the previously slide is more likely to be sick. Ask your audience another question: Knowing this to be the case, why do most of us not take better care of ourselves? Why is it that we choose to eat poorly, especially when we all know that foods like fruits and vegetables should be consumed rather than grease burgers and desserts? To answer this question honestly is very difficult. Most people will make a lighthearted comment and state that they just cannot help themselves. I believe most people eat poorly because they have yet to be given a good reason to eat properly.

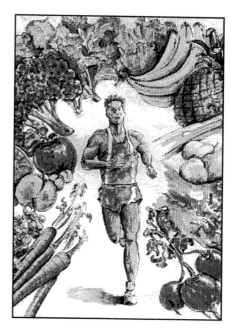

The point to get across to your audience before moving to the next slide is that the more healthy, fit and trim we are, the less likely we are to have aches, pains and other ailments. Ask your audience: "Speaking of health and fitness, raise your hand if you believe that you are basically healthy?" In response to this question, you will see some of the sickest looking people raise their hands.

Go to the next slide.

NOTES:

#6 – WHAT IS HEALTH?

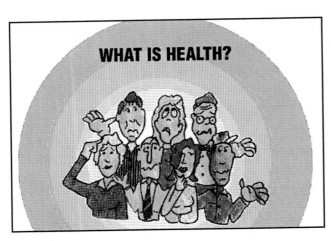

Ask your audience: What is health? Then, ask those who raised their hands to define the word "health" for the rest of the audience. You will find out that virtually no one knows the correct definition of health.

Most people say that health is freedom from disease and/or feeling good. State that, no one has given us the correct definition of health, yet many people claim that they are healthy. Then ask your audience another question: "If we do not know the definition of health then how can we claim to be healthy?" Let this one sink into their minds for a little while. You will probably get many blank stares.

Continue by stating that very few of us have been given accurate information about health, and therefore, we should not assume that we are healthy, especially if we do not know what the word means. Before moving to the next slide, explain that your reason for discussing the topic of health is that only unhealthy people are in pain, and this will become more clear as your presentation continues.

Go to the next slide.

♦For the Doctor♦

In the past several years, I have personally asked thousands of lay people and many doctors to define the word health, and no one has **EVER** given me the correct definition as stated by the World Health Organization or Dorland's Medical Dictionary. Do you know the correct definition? This brings up a very important point. If we as so-called health-care practitioners cannot properly define the word health, then is it really accurate to characterize ourselves as health-care practitioners?

As painful as it is to admit, we are all predominately disease-care doctors, and this is especially true if we do not recommend life-style management to our patients. For years, we as chiropractors have stated that medical treatment (i.e., drugs and surgery) only masks a patients symptoms and never gets to the cause. At the same time we tend to glorify ourselves and claim that chiropractic eliminates the cause of ill-health. Unfortunately, in many cases, nothing could be further from the truth. An interesting case report by Drs. Dyck and Embree will bring this fact to light for us. What follows is quoted from the abstract of their paper.

> "In the case presented, a right lower quadrant pain due to appendicitis was intensified by lateral pressure on the L4 spinous process, and temporarily eliminated by manipulation of L4, L5 and right sacroiliac articulations. Following surgical removal of the appendix, the right lower quadrant pain was reproducible by lateral pressure of the L4 spinous process. It was concluded that if spinal manipulation can, in fact, reflexly modulate such visceral pains, practitioners should be alerted to the possibility that manipulation of the spine may mask the pain of an ongoing pathology, and reductions of symptoms following manipulative procedures does not necessarily imply removal of the cause of those symptoms."

From: Dyck, G & Embree, B., *"The enigma of referred abdominal pain in chiropractic practice: literature review and case report,"* JMPT 4(1):11-14, 1981

The point to appreciate is that the chiropractic adjustment may help to eliminate a patient's symptomatic picture; however, an underlying disease process may be present. Whatever the underlying pathology may be, a patient will have a better chance at battling a disease if a doctor were to provide proper dietary recommendations. More on this topic later.

#7 – THE DEFINITION OF HEALTH

Read this definition to your audience; then read it a second time and have them read it with you. Explain to your audience that, health by definition is a state of complete well-being. Ask your audience, how many people in this room live in a state of complete physical, mental and social well-being, or in other words, how many in this room are completely well and have absolutely no problems? How many in

---

HEALTH

A state of complete physical, mental and social well-being and NOT merely the absence of disease and infirmity.

Dorland's Illustrated Medical Dictionary (25th ed.), p.683, W.B. Saunders Co., Philadelphia, 1974

---

this room are perfect? Believe it or not some people will say that they are completely well and perfect. These people should be referred for psychotherapy...just kidding. Most people will swallow their pride and admit that they are not healthy.

At this point, explain to your audience that health is an ideal, and one that is probably impossible to achieve in this day and age because of all the pollution, etc. What can we do to make this unattainable ideal called health one of our main goals in life? Everyday we must make choices that will bring ourselves closer to experiencing the ideal. Explain that, "although we may never achieve the goal of true health, everyday we can set achievable goals that bring us closer to the ideal. Step by step, everyday, observable improvements can be made, which is exceedingly fulfilling. Furthermore, by doing this you may help to motivate your friends and family members to do the same.

Conclude your discussion of this slide by stating that, because health is a state of complete well-being, it would be impossible to experience aches and pains if you were healthy by definition. In this way, aches and pains are good because they let you know that you need to improve your physical and mental condition. And at the same time, just because you may become symptom-free, it does not mean that you are healthy. It only means that tissue damage within your body is not reaching your conscious awareness, and this will be illustrated in the following slides.

Go to the next slide.

♦For the Doctor♦

You can also tell your audience that terms such as complete health, optimal health and total health are oxymorons. Health by definition is complete, optimal and total. How can something be completely complete, optimally optimal or totally total? It can't be. People who characterize health in this fashion actively demonstrate their ignorance about the subject. I realize that many of you may use the terms complete health, optimal health and total health, and I did too until I learned the correct definition and subsequently developed a greater appreciation for the meaning of the word. If you currently use inaccurate terminology - stop today.

#8 – THE NATURAL HISTORY OF DISEASE

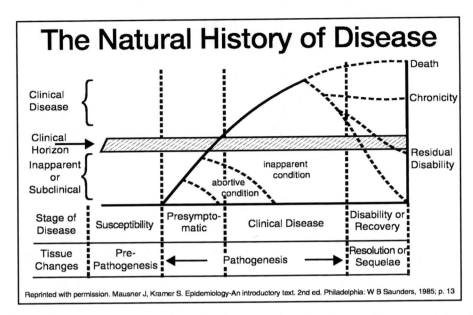

Reprinted with permission. Mausner J, Kramer S. Epidemiology-An introductory text. 2nd ed. Philadelphia: W B Saunders, 1985; p. 13

This chart provides a visual tool that you can use to demonstrate the concept of health as you described it in the previous slide. I personally like to describe it in the following manner.

As you can see on the left side of the chart, the manifestation of disease is divided into two categories: inapparent or subclinical, and clinical disease. These two categories are separated by a crossover point called the clinical horizon. On the bottom of the chart you can see that there are four stages of disease: susceptibility, presymptomatic disease, clinical disease and disability or death.

Notice that Stage I, the stage of susceptibility, is characterized as a pre-pathogenic and symptom-free state. This is where we should all be, however, most of us occupy the second or third stage.

Stage II, the stage of presymptomatic disease is also a symptom-free stage. However, look on the bottom of the chart where it describes tissues changes and you can see that in the pre-symptomatic stage actual pathology may exist. In other words, you can be pain-free and have cancer.

Stage III, the stage of clinical disease, refers to the stage in which the disease process is more readily detectable. Specific signs and symptoms are present which help to make a diagnosis.

Stage IV, the stage of disability or death, should be clear to most in the audience. The patient is either disabled from the disease or they are deceased.

Lets take a closer look at the topic of presymptomatic disease.

Go to the next slide.

This slide is an adaptation of a chart from: Mausner, J & Kramer, S., <u>Epidemiology- An Introductory Text</u> (2nd ed.), p.13, W.B. Saunders, Philadelphia, 1985. We thank W.B. Saunders for granting us permission to use this chart.

NOTES:

#9 – PRESYMPTOMATIC DISEASE

Read the slide to your audience and then ask for someone to explain what the statement means. Go around the room and get some answers...and push to get people to respond. Try to get people to feel the weight of the fact that just because they are symptom-free, or only have a couple of complaints, does not mean that they are in good shape.

Go to the next slide.

Presymptomatic Disease

At this stage there is no manifest disease and no signs or symptoms of illness, but usually through the interaction of a variety of risk factors, pathogenic changes have started to occur. An example of presymptomatic disease is premalignant (and, unfortunately, sometimes malignant) alterations in tissue.

Mausner, J. & Kramer, S., Epidemiology - An Introductory Text (2nd ed.), p.7, W.B. Saunders Co., Philadelphia, 1985

♦For the Doctor♦

Being that the topic of this slide is Presymptomatic Disease, it is an excellent time to complete our discussion [which we started in Slide # 6] about how the chiropractic adjustment can mask the symptoms of disease. Recall that we talked about the report by Dyck and Embree that described how the chiropractic adjustment masked the pain of appendicitis. With this in mind, consider the following diseases which can ultimately lead to death or disability: Coronary heart disease, stroke, high blood pressure, cancer, diabetes mellitus, obesity, osteoporosis, dental diseases and diverticular disease. All of these diseases develop asymptomatically over time, and all of these diseases have been intimately linked to inappropriate dietary practices[1].

Every week, hundreds of patients walk into your office in the stage of presymptomatic disease. Many have pathological tissue changes that are not at all characterized by the condition that brought them to your office, i.e.. their musculoskeletal ache or pain. You provide them with appropriate adjustments, and they walk out of your office feeling more healthy and alive. However, despite a patient's restored sense of well-being, a subclinical pathological process may be marching on toward the future clinical manifestation of coronary heart disease, stroke, high blood pressure, cancer, diabetes mellitus, obesity, osteoporosis, dental diseases or diverticular disease and such. Many of these people enter our offices at a time where dietary intervention might help reverse the progression of disease and promote the reestablishment of healthy tissues.

What should we tell our patients? It is very simple. Eat a diet that consists mostly of fresh vegetables and fruits. Gladys Block, Ph.D., who worked at the National Cancer Institute and is currently a professor at the University of California at Berkeley states, "...the nutrients in fruits and vegetables, particularly the antioxidant micronutrients, are associated with real and substantial disease protection"[2].

Not only should we provide our patients with the chiropractic adjustment, all of our patients should also be made aware of the fact that eating mostly fruits and vegetables can prevent a host of diseases. If our patients are foolish enough to not take such advice about their diet, at least we offered the information that all patients need to hear from a health-care practitioner.

There is one more point I would like to make about the adjustment. The chiropractic adjustment is a powerful therapeutic and diagnostic tool. In and of itself, the adjustment alone can provide the patient with a profound sense of well-being and vitality. So much so, that if we do not recommend appropriate life-style changes, nutrition in particular, a patient may utilize his/her new found energy to more fervently practice the bad habits that brought them into the chiropractic office in the first place. From this perspective, the chiropractic adjustment can ultimately be detrimental to a patient's well-being.

1. The Surgeon General's Report on Nutrition and Health, US. Dept. Health & Human Services, US. Government Printing Office, Wash., DC., 1988
2. Block, G., *"Dietary guidelines and the results of food consumption surveys,"* Am J Clin Nutr 53:356S-57S, 1991

#10 – THE NATURAL HISTORY OF DISEASE
(PICTORIAL VERSION)

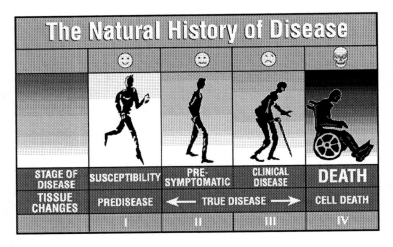

This is a pictorial version of the chart in Slide #8, that was adapted from <u>Epidemiology-An Introductory Text</u> (2nd ed.). In this way, patients can better see the progression from a state of physical fitness to an ultimate state of physical disability and death. Explain this process step by step. Emphasize that the factor which most powerfully influences an individual's progression down the road of physical degeneration is what they eat. In 1988, the Surgeon General said it best: "...one personal choice seems to influence long-term health prospects more than any other: what we eat"[1].

Explain to your audience that it is not just poor nutrition that promotes the development of disease. A variety of factors are responsible. Ask your audience if they can think of a word that would best collectively characterize the factors (i.e., poor nutrition, alcohol, pollution, urban life, etc.) that promote the development of disease. The best answer is STRESS. Ask your audience: "What is STRESS?" Spend some time on this question and get as much feedback as you can. You will probably hear things that have to do with mental tension. See if anyone knows the difference between stress and a stressor. Find out what people think and...

Go to the next slide.

1.   <u>The Surgeon General's Report on Nutrition and Health</u>, US. Dept. Health & Human Services, US. Government Printing Office, Wash., DC., 1988

◆ For the Doctor ◆

What we as chiropractors should appreciate is that we basically have two choices as it relates to influencing a patient's journey down the road of physical degeneration toward chronic disease. We can provide only the chiropractic adjustment, which can help to make our patients more functional and comfortable during the development of chronic disease, or we can provide the chiropractic adjustment and recommend proper nutrition and exercise so that our patients can be more functional and comfortable during a longer, healthier and more productive life.

The topic of presymptomatic disease should be of special interest to chiropractors. During our first year of chiropractic college we typically learn a great deal about the philosophy of chiropractic according to D.D. and B.J. Palmer. The concept of dis-ease is usually discussed at great length. Unfortunately, most of the unique chiropractic terms, such as dis-ease, were not translated into more contemporary terms for us so that we could more effectively communicate chiropractic with others. When I first saw Mausner and Kramer's chart depicting **The Natural History of Disease**, the concept of dis-ease popped into my mind. I believe the stage of presymptomatic disease, when a patient is not healthy and also not clinically manifesting a disease process, to be equivalent with the state of dis-ease as described by chiropractors.

#11 – STRESSORS

Begin your discussion about stress by stating that this slide provides a list of stressors. STRESS is the reaction or response the body has to a stressor. There is only one stress reaction, known as the General Adaptation Syndrome (GAS), and each of the many stressors is capable of initiating the reaction. If you would like to obtain more information about the particulars of the stress reaction pick up a copy of <u>The Stress of Life</u> by Dr. Hans Selye. Selye was the pioneering researcher in the field of stress.

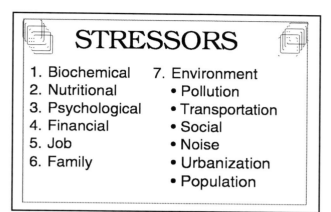

There is a very important point to appreciate about stress. The stress reaction is ultimately characterized by the formation of gastrointestinal ulcers, hyperactivity of the adrenal gland and weakening of the immune system. Remind your audience that such a reaction is stimulated by stressors, and then state that most diseases known to man can be related to gastrointestinal, adrenal and immune system problems (such relationships are described in Selye's book). Explain that a logical way to reduce the stress reaction would be to eliminate those stressors over which you can exert an influence. Then read the list of stressors aloud. Ask your audience which stressors they think they can control. Find out what they think and then state that, for all intents and purposes, we can only influence the first three stressors to any appreciable degree. These, as you can see, include biomechanical, psychological, and biochemical or nutritional stressors. In other words, the way to improve the health status of the human body is to make it physically, mentally and nutritionally strong. To keep this in mind, we can create a visual image that is easy to remember.

Go to the next slide.

♦ *For the Doctor* ♦

To gain an appreciation for the field of stress and the work of Dr. Hans Selye, I highly recommend reading <u>The Stress of Life</u> (McGraw Hill, New York, 1978). There are almost 500 pages in this book so I decided to highlight the most important points to save you time.

STRESSOR - Any nonspecific factor (an agent or condition) which produces stress (p.78-79). Joint complex dysfunction probably acts as a stressor that induces the GAS.

STRESS - The nonspecific response of the body to any demand, whether it is caused by, or results in, pleasant or unpleasant conditions (p.74). Selye delineates the difference between distress and eustress. "During both eustress and distress the body undergoes virtually the same nonspecific responses to the various positive or negative stimuli acting upon it. However, the fact that eustress causes much less damage than distress graphically demonstrates that it is *how you take it* that determines, ultimately, whether one can adapt successfully to change (p.74)."

Continued on next page

Slide # 11 "Stressors" -- Continued

STRESS SYNDROME - The stress syndrome, also called the General Adaptation Syndrome (GAS), is specific in its manifestation although it [the GAS] is induced by nonspecific agents and conditions known as stressors (p.64).

The specific biologic changes associated with the GAS include the following (p.25):

a) Adrenal enlargement
b) Thymicolymphatic involution
c) Ulceration of intestinal tract

There are three stages of the GAS (p.36-38):

(1) The Alarm Reaction: This is the generalized call to arms of the defensive forces of the body in response to a stressor(s). The biologic changes (a, b & c) described above can begin to develop in this stage.
(2) The Stage of Resistance: The body adapts to the presence of the stressor and is able to function in an apparently normal manner, despite the continued presence of the stressor. The biologic changes (a, b & c) return toward normal in this stage.
(3) The Stage of Exhaustion: The body loses its ability to adapt to the presence of the stressor and eventually dies. The biologic changes (a, b & c) return and progress until the death of the organism.

NOTES:

#12 – THE TRIANGLE OF HEALTH

The Triangle of Health is the visual image that can help remind us about the three main stressors we can influence. As you can see, biomechanics (i.e.., body structure) forms the foundation of the triangle and psychology and biochemistry (nutrition) form the two sides. As you can see, this is an equilateral triangle - all sides are equal in length and therefore, the triangle is balanced in appearance.

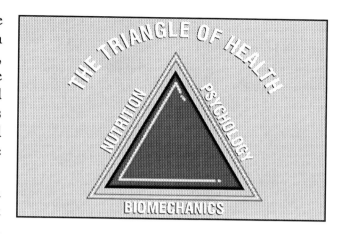

For us to improve our physical condition and move closer to the ideal of health, we must keep our personal triangle of health balanced. We must take care of our structure, our body chemistry (nutrition) and our minds. If we neglect any of the three aspects, our triangle will be unbalanced and we will become less fit.

To take care of our structure/biomechanics, we should be checked by a chiropractor on a regular basis and we should maintain a disciplined schedule of daily exercise. To maintain the integrity of the psychological side of our triangle we must program ourselves with positive thoughts and ideas. I believe that <u>The Road Less Traveled</u> by M. Scott Peck, M.D. is very helpful in this regard. And finally, to keep our biochemical or nutritional side of the triangle balanced, we must eat properly and take appropriate nutritional supplements when necessary.

Remind your audience that taking care of our biomechanics, our psychology and biochemistry is not new. Most everyone has heard that the way to stay healthy is to get regular exercise, think positive thoughts and eat properly. The concept of the triangle of health provides us with a visual image to remind us of what we already know.

Of course, this presentation is about the nutritional side of the triangle. A common question that I have been asked is, "just how important is nutrition; do I really have to eat properly?" And the answer is: nutrition is of the utmost importance and you must eat properly if you want to feel better. Consider the following information about the importance of nutrition.

Go to the next slide.

NOTES:

#13 – CAN OUR CELLS LIVE FOREVER?

Nutrition & Longevity

At all levels of organization, in the body of a cell or in that of man, physiological time depends on modifications of the medium produced by nutrition, and on the response of the cells to those modifications...Colonies obtained from a heart fragment removed in January, 1912, from a chick embryo, are growing as actively today as twenty-three years ago. In fact, they are immortal.

Carrel, A., Man The Unknown, p.172-173,
Harper & Brothers Pub., New York, 1935

After reading the title of the slide, state that our cells are not really immortal. Then read the slide which explains why this particular title was chosen.

In actuality, Carrel kept those heart cells alive for over thirty years. The cell culture supposedly died when a new laboratory attendant incorrectly changed the fluid medium in which the cells lived. In other words, the nutrient medium from which the cells maintained their viability was altered and the cells died. Carrel and this aspect of his research has been scrutinized over the years, but nonetheless, think about the life-enhancing implications of this research.

Before moving to the next slide, make sure to tell your audience a little more about Dr. Alexis Carrel. This will help your audience to better appreciate the information in this slide. Dr. Carrel spent most of his life conducting research at the Rockefeller Institute for Medical Research in New York City. During that period of history the Rockefeller Institute was one of the most well respected research facilities in the world. Carrel won the Nobel Prize in 1912 for his work that demonstrated how blood vessels could be sutured together. The development of his technique laid the foundation for vascular surgery, heart surgery and transplantation of organs. The point to appreciate is that the mind of Dr. Alexis Carrel was deeply rooted in science. He would not have stated that cells had the potential to live forever unless there was some truth in the statement.

Dr. Carrel was not the only person who believed that living tissues had the potential to live forever.

Go to the next slide.

♦ For the Doctor ♦

If you would like to read more about Dr. Alexis Carrel, consult the following books:

Carrel, A., Man, The Unknown, Harper & Brothers Publishers, New York, 1935

Malinin, T., SURGERY AND LIFE, The Extraordinary Career of Alexis Carrel, Harcourt Brace Jovanovich, Inc., New York, 1979

NOTES:

#14 – YES, OUR CELLS LIVE FOREVER?

This quote came from the 1991 edition of Guyton's <u>Textbook of Medical Physiology</u>, which is one of the most well respected physiology books in existence. In addition to authoring eight editions of this text, Dr. Guyton, as a research scientist, also helped to unravel the complex relationship between heart function and blood flow, and pinpointed the crucial role of the kidneys in controlling blood pressure. With this information about Dr. Guyton in mind, consider what he has to say about the potential longevity of the cells in our

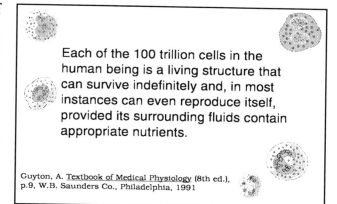

Each of the 100 trillion cells in the human being is a living structure that can survive indefinitely and, in most instances can even reproduce itself, provided its surrounding fluids contain appropriate nutrients.

Guyton, A. <u>Textbook of Medical Physiology</u> (8th ed.), p.9, W.B. Saunders Co., Philadelphia, 1991

bodies. Then read the quote on this slide. Wait for a moment to let this information sink in and then...

Go to the next slide.

NOTES:

#15 – THE HEALTHY CELL

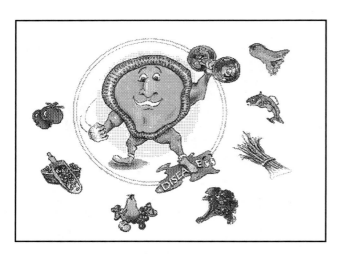

This slide is an artist's interpretation of a cell that has been bathed in proper nutrients. The foods that nourish this cell include fruits, vegetables, and fresh fish. These are the foods that we have all been told to eat like mad if we want to be strong and healthy.

Notice the beautiful golden-yellow color of the cell membrane. This cell can fight off disease like a champion. Theoretically speaking, this is how all of our cells should look. Unfortunately, this is not the case.

Go to the next slide.

NOTES:

#16 – THE UNHEALTHY CELL

Unfortunately, most of our cells look like this one. And most people who have cells like this, have complaints similar to this cell's — "oh, won't someone HEAL ME." This cell's groan for help accurately characterizes how a significant percentage of people in our nation view the issue of health care. Many, many people expect that others should be responsible for making them well. Generally speaking, people do not want to take responsibility for their physical condition. With rising insurance costs, we must start taking better care of ourselves.

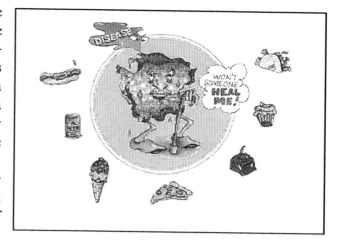

Notice what these cells have been fed. Hot-dogs, cupcakes, ice cream and candy. These are the foods that we have all been told not to eat.

Look at the cell membrane of this cell. It is disrupted, it is defenseless against invaders, and its golden-yellow color has turned brown. Cells actually turn this color as they age and degenerate. The brown pigment is called lipofuscin.

In the last few slides, we have talked about the potential for unparalleled longevity and showed slides of an artist's interpretation of healthy versus sick cells. If I were listening to this presentation, I would be wondering what happens to our cells in real life. The next two slides demonstrate how the quality of our food determines the quality of our physical appearance.

Go to the next slide.

NOTES:

#17 – HEALTHY MELANESIAN WOMAN

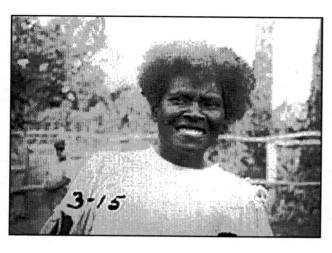

This slide, as well as the next one, are just two of some 400 slides from a collection that was put together by Dr. Weston Price. During the 1930s, Dr. Price traveled the world to see how westernized eating habits might affect those cultures that subsisted on only natural foods. This woman represents someone who did not eat the pastries, sweets, canned food, white rice and white flour products brought in by Westerners. She ate only the local natural foods. Her beauty and obvious physical strength are reminiscent of all native people who ate only the local natural food.

As you can see, this is slide #15 from lecture #3. The woman pictured is Melanesian and her physical stature and beauty are characteristic of those individuals who adhere to the indigenous, traditional method of eating. The traditional diet consisted of fresh plants and seafood.

In contrast, at ports where modern foods were received, the traditional fresh foods were replaced by imported foods such as white-flour products, sugar and sweetened foods, canned foods and polished rice. The consumption of such foods consistently result in marked physical degeneration and loss of beauty. The following slide illustrates a woman who lived on imported processed foods.

Go to the next slide.

NOTES:

#18 – UNHEALTHY MELANESIAN WOMAN

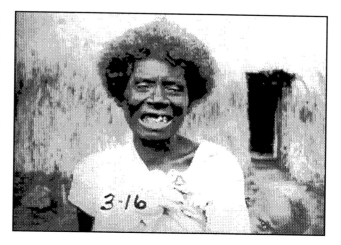

Notice that this slide is labeled #3-16. There is quite a difference in appearance between the woman in this slide (#3-16) versus the woman in the previous slide (#3-15). Bring up the point that these two woman look like they are probably about the same age. Let your audience look at this slide for a couple of moments and get some feedback.

I would suggest asking your audience some or all of the following questions about the two women:

- **Which woman would be more likely to have aches and pains?**

- **Which woman is probably less happy about life?**

- **Which woman, if both were alive today, would probably be a greater economic burden on our collapsing disease-care system?**

- **Which person would you rather be?**

- **Which person do you most likely resemble?**

- **Which person does the average person on the street resemble?**

Tell your audience to think about these questions and their answers. Then explain that for those who desire to improve their health status, it is very important that they understand how the body degenerates.

Ask your audience if anyone knows how the degenerative process works? How is it that our cells degenerate? How is it that they are degenerating this very moment? Find out what your audience knows and then state that these questions can be answered with an apple.

Go to the next slide.

♦ *For the Doctor* ♦

Both slide #17 and #18 were reprinted with permission from Price-Pottenger Nutrition Foundation (PPNF). PPNF is a non-profit organization that maintains itself through Foundation memberships, a doctor/patient referral system, and by the sales of a variety books and tapes. I urge you to support PPNF by becoming a member. If PPNF is unable to maintain itself, people will no longer be able to obtain the famous and important works of both Drs. Price and Pottenger.

> Price-Pottenger Nutrition Foundation
> PO Box 2614
> La Mesa, CA 91943-2614
> 619-582-4168

All of Dr. Price's slides, as well as his book entitled <u>Nutrition and Physical Degeneration</u>, can be purchased from PPNF. A book entitled <u>POTTENGER'S CATS: A Study in Nutrition</u>, as well as all of the scientific articles published by Dr. Francis Pottenger, Jr., are also available from PPNF. Dr. Pottenger found that the consumption of cooked food causes a multitude of degenerative conditions in experimental animals. He studied the effect of cooked meat and pasteurized milk versus their raw counterparts. The results demonstrated that the cats fed cooked food developed significantly more diseases compared with those eating raw food and milk.

#19 – FREE RADICAL PATHOLOGY - APPLE

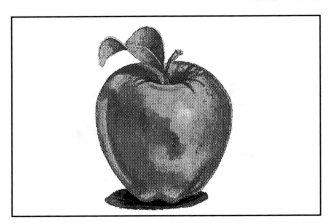

Why an apple? Because for this example we are going to pretend that all of the cells in the human body are apples. Have audience members close your eyes for a moment and picture, in their minds, that all the cells in the body are made up of apples. Ask for a show of hands of those people who find this difficult to do.

Go to the next slide.

♦ For the Doctor ♦

An explanation of free radical pathology can be found in *Chapter 5, pages 76-79.*

#20 – FREE RADICAL PATHOLOGY - APPLE MAN

This is the image that everyone should have in their mind. Find out if this was what everyone was visualizing? Now see if anyone knows how many cells exist in the human body. The answer is 100 trillion. This was already told to them in Slide #14. For this explanation, all 100 trillion cells in the body are apples.

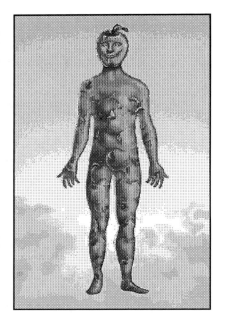

Now have your audience think about diseases such as cancer, heart disease, diabetes, cataracts, arthritis and immune disorders. What is it that causes these conditions? Do they just happen? Or is their development part of a process that can be either inhibited or promoted? Find out what your audience thinks about these questions.

The fact is that the diseases mentioned above, as well as most other diseases, are promoted [in part] by certain agents. See if anyone knows what these agents are? The correct answer is free radicals or oxidants. Find out if anyone knows how free radicals damage cells.

Go to the next slide.

NOTES:

#21 - FREE RADICAL PATHOLOGY - OXIDANTS

Free radicals/oxidants have the ability to literally take bites out of our cell membranes, just like the teeth you see in the upper right part of this slide. There are many sources of oxidants, but some of the most common include air pollution, water pollution, normal metabolic reactions, radiation, drugs and cigarette smoke.

The point to appreciate is that, even if our environment was oxidant-free, we would still be at risk of oxidant damage because our body produces oxidants during normal metabolic reactions.

Go to the next slide.

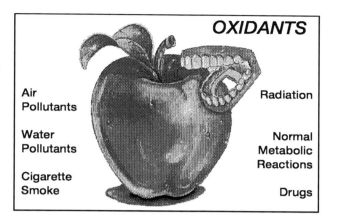

#22 – FREE RADICAL PATHOLOGY - BITTEN APPLE

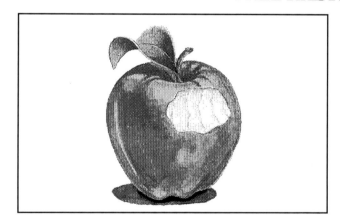

As stated earlier, oxidants take bites out of cell membranes. Remind everyone that, for this example, all of the cells in the body are apples.

Ask what happens when you take a bite out of an apple and let it sit for an hour? The answer will be, "it turns brown."

Go to the next slide.

NOTES:

#23 – FREE RADICAL PATHOLOGY - OXIDATION PROCESS

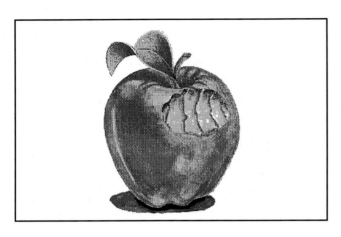

See if anyone knows what the browning process is called? Many will give the correct answer - "oxidation," and you can say that the apple becomes oxidized.

In real life, our cells become oxidized when they are exposed to pollutants, drugs, cigarettes, and during normal metabolic reactions. Explain that our cells should be able to repair themselves after an attack by oxidants. If our cells are unable to repair themselves, then an oxidized cell will become a free radical or oxidant. And now our cells can literally attack each other.

How do you suppose our cells repair themselves? Make sure you get some responses. It doesn't matter if the answers are right or wrong; the important point is that your audience is forced to think and respond.

Go to the next slide.

#24 – FREE RADICAL PATHOLOGY - ANTIOXIDANTS

Our cells are repaired by antioxidants. Antioxidants include various nutrients which either act as antioxidants or support antioxidant enzyme systems. Some of these nutrients include vitamin E, zinc, copper, cysteine, manganese, glutathione, vit C, vit B2 & B3, taurine, selenium and beta-carotene. When these nutrients are present, our cells have the where-with-all to repair themselves.

The next slide lists some diseases that are associated with inadequate antioxidant intake.

Go to the next slide.

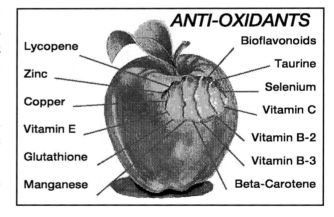

ANTI-OXIDANTS

Lycopene
Zinc
Copper
Vitamin E
Glutathione
Manganese
Bioflavonoids
Taurine
Selenium
Vitamin C
Vitamin B-2
Vitamin B-3
Beta-Carotene

NOTES:

#25 – CONDITIONS ASSOCIATED WITH AN INADEQUATE INTAKE OF ANTIOXIDANTS

Conditions associated with an inadequate intake of antioxidants:

Cancer	Heart disease
Cataracts	Macular degeneration
Aging	Parkinson's disease
Altered immunity	Alzheimer's disease
Diabetes	AIDS
Liver disease	Arthritis
Multiple Sclerosis	

Cancer, cataracts, aging, altered immunity, diabetes, liver disease, multiple sclerosis, heart disease, macular degeneration, Parkinson's disease, Alzheimer's disease, AIDS and arthritis are all associated with an inadequate intake of antioxidants. Make sure that your audience appreciates the fact that some of these diseases are the leading killers of Americans.

Ask if anyone in the audience knows the best way to insure appropriate antioxidant intake. The answer is fruits and vegetables; however, if no one gets the answer right, ask your audience what we all need to eat more of. Hopefully they will say fruits and vegetables. Before you go to the next slide, make sure your audience is thinking about fruits and vegetables.

♦ *For the Doctor* ♦

Below is a list of articles which discuss the relationship between antioxidants and the diseases mentioned in this slide.

For cancer, cataracts, aging, altered immunity, heart disease, Parkinson's disease and arthritis see:

Am J Clin Nutr Suppl to 53(1):Jan/1991

*All the articles in this entire supplement are devoted to antioxidants

For AIDS, diabetes, macular degeneration, Alzheimer's disease, Multiple Sclerosis, and liver disease see:

1) Baker, D., *"Cellular Antioxidant Status and Human Immunodeficiency Virus Replication,"* Nutr Rev 50(1):15-18, 1992
2) Slonim, A., *"Modification of Chemically Induced Diabetes in Rats by Vitamin E: Supplementation Minimizes and Depletion Enhances Development of Diabetes,"* J Clin Invest 71:1282-1288, 1983
3) Gerster, H., *"Review: Antioxidant protection of the aging macula,"* Age Aging 20:60-69, 1990
4) Jesberger, J., *"Oxygen radicals and brain dysfunction,"* Inter J Neurosci 57:1-17, 1991
5) Mai, J., "High dose antioxidant supplementation to MS patients: Effects on glutathione peroxidase, clinical safety, and absorption of selenium," Bio Trace Element Res 24:109-17, 1990
6) Feher, J., *"Free radicals in tissue damage in liver diseases and therapeutic approach,"* Tokai J Exp Clin Med 11(Suppl):121-34, 1986

NOTES:

#26 – ANTIOXIDANT NUTRIENTS

ANTIOXIDANTS

It is clear that the nutrients in fruits and vegetables, particularly the antioxidant micronutrients, are associated with real and substantial disease protection. And it is clear that in the United States the population's intake of these foods is remote from the recommended levels.

Block, G., "Diet Guidelines and the Results of Food Consumption Surveys," Am J Clin Nutr 53:356S-57S, 1991

After you read this slide, it should be pretty clear as to why our population is overcome by degenerative diseases. Ask your audience if they know people who are afraid of getting cancer, heart disease or any of the other diseases mentioned on the previous slide. Then ask how many of them are afraid for themselves and for family members. Many people will probably raise their hands.

Now find out how many people eat massive amounts of fruits and vegetables. Most will say that they do not. Make sure that the audience realizes that such dietary habits can lead to the development of a debilitating disease. In actuality, such a diet is really a request for a disease.

At this time, I would introduce the topic of nutrition for pain control. Explain that eating lots of fruits and vegetables can also help reduce aches and pains. In other words, the diet that can prevent the development of degenerative diseases can also help to fight pain.

Ask your audience if anyone understands the nature of pain (How many people here know what pain is?). Wait for their responses and then ask: What is the difference between back pain, neck pain, headaches or leg pain? Wait for their responses and then ask: How many people have taken, or heard about taking, different pain medications for pain in different locations? Wait for their responses and then state: "Well, for the most part, the treatment of pain doesn't make much sense and here's why."

Go to the next slide.

NOTES:

#27 – THE IRRITATION OF PAIN NERVES

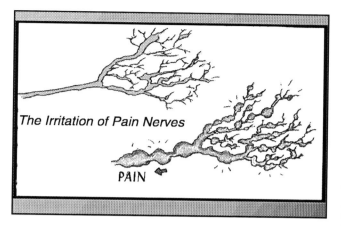

The Irritation of Pain Nerves

PAIN

To begin with, we all must appreciate that fact that pain is caused by the irritation of pain nerves. This is no big brainstorm when you think about it and makes complete sense. The problem is that pain is not addressed from this perspective in clinical medicine. Pain certainly isn't described like this on TV commercials for pain medication. But nonetheless, pain is merely the irritation of pain nerves. And what you will learn in the remainder of the presentation is how taking certain supplements and eating large amounts of fruits and vegetables can help to reduce pain, relax tight muscles, and reduce joint restriction. Before we go any further, we must blaze into our minds the fact that...

Go to the next slide.

#28 – NEUROLOGICALLY SPEAKING PAIN IS PAIN

...neurologically speaking PAIN is PAIN. This means that regardless of the location of pain, the pain itself is due to the irritation of pain nerves. So, regardless of where your pain is located, as long as we can remove the irritation, pain, stiffness and other associated symptoms, it should be easy to reduce. Ask your audience if this makes sense to them. Although this concept is new to many, it is still very simple to understand.

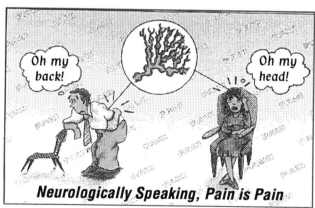

Neurologically Speaking, Pain is Pain

Regarding treatment, if we knew what stimulates pain nerves we could conceivably learn to reduce pain nerve irritation. And fortunately, we know what irritates pain nerves.

Go to the next slide.

NOTES:

#29 – PAIN NERVES ARE IRRITATED BY:

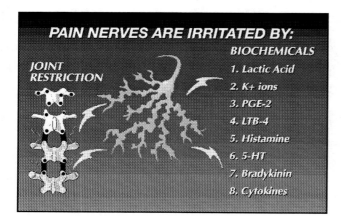

Pain nerves are irritated by joint restriction and by direct trauma. Pain nerves are also irritated by certain biochemicals including lactic acid, PGE-2, LTB-4, potassium ions, histamine, serotonin, bradykinin and cytokines. It is not important that the people in your audience remember all of these biochemicals. Your audience should remember that these are the biochemicals that are released from injured tissues to cause inflammation and pain.

Go to the next slide.

#30 – FOOD, CONSUMED, DIGESTED, CONVERTED, BIOCHEMICALS

Our discussion today centers around how proper nutrition can help to reduce the production of the biochemical irritants. This slide demonstrates why we all need a healthy diet. All the food that we eat is digested and converted into biochemicals. When foods like meat, dairy and cheese are consumed in excess, the associated animal fats are digested and converted into PGE-2, LTB-4 and help to promote the release of 5-HT. This does not occur to the same degree when we eat large amounts of fruits and vegetables in addition to the aforementioned animal products.

What do most Americans eat too much of? Your audience will tell you that we eat too much meat, dairy, cheese, desserts and **NOT enough** fresh fruits and vegetables. It should be clear to your audience that the same diet (too much meat and other fatty foods) that causes cancer and heart disease can also cause aches, pains and joint complex dysfunction.

Now we will look at how these biochemicals cause pain, spasm and other associated symptoms (autonomic concomitants).

Go to the next slide.

♦ For the Doctor ♦

We as chiropractors all know that one of the biggest complaints directed our way is the fact that we tell people that they must be adjusted "so" many times. How many times have you yourself heard the following statement? "The bad thing about chiropractors is that once you start going they tell you that you have to keep going forever if you want to feel good."

My experience, as well as that of many other chiropractors, has demonstrated that this complaint is true only when exercise (rehabilitation and/or for general fitness) and proper nutrition are not part of a patient's treatment plan. Chapter 5, A Diet Induced Pro-inflammatory State, describes how we eat ourselves into a pain and dysfunction-ridden state.

#31 – NOCICEPTIVE RECEPTOR (WINE GLASS MODEL)

Believe it or not, with this wine glass we can visualize the manner in which pain nerves function. The stem of the glass represents the pain nerve. The base of the glass is where potentially painful or unpleasant information is transferred to another nerve, or to a collection of nerves such as the brain. The glass itself, or the receptacle for the wine, illustrates a nerve receptor. There are all different kinds of receptors. Some sense pressure, movement, vibration, etc., and some sense painful stimuli.

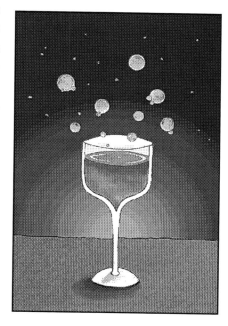

Remember that pain receptors can be stimulated by mechanical trauma or by biochemical irritants. As you can see in the illustration, the different biochemicals are around the receptor and some are filling up the receptor. The critical point to appreciate is that the nerve cannot be activated [or fired] unless the receptor is filled to the top. The closer the receptor is to being filled to the top, the easier it will be for the nerve to start firing impulses.

At this point in the discussion you can give a real-life example that most people can appreciate. Ask your audience if they ever met anyone who was very sensitive to the touch and experiences pain easily. Many people experience pain in situations that would normally not be painful. For example, when these people are seated or engaged in non-stressful activities such as walking, they do not experience pain. However, if they walk through a door and just lightly graze their shoulder on the door frame, pain results. Pain can occur even if they are gently patted on the back or hugged. These people are everywhere and many are probably in the audience. Ask if anyone in the audience knows someone like this. Generally speaking, the typical patient who is compromised by excessive chemical irritant production is one that consumes large quantities of aspirin, Tylenol and other ache & pain medications. Many of your audience members and people they know liberally consume such medications. Get a show of hands from the audience to verify that they or someone they know is in this situation.

Remember that there are different degrees of tenderness. The point is that most people have varying degrees of increased sensitivity to normal stimulation, and to this degree these people need to empty their nociceptors of chemical irritants. Upon palpation, these folks generally have tissues that feel boggy, sensitive and subtly inflamed.

Now tell your audience to look at the pain receptor and think about the people who experience pain very easily. Ask your audience: "If the receptor is filled to the top with these biochemicals, do you think someone will be more or less likely to feel pain during minor physical strain?" The answer should be **more** likely.

Ask a similar question: "If the receptor is only one quarter full, do you think someone will be more or less likely to feel pain during minor physical strain?" The answer should be **less** likely.

Ask another question: "If you had the choice, would you like your receptors filled with biochemical irritants or empty?" Most will, of course, say empty.

Continued on next page

Slide # 31 "Nociceptive Receptor" – Continued

Ask still another question: "How many here live on meat (i.e., bacon, sausage, lunch meat, burgers, steak, etc.), dairy, cheese and white flour products (i.e., white bread, rolls, etc.) and also love to munch on desserts? How many of you eat massive amounts of fruits and vegetables?" Wait for their answer.

Because most Americans have horrendous diets and do not eat enough fruits and vegetables, most of your audience members, if they are average Americans, do not eat enough fruits and vegetables. Some may not wish to admit that they eat poorly and live on burgers, franks, donuts and coffee. If this is the case, joke around with them until they feel comfortable enough to admit it.

Generally speaking, the way you can be fairly sure that someone does not eat enough fruits and vegetables is by their weight. People rarely gain weight when they eat lots of fruits and vegetables.

End by stating the following: "For those of you who eat a lot of meats, dairy, cheese, white bread and desserts, and not enough fruits and vegetables, your pain nerve receptors may be filling up as I speak. If you want to decrease the amount of biochemicals in your receptors, you must consume more fruits and vegetables. Let's look more closely at a couple of the biochemicals listed in this slide and see how we can reduce their production."

Go to the next slide.

NOTES:

#32 – TO REDUCE LACTIC ACID

State that, nearly everyone has heard of lactic acid and understands that it is in some way related to muscle function and exercise. However, all of the cells in the body are capable of producing lactic acid, including the cells (i.e., chondrocytes) that make up the discs and the joints of the spine. Studies have shown that the more acidic the tissues are in the low back, the more likely a patient is to experience pain.

Before going any further it should be re-stated that biochemical irritants are known to be involved in the body's inflammatory process.

> To reduce the production of
>
> # Lactic Acid:
>
> - B-complex
> - Antioxidant micronutrients
> - Minerals (Mg, Mn, Fe)
> - Eat large amounts of fruits and vegetables

Thus, if a body produces a lot of these biochemicals, then the body's biochemistry can be defined as "pro-inflammatory." Such a pro-inflammatory state promotes pain and joint restriction, whereas an anti-inflammatory state would reduce the development of pain and joint restriction. People who consume mostly meats, dairy, cheese and white flour products are prone to developing a pro-inflammatory state.

Lets look at those factors which help to reduce the production of lactic acid and thereby increase ATP synthesis and energy production. Read through the list and emphasize the last recommendation (eat large quantities of fruits and vegetables) and reiterate that the consumption of fruits and vegetables helps to create an anti-inflammatory state.

Ask your audience what they think is the best source of B-complex vitamins, antioxidant micro nutrients and minerals. Wait for their response, and then state, once again, that the answer is fruits and vegetables.

Go to the next slide.

♦ For the Doctor ♦

See the section on lactic acid in Chapter 8 for a list of supplements that may help increase ATP synthesis and reduce lactic acid production.

NOTES:

#33 – TO REDUCE PGE-2

To help reduce the production of

Prostaglandin E-2:

* Reduce intake of meat and dairy

* Omega-3 fatty acids (fish, fish oils, flaxseed oil, green leafy vegetables)

* Ginger, turmeric, bromelain and bioflavonoids

* Eat large amounts of fruits and vegetables

What is prostaglandin E-2? See how many people know. See if anyone knows what drugs are used to inhibit PGE-2. The answer is aspirin and nonsteroidal anti-inflammatory drugs (NSAIDS). NSAIDS include drugs like Advil, Nuprin, Motrin, Naprosin, Feldene, Indomethacin and Ibuprofen. As many may know, these drugs are used to treat pain and inflammation.

Find out how many people in your audience currently take aspirin or NSAIDS. Find out how many people know someone who regularly takes aspirin or NSAIDS. Wait for their answer and state that around 3 billion dollars are spent each year on over-the-counter (OTC) pain medications (*see below*) and billions more are spent on prescription drugs.

What you have just demonstrated is that many people have problems with excessive PGE-2 production. Now read off the list of nutritional factors that can help to reduce PGE-2 production.

You can divide and describe the list in the following manner:

1. Reduce intake of meat and dairy products because they contain arachidonic acid, the direct precursor of PGE-2.

2. Consider supplementing the diet with EPA, ginger, turmeric, and bioflavonoids. All of these help to inhibit the production of PGE-2.

3. Eat large amounts of fruits and vegetables. They contain a lot of the nutrients needed to inhibit the production of PGE-2.

Let your audience think about this information for a moment or two. Let them see that the foods that most of them currently consume are the ones that help promote pain. Make sure they see this and also make sure that they know that the foods that they are not eating are the ones they need to eat to help fight pain.

Go to the next slide.

Slide # 33 "To Reduce PGE-2" – Continued

◆ *For the Doctor* ◆

Below is a breakdown of the estimated costs for OTC and prescription pain relieving drugs. I received this information from Michael Perlmutter during a phone conversation in 1992. He works for Kline and Company, a group that charts drug consumption (New Jersey; 201-227-6262). The numbers reflect costs for 1991.

Aspirin:	921,250,000
Acetaminophen:	1,113,750,000
Ibuprofen:	715,000,000
Total for general pain OTC costs:	$ 2,750,000,000
Arthritic meds (aspirin) OTC:	$135,000,000
Menstrual meds OTC:	$ 75,000,000

While this slide is up, you may want to mention the side-effects of aspirin and NSAIDS, and then suggest that eating properly is probably the safer alternative. See Chapter 4 for a thorough discussion about NSAIDS and their side effects.

NOTES:

#34 – TO REDUCE 5-HT

```
To help reduce the production of

                5-HT:

❀ Greatly reduce intake of saturated fat & sugar
❀ Omega-3 fatty acids
❀ Vitamin C
❀ Antioxidant micronutrients
❀ Ginger, turmeric, garlic, onions, & olive oil
❀ Eat large amounts of fruits and vegetables
```

Ask how many people here have heard of 5-HT? Most have never heard of it. How many have heard of serotonin? Many people have heard of serotonin; however, most will not be aware of the fact that when serotonin is released from blood platelets, it causes pain and is implicated in arthritic disease. Most people will instead associate serotonin with tryptophan's ability to reduce pain and promote sleep.

Some may also be aware of the tryptophan-EMS (Eosinophilia Myalgia Syndrome) scandal of 1989[1]. People may ask you about it. The consensus is that the EMS problem was due to a contaminated batch of tryptophan and not the amino acid itself[2].

While this slide is up I would suggest that you explain the functional difference between 5-HT/ serotonin in the brain and spinal cord versus platelet 5-HT. Explain that, in the brain and spinal cord, 5-HT promotes sleep and inhibits pain; however, in the periphery, such as around the spine and other joints, 5-HT causes pain. Make sure your audience gets this point and then continue.

In the peripheral circulation, 5-HT is found in platelets. Ask how many have heard of blood platelets and what they know about them? Let your audience tell you what they know and then explain that, generally speaking, there are three types of blood cells.

There are red blood cells (for oxygen delivery, etc.), white blood cells (for defense, etc.) and there are platelets. Platelets are involved in more than just 5-HT release. Platelets are a required component of the blood clotting mechanism and thus, are very important in preventing excessive bleeding. Therefore, if we were to have inefficient platelet activity, we could potentially bleed to death.

On the other hand, if we were to have excessive platelet activity, then platelets would clump together and blood flow to vital tissues could stop and the tissue would die, which is very often the case with a heart attack or stroke.

With respect to platelet function, which of the two problems, either excessive bleeding or excessive clumping, do you think most Americans are more prone to developing? The answer is excessive clumping. Aspirin is known to prevent platelets from clumping and this is why we are told that an aspirin-a-day will keep the heart attackk[3] and stroke away[4]. Flavonoid-rich alcoholic products are also known to prevent platelet clumping, and this is thought to be a reason why the wine-drinking French have a low death rate from heart disease, despite an extremely high fat diet which is otherwise known to cause platelet clumping and heart disease[5].

Now have your audience look at the slide and state that all of these nutritional guidelines listed on this slide will help to prevent platelet clumping. Remember that we want to prevent excessive clumping, because when platelets clump they cause heart attacks, strokes, impotence, and in the periphery, clumped platelets release 5-HT which causes pain, muscle spasm and joint restriction.

Slide # 34 "To Reduce 5-HT" – Continued

Obviously, for many health reasons we must stop our platelets from clumping. Ask your audience what they think is the safest and healthiest way to stop platelets from clumping. By consuming large quantities of aspirin and wine? Or by eating properly? Most will hopefully say eating properly. Now go through the list on the slide.

State that the list of nutritional recommendations to reduce the production of 5-HT is very similar to the list for PGE-2. Let's take a look at a list of general nutritional recommendations that help reduce the production of all the chemical irritants. These include...

Go to the next slide.

♦ For the Doctor ♦

Below is a list of references which help to support a discussion about tryptophan-EMS, the platelet-aspirin inhibitory connection to heart attacks and strokes, and the wine-rich diet of the French and improved platelet function.

1.   Duffy, J., The lessons of Eosinophilia-Myalgia Syndrome, Hosp Pract 4/30/92, p.65-90
2.   Jaffee, R., Eosinophilia Myalgia Syndrome secondary to contaminated tryptophan—Clinical experience, J Nutr Med 2(2):195-200, 1991
3.   Willard, J., The use of aspirin in ischemic heart disease, NEJM 327(3):175-81, 1992
4.   The Merck Manual (15th ed), Volume 1 - General Medicine, p.1066-67, Merck & Co., Rahway, NJ, 1987
5.   Craig W. Phytochemicals: Guardians of our health. J Am Diet Assoc 1997;97(10 suppl 2):S199-S204

NOTES:

#35 – NUTRITIONAL RECOMMENDATIONS

Nutritional Recommendations

- Moderate protein intake [meat, fish, chicken, eggs, etc.]
- Greatly reduce saturated fats & sugar [in particular those found in desserts]
- Eliminate refined [fiberless grain/grain products]
- Enjoy large quantities of fruits and vegetables
- Drink at least 1 pint to $1^{1/2}$ quarts of water/day
- If possible, drink at least 1 pint of fresh vegetable juice/day
- Take appropriate nutritional supplements
- RELAX, don't be a calorie counting worry wart

Read the list to your audience and then ask how many people can see that the general nutritional recommendations listed here are the same as the ones we are told to follow if we want to be healthy and prevent disease? Let your audience know that this is a great thing that we can do for ourselves; we can eat to fight pain, help reduce joint restriction and, at the same time, become healthy and prevent the development of chronic disease.

I would suggest that you go through the list and briefly comment on each recommendation.

• Enjoy moderate amounts of meat, eggs, fish, and other proteins

Many people mistakenly believe that eating healthy means that you must give up animal proteins. This notion is incorrect. Animal protein offers the highest quality protein, and most people do very well when they regularly consume moderate amounts.

• Greatly reduce saturated fat and sugar (in particular those found in desserts)

High sugar diets are typically deficient in the nutrients needed to prevent the release of most of the chemical irritants. The average American consumes about 100 pounds of sugar each year. Saturated fat is also be associated with heart disease and diabetes. Dessert foods also contain n-6 fatty acids which are pro-inflammatory.

• Eliminate refined [fiberless] grains/grain products

Refined/processed grains and flours are deficient in vitamins, such as the B-complex, and minerals, such as magnesium and iron. Deficiencies in these nutrients can promote pain and inflammation. Refined grains/flours are also fiberless, so they promote constipation which is associated with colon and other types of cancer. Additionally, grain products are rich in n-6 fatty acids. Because of their n-6 fatty acid content, whole grain products should be kept to a minimum as well. Additionally, gliadin sensitivity is common and the most frequently eaten grains are gliadin-rich, i.e., wheat, rye, oats, and barley.

• Enjoy large quantities of fruits and vegetables

All of the nutrients that help to reduce the production of chemical irritants are found in fruits and vegetables. However, as stated in Slide #26, the consumption level for Americans as a whole is REMOTE from that which is recommended. Because of this fact, we as a people are automatically prone to pain and inflammation. No wonder why we find ourselves in need of taking billions of dollars worth of pain medications annually.

Slide # 35 "Nutritional Recommendations" – Continued

• Drink at least 1 to 1¹ᐟ² quarts of water per day

40% to 60% of an individual's body weight is water[1]. Obviously, water intake is very important to maintain a fit body. One study demonstrated that a deficiency in water intake could promote pain syndromes[2].

1. McArdle, Katch & Katch, Exercise Physiology (3rd ed), p.60, Lea & Febiger, Philadelphia, 1991
2. Bathmanghelidj, F., Pain: A Need for a Paradigm Change, Anti Cancer Research, 7:971-990, 1987

• If possible, drink at least 1 pint of fresh vegetable juice per day

This is the best way to get a healthy supply of vitamins and minerals. Carrots, celery, a beet, a little kale, and some ginger is a wonderful combination. For more information about juicing and juice recipes, consult your local health food store where many juicing books are sold.

One of the most ridiculous criticisms against juicing that I ever heard was that drinking fresh fruit and vegetable juices can be dangerous because juices lack dietary fiber which is needed for proper colon function. This would be true only if you lived solely on juice and did not eat solid food.

• Take appropriate nutritional supplements

What you say here depends upon how you choose to provide your patients with supplements. Chapter 8 contains a list of various supplements that can inhibit the production of chemical irritants.

• RELAX, don't be a calorie counting worry wart

Everybody worries about food whether they say so or not. Some worry about what they eat and others worry that if they start eating properly, they will never be allowed to eat desserts again. Still others eat as much and as fast as possible, as if it is their last meal, and their worry is that someone will try to stop them. On one level or another, we all have our own personal "diet neurosis," and we would all be better off if we could just RELAX a little when it comes to the subject of eating.

A very important point to appreciate and to describe to your audience is that it is very possible to eat a diet with too few calories. Consider the following information:

"Many essential nutrients especially minerals, are distributed widely in our food supply, but in low concentration. It is, therefore, difficult and often impossible to assure nutritional adequacy of diets that are low in energy content. Adequate essential nutrients may not be available in diets of less than 2,000 kcal for adults and adolescents." (Diet and Exercise: Synergism in Health Maintenance, White, P & Mondeika, T., p.32, Am Med Assoc, Chicago, Ill., 1982)

The point to appreciate is that, based on this information, very few Americans come close to nutritional adequacy for a variety of essential nutrients. So, the last thing that we want to turn our patients into are calorie counting worry warts. Let them eat as much as they want [within reason], as long as they are eating large quantities of fruits and vegetables in addition to their protein foods.

I would end this slide by appealing to people's sense of logic and reason. Most people are intelligent enough to know the difference between healthy and unhealthy food. Everyone knows they should eat more fruits and vegetables and less soda and candy bars. I would also discuss some of the visual eating guidelines discussed in Chapter 10. The plate explanation is very helpful.

Go to the next slide.

#36 – THE JUICER-DIGESTIVE TRACT

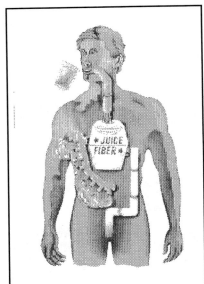

This slide is a fun way to illustrate the best way to eat. It shows our digestive system as a vegetable juicer and pipes.

When we drink juice, it goes down our throat, into our juice machine, and out the pipes that send the nutrients to our cells. If we were to eat a big helping of carrots and greens, they would travel down our throat to enter our juice machine. Our juicer would separate the liquid and the fiber. The nutrient-filled juice would nourish our tissues, and the fiber would travel down our digestive pipes [our small intestine and colon] and be expelled. The fiber of course keeps our digestive tract clean and prevents the development of colon and other forms of cancer.

This is basically how our digestive system works, it really does function like a living juicer. It receives food and separates the nutrients from the fiber.

Now ask your audience to call out some of the different fruits and vegetables that we could put in a real juicer or in our juicer digestive system. Then ask how well white bread and a danish would be digested in our juicer system.

Who would put white bread or a donut in a real juicer? No one in your audience would do that. Ask, why not? The response you are looking for is something to the effect that white bread and donuts would clog up a juicer. As you point to the screen, ask how many think it would be a good idea to put white bread, donuts, a cheeseburger and french fries into the body's juicer digestive system? Ask, why not? The answer will be that the digestive juicer will get clogged up.

Now ask your audience, how many people do you know who regularly put white bread, donuts, cake, candy and french fries [or something similar] into the body's digestive juicer? What do you think happens when we do this? Clearly, these foods will clog up the digestive system and cause constipation.

Go to the next slide.

NOTES:

#37 – BIOCHEMICAL IRRITANTS AND JOINT RESTRICTION

Up to this point we have discussed diet as it relates to pain, health, and disease prevention. This slide provides you with an excellent opportunity to relate diet to joint complex dysfunction.

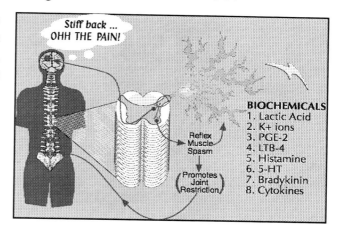

The various biochemical irritants activate pain nerves which enter the spinal cord and stimulate two different nerves. One of the nerves takes this information to the brain where it allows you to consciously experience pain. The second nerve leaves the spinal cord to stimulate muscles to tighten and contract, which results in muscle spasm. This causes different vertebrae throughout the spinal column to become restricted, i.e. different joints stop moving properly.

Ask your audience an important question: How many here think that if the body's production of biochemical irritants was greatly reduced, then the need to see a chiropractor for pain, stiffness and muscle spasms would also probably be reduced? Their answer should be yes, and the answer is yes. Respond by saying, "this is exactly why I want you all to eat properly. If you would all make an effort to eat properly, you would not need to see me as often or as long. This could save you a substantial amount of time and money."

Create another scenario for your audience. Let's say that for the past six months they have all been eating properly and taking proper supplements. Then one day someone lifts something heavy or bends the wrong way and they injure their back and develop a restricted vertebral joint..

Go to the next slide.

NOTES:

#38 – RESTRICTED VERTEBRA

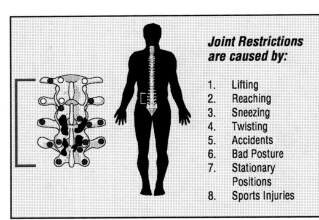

Joint Restrictions are caused by:

1. Lifting
2. Reaching
3. Sneezing
4. Twisting
5. Accidents
6. Bad Posture
7. Stationary Positions
8. Sports Injuries

Point to the black marks between the vertebrae and explain that this is a restricted joint and it is not moving properly. Look at all the red dots? These are pain nerves. Remember that mechanical trauma/injury and biochemical irritants can stimulate pain nerves.

Point to the blue dots on the vertebrae above the restriction and explain that the blue dots are called mechanical nerves and their function is to relax tight muscles, improve coordination and inhibit pain. These blue mechanical nerves can do that only when a vertebra is moving properly. A chiropractic adjustment is needed to restore motion to a restricted joint.

Who do you think is going to need more adjustments, someone who eats properly and has reduced the production of chemical irritants, or someone who lives on pizza, beer and soda? Their answer should be the person who lives on pizza, beer and soda.

Point to the blue mechanical nerves and reiterate the fact that mechanical nerves work only when the joints move properly, and when there is an excessive production of chemical irritants, pain nerves will be stimulated which promotes muscle spasm and joint restriction. Make sure that everyone understands that we need proper mechanical nerve function and that an excess of biochemical irritants can damage such normal function.

Go to the next slide.

NOTES:

#39 – PROPER NUTRITION AND NORMAL JOINT FUNCTION

Just read through the points on this slide. When you have proper nutrition, you reduce the production of chemical irritants which in turn reduces pain nerve irritation. The result is no joint restriction and normal mechanical nerve function. And remember, we want normal mechanical nerve function because mechanical nerves relax tight muscles, improve coordination and inhibit pain.

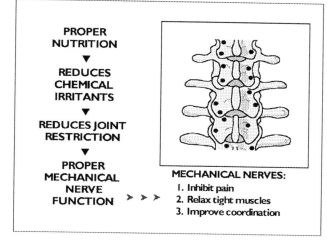

Eating properly [and taking appropriate supplements] can serve as a biochemical adjustment. This is very important to know because, in this way, you can get rid of your aches and pains faster. A nice side-benefit from eating properly is that you will probably reach your desirable weight and prevent the development of a host of diseases.

Go to the next slide.

NOTES:

#40 – THE COMPREHENSIVE TREATMENT OF PAIN

Although we are calling this approach The Comprehensive Treatment of Pain, we really mean, The Comprehensive Approach to Health Restoration. Explain to your patients that you are interested in their welfare beyond just merely relieving their pain. You want your patients to pursue health and prevent the development of disease. State that you do not want your patients to become dependent on doctors, pills or surgery. One of the best ways to help achieve this end is to eat properly.

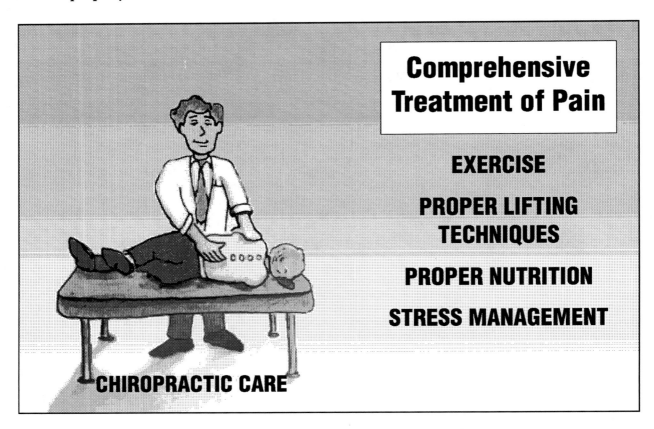

NOTES:

APPENDIX B

Appendix B contains three articles that were recently published in the Journal of Manipulative and Physiological Therapeutics (JMPT):

Proprioceptor: An obsolete, inaccurate word

Joint complex dysfunction, a novel term to replace subluxation/subluxation complex: Etiological and treatment considerations

Dysafferentation: a novel term to describe the neuropathophysiological effects of joint complex dysfunction. A look at likely methods of symptom generation

Each is devoted to conceptual and theoretical issues related to spinal joint dysfunction. JMPT regularly publishes theoretical, clinical, and research papers related to chiropractic care. For those who do not have access to a library, subscribing to JMPT is an excellent way to keep up to date with the chiropractic literature.

A special thanks to Dr. Dana Lawrence, Editor of JMPT, for granting permission to reprint these articles.

Reprinted by permission of the Journal of Manipulative and Physiological Therapeutics

Journal of Manipulative and Physiological Therapeutics   279
Volume 20 • Number 4 • May, 1997

Commentary

COMMENTARY

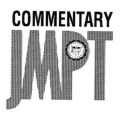

Proprioceptor: An Obsolete, Innacurate Word

Should We Stop Using the Word Proprioceptor?

Every text on neurology discusses the somatosensory system, some in more detail than others. Each indicates that somatic receptors act as biological transducers; they transform environmental stimuli into action potentials in the associated afferent fiber (1-8).

The two main categories of somatosensory receptors include mechanoreceptors and nociceptors (9). Mechanoreceptors are stimulated by innocuous mechanical deformation of the skin, muscles, and joints, which occurs, for example, when pressure is applied to the body and during body movement (10). Nociceptors are stimulated by noxious stimuli that can be either overtly damaging to tissues or potentially tissue damaging (11).

Notice that "proprioceptors" are not considered a category for receptors. One of the main reasons for this is that "proprioceptor" is an inaccurate word that engenders confusion. In fact, it is the rare chiropractic or medical doctor who can adequately describe the difference between a mechanoreceptor, proprioceptor, and nociceptor. Many contend that mechanoreceptors and nociceptors are subcategories of proprioceptors. Others maintain that proprioceptors can encode tissue injury. Still others claim that proprioception occurs at the level of the sensory receptor. None of these notions are accurate.

This commentary is offered because the chiropractic profession has begun to move away from explanations such as "bones out of place" and "pinched nerves" to describe subluxation/joint dysfunction and the neurologic effects of the chiropractic adjustment. Most contemporary chiropractic texts now discuss proprioceptors, mechanoreceptors, and nociceptors, and their relationship to joint function (12-18). Unfortunately, the details of receptor function and classification systems have yet to be clearly defined. As a consequence, we do not adhere to a common "neurological language" when discussing joint function, subluxation and related research topics. It is my contention that we should stop using the term proprioceptor and *only* use the term *mechanoreceptor* when discussing the category of receptor that is involved in the neurological reception of mechanical-induced tissue deformation which occurs during physical contact and body movement.

The Origin of Proprioceptors

Sherrington should be credited for providing us with the terms interoceptors, exteroceptors, and proprioceptors (19). Whereas interoceptors refer to receptors activated by stimuli inside the body, exteroceptors are receptors which receive stimulation from outside the body (20). Interoceptors include receptors, such as nociceptors, mechanoreceptors, chemoreceptors and baroreceptors, which are found in the walls of viscera, glands, and blood vessels (8). Exteroceptors include non-encapsulated (nociceptors) and encapsulated (mechanoreceptors) receptors in the skin and around hairs, and special sensory receptors of smell, vision, hearing, and taste (8). Proprioceptors include encapsulated receptors (mechanoreceptors) found in the deeper tissues of the musculoskeletal system, such as Golgi tendon organs and Pacinian corpuscles, which respond to body movements (8).

"Proprioceptor," an Obsolete Word

As stated above, mechanoreceptors are found in the interoceptor, exteroceptor and proprioceptor categories. Notice further that nociceptors are only found in the interoceptor and exteroceptor categories, and that the proprioceptor category contains only mechanoreceptors. At first glance, it may not be clear why there would be a problem with this classification system. However, there are two main reasons, which will become quite obvious.

First, within this system of receptor classification, there is no category for deep tissue nociceptors found in muscles and connective tissue, despite the fact that their anatomical presence is well-known (2, 8). This is an enormous problem because it is well known that deep tissue nociceptors are involved in the generation of spinal pain and dysfunction (2). Second, this system of classification only allows the deep tissue mechanoreceptors (so-called proprioceptors) to play a role in proprioception. This exclusion is completely inappropriate as it is well-known that cutaneous mechanoreceptors (so-called exteroceptors) are also involved in the generation of proprioception (9). These inherent limitations demand that we pronounce the interoceptor, exteroceptor, proprioceptor system of receptor classification as obsolete and focus on mechanoreceptors and nociceptors.

What Is Proprioception?

Sherrington referred to proprioceptors as the type of receptor involved with proprioception.

The term proprioception was derived by Sherrington (1906) from the Latin *proprius* to refer to perception of sensations that originate in receptors that are stimulated by an organism's *own* movement (21).

Current authors provide similar definitions for proprioception. For example, proprioception has been defined as, "the awareness of posture, movement and changes in equilibrium and the knowledge of position, weight and resistance of objects in relation to the body (20)." Another author states that

Commentary

limb proprioception is the sense of position and movement of the limbs. There are two submodalities of limb proprioception: the sense of stationary position of the limbs (limb position sense) and the sense of limb movement (kinesthesia) (9).

It should be clear that proprioception refers to the conscious awareness of body position and body movement. Thus, we can safely state that proprioception is a conscious cortical experience, and not a peripheral sensory phenomenon. Indeed, proprioception could not occur if the cortical centers were not intact.

'Proprioceptor': an Inaccurate Word

The prefix *proprio* implies that proprioception, the conscious awareness of body position and movement, is the function of a receptor. This is misleading because proprioception does not and cannot occur at the level of the receptor. For example, it is well known that mechanoreceptors, found in muscles, skin and joints, are not depolarized by "cortical awareness." Rather, these mechanoreceptors are depolarized by pressure against the body and by body movements (10). After such depolarization, there are first-, second- and third-order neurons that must first transmit mechanical stimuli to the cerebral cortex before the experience we call proprioception can occur.

The word proprioceptor also implies that the receptor's function is limited to its relationship to the experience of proprioception, which is inaccurate. Mechanoreceptors have many additional functions besides receiving and transmitting information about mechanical tissue deformation to the cerebral cortex where proprioception occurs. For example, mechanoreceptor depolarization results in the inhibition of nociception at the level of the spinal cord (22-24). Mechanoreceptors from skin, muscles and joints are also involved in the modulation of segmental somatomotor output (25-27) and segmental autonomic output (26,28). It is also known that normal suprasegmental motor control is dependent, in part, upon mechanoreceptor input (29).

Another point of confusion generated by the word proprioceptor is related to the all too common use of the terms "proprioceptive insult hypothesis" or "proprioceptive insult" when discussing the neurology of subluxation. These terms incorrectly imply that proprioceptors (i.e., mechanoreceptors,) can encode noxious stimuli.

Mechanoreceptors do not encode noxious stimuli. Mechanoreceptors are thought to respond only to weak mechanical stimuli, do not respond with higher frequencies to nociceptive mechanical stimuli and, in fact, many are actually suppressed by noxious stimulation, particularly noxious heat (30). A recent paper states that mechanoreceptors are probably not involved in joint nociception and pain; rather, they are excited by gentle local stimuli and joint movement within the *normal* range (31). Schmidt et al. state that

> although they encode pressure and particularly movement stimuli up to the noxious range, their responses are more closely related to the particular type of stimulus (e.g., movement in a specific direction) than to intensity (innocuous vs. noxious) (31).

It is known that repetitive stimulation of a pacinian corpuscle afferent i.e., a mechanoreceptor afferent results in the sensation of vibration. When this afferent is stimulated with in- creased intensity, the result is an increase in the apparent rate of vibration and not pain (32). Similarly, the stimulation of the afferent fiber of a Merkel cell ending results in the sensation of pressure. Increased stimulation results in increased pressure, not pain. Under normal circumstances, mechanoreceptor depolarization never becomes painful whatever the frequency of stimulation (32).

At the present time, a great deal more is understood about the nature of mechanoreceptors and nociceptors, compared with what was known at the turn of the century when the exteroceptor, interoceptor and proprioceptor categories were originally put forth. This new information has a considerable impact on how we should study and research the vertebral subluxation complex and the chiropractic adjustment in years to come.

Mechanoreceptors and the chiropractic adjustment. As described above, mechanoreceptor depolarization may result in proprioception, nociceptive inhibition, segmental somatomotor modulation, segmental autonomic modulation and normal suprasegmental motor control. The existence of such a relationship between mechanoreceptors and nervous system function is very important for the chiropractic profession. This is because many authors agree that mechanoreceptor stimulation is a mechanism by which the spinal adjustment influences the nervous system (12, 18, 22, 23, 25, 33-36).

There is also evidence to suggest that the adjustment stimulates mechanosensitive nociceptors, which results in the activation of a suprasegmental analgesic mechanism involving powerful descending inhibitory pathways which travel from the brain stem to the spinal cord (23, 37). At first, the idea that nociceptive input can reduce nociception and pain may seem paradoxical; it is not [see Gillette (23, 37) for details regarding this mechanism]. The suprasegmental analgesic mechanism induced by nociceptor stimulation has been called "diffuse noxious inhibitory control."

Unfortunately, the outcome of mechanoreceptive and nociceptive stimulation has not been investigated sufficiently in the academic and clinical chiropractic setting and consequently, this topic is poorly understood. Indeed, recently, a renowned chiropractor suggested recently that mechanoreceptors and nociceptors should not be discussed until more is known about their functions. However, "more" is already known, such that certain medical researchers feel confident enough to state that

> manipulations performed by chiropractors excite somatic afferent fibers in musculoskeletal structures of the spine. These afferent excitations may, in turn, provoke reflex responses affecting skeletal muscle, autonomic, endocrinologic and immunologic functions (38).

It is clear that we should more thoroughly investigate what is *already* known about mechanoreception and nociception. If we do not, the majority of our profession may forever explain subluxation and the chiropractic adjustment with the antiquated pinched nerve model.

I propose that there are three distinct time periods by which the application of an adjustment can help to stimulate mechanoreceptors. First, the pre-adjustment setup requires that pressure is placed upon the skin, muscles, and joints. This pressure will activate a population of cutaneous, muscle and, perhaps, joint mechanoreceptors.

Second, the dynamic thrust of adjustment is known to increase joint motion, which will stimulate additional joint receptors that are not stimulated by the pressure associated with the preadjustment setup.

Third, mechanoreceptor stimulation will continue to occur after the administration of the adjustment, so long as the improved mobility is maintained. In other words, the adjustment probably improves joint and muscle function so that the "normal mechanical function" will naturally stimulate the resident mechanoreceptor population, which will then subsequently derive the five-fold benefit of mechanoreceptor stimulation.

Compared to mechanoreceptors, nociceptors are probably only activated once (i.e., during the dynamic forceful thrust). Whereas the force associated with a dynamic thrust can exceed the threshold of almost all spinal mechanoreceptors and nociceptors (37), the force associated with spinal palpation and normal joint motion is only sufficient to activate mechanoreceptors. It is likely that the force of the adjustment can momentarily stimulate nociceptors without causing actual tissue injury and thus derive the antinociceptive benefits of the diffuse noxious inhibitory control system.

Based on the information in this section, it should be apparent that the word "proprioceptor" is inaccurate and limits our ability to discuss the neurology of the adjustment. There is, in fact, a growing body of information that supports the elimination of the use of proprioceptor when discussing human physiology.

More Evidence to Support the Elimination of the Use of the Word 'Proprioceptor'

The proposal to eliminate the use of the term "proprioceptor" is based on the fact that many well-respected neurology texts do not use "proprioceptor" to describe a category of somatic receptors (3, 9, 10, 39-46). It should be understood that this proposal is not arbitrary or capricious in any way. In fact, *Gray's Anatomy* states that the interoceptor-exteroceptor-proprioceptor classification system *is* arbitrary.

The 36th edition of *Gray's Anatomy* introduces the classification of receptors by explaining that, "receptors can be classified in various ways, for example, by the particular energy forms or modalities to which they are especially sensitive (8)." The classifications include mechanoreceptors, chemoreceptors, photoreceptors, thermoreceptors, osmoreceptors and nociceptors. The authors continue by stating that,

> another widely used (but rather arbitrary) classification divides receptors on the basis of their distribution and role in sensory activities of the body, into three main groups, namely exteroceptors, proprioceptors and interoceptors (8).

The 37th edition of *Gray's Anatomy* refers to this particular classification system as "somewhat arbitrary (47)."

Unfortunately, both editions of *Gray's Anatomy* then go on to use this arbitrary and outdated system of classification in the text, and many other respectable books continue to follow suit

(1, 2, 48, 49). Other authors choose to mention the proprioceptor classification system and then state their reservations. For example, Burt states that, "this classification system reveals little of the sensory modality of the general somatic afferent receptors (40)," which clearly suggests that the proprioceptor classification system is nonphysiological. Nolte explains that, "a more commonly used classification system subdivides receptors on the basis of the type of stimulus to which they are most sensitive (called the adequate stimulus)" (50, 51).

In many texts, there are inconsistencies in the manner in which receptors are described. For example, many texts provide tables which categorize sensory receptors (3, 7, 10, 42) and none use "proprioceptors" as a category of receptors. Interestingly enough, some of these authors still use the term "proprioceptor" in the body of the text (7, 10, 42).

There are many other ways in which the term "proprioceptor" is used in an inconsistent fashion. Some authors do not include "proprioceptor" in the index and then discuss them in the body of the text (10, 42, 46). On the contrary, Burt lists "proprioceptors" in the index and then on certain indicated pages of text, the term mechanoreceptor is used instead of proprioceptor (40). Other authors state that mechanoreceptors can be proprioceptors, and then go on to mention nociceptors in the proprioceptor section under the heading of mechanoreceptor, which suggests that nociceptors and mechanoreceptors are the same (2). Another author uses the terms proprioceptor and kinesthetic receptors interchangeably (17); however, there are no known peripheral somatic receptors that encode kinesthesia. All of this "mixing and matching" of terms and blatant inaccuracies can be very confusing to students, chiropractors, allopaths and researchers, which further illustrates why the term mechanoreceptor should be used instead of proprioceptor.

Based on the fact that the proprioceptor-interoceptor-exteroceptor classification system is obsolete, inaccurate, arbitrary (8, 47), nonphysiological (40), a less commonly used system (50, 51) and a source of great confusion, we are led to ask the question: Why is the system used at all? The answer probably has do to with the difficulties related to breaking with convention. Fortunately, this is changing.

A Solution

As mentioned above, several well-known texts have curtailed or eliminated the use of the interoceptor-exteroceptor-proprioceptor system of receptor classification. Recently, there was an International Symposium on Mechanoreceptors, during which the participants discussed muscle spindles, Golgi tendon organs, joint receptors and cutaneous receptors. The term proprioceptor was not used when discussing the various mechanoreceptors (52).

Principles of Neural Science is a very well-known neurology text that is used in both medical and chiropractic schools; it has never considered proprioceptors to be a category of receptors. The third edition (9) provides a table that lists the various classes of receptors (nociceptors, cutaneous and subcutaneous mechanoreceptors, and muscle and skeletal mechanoreceptors see Table 1). This table from *Principles of Neural Science* is

282 Journal of Manipulative and Physiological Therapeutics
Volume 20 • Number 4 • May, 1997
Commentary

Table 1. *Classes of receptors*

Receptor type	Fiber Group	Quality
Nociceptors		Pain
Mechanical	A-delta	Sharp, pricking pain
Thermal and mechano-thermal	A-delta	Sharp, pricking pain
Thermal and mechano-thermal	C	Slow, burning pain
Polymodal	C	Slow, burning pain
Cutaneous and subcutaneous mechanoreceptors		
Meissner's corpuscle	A-beta	Touch
Pacinian corpuscle[a]	A-beta	Flutter
Ruffini corpuscle	A-beta	Vibration
Merkel's receptor	A-beta	Steady skin indentation
Hair-guard, hair-tylotrich	A-beta	Steady skin indentation
Hair-down	A-beta	Flutter
Muscle and skeletal mechanoreceptors		
Muscle spindle primary	A-alpha	Limb proprioception
Muscle spindle secondary	A-beta	
Golgi tendon organ	A-alpha	
Joint capsule mechanoreceptors	A-beta	

[a]Pacinian corpuscles are also located in the mesentery, between layers of muscle and on interosseous membranes.

Reprinted by permission of Kandal, E., Principles of Neural Science, 3rd ed., Appleton and Lange, 1991:342 (Table 24-1).

offered because the text is well-respected by both the medical and chiropractic professions. For a more detailed table see Willis and Coggeshall (10).

Table 1 illustrates two main facts about somatic receptors. First, proprioceptors are not considered to be a class of receptor; and second, nociceptors and mechanoreceptors are the two classes of somatic receptors which deserve our attention. We are also provided with the type of nerve fiber that is associated with each type of receptor and the sensation, or conscious experience, that occurs when a given receptor is activated. It should not be a surprise that such a table does not provide us with significant functional information that we can apply clinically. This is because typical classification tables have inherent functional limitations. It is our job as practitioners and/or researchers to bring clinical correlations to such tables. I will attempt to do this by briefly discussing each type of receptor.

Nociceptors. Table 1 does not mention that nociceptors are found in the skin and numerous musculoskeletal structures. This is not uncommon; most tables that classify sensory receptors do not provide detailed lists regarding their anatomical location (3, 10, 42). Consequently, we are unable to appreciate the fact that nociceptor distribution in musculoskeletal tissues is almost ubiquitous, which suggests that numerous tissues may be responsible for generating nociceptive input after injury. Except for joint cartilage, synovial membranes, the nucleus pulposus and the inner layers of the annulus fibrous, every other musculoskeletal, connective tissue, and vascular structure within the spine is thought to contain nociceptors (35, 53-57).

Please note that typical classification tables for receptors do not emphasize the ratio of receptor distribution within musculoskeletal tissues (3, 9, 10, 42). Thus, it is important to mention

that fact that numerous researchers believe that the number of nociceptors greatly exceeds that of mechanoreceptors. A recent paper demonstrated that the majority of afferent fibers innervating the knee joint of the cat are those which are most commonly associated with nociception, namely A-delta and C fibers (31). In the medial articular nerve, 21% were found to be A-delta fibers and 70% were C fibers. In the posterior articular nerve, 14% were found to be A-delta fibers and 60% were C fibers. Whether this distribution is consistent within all joints of the cat, and in other species such as humans, has yet to be determined. We also do not know the exact number of A-delta and C fibers which are involved in nociception. Evidence suggests that not all of such fibers function as nociceptive afferents (31). Zimmerman has estimated that about half of the afferent fibers entering the spinal cord via the dorsal roots are nociceptive (58). Fields presents evidence that indicates that approximately 55% of afferents in typical cutaneous nerve are nociceptive C fibers (59). Charman maintains that C fibers form about 70% of all dorsal root afferents (57).

Receptor classification tables also do not discuss the outcome of nociceptive input (3, 9, 10, 42). Research has demonstrated that nociceptive input can dramatically influence the nervous system, resulting in the generation of numerous physiological responses and symptomatic presentations. For example, nociceptive input can result in segmental responses as muscle spasm and sympathetic hyperactivity (60-62). It is quite conceivable that such activity will result in reduced joint mobility, which may set the foundation for the development of the various pathological components of the subluxation complex and perpetual nociceptive stimulation.

Suprasegmental responses are also known to occur due to nociceptive input. Pain is the most well-known response; however, nociceptive input can result in many additional symptoms. For example, nociceptive input can stimulate areas in the hypothalamus and medullary reticular formation (62), resulting in seemingly bizarre symptoms such as nausea, pallor, sweating, subjective faintness, and syncope (63). Changes in heart rate, blood pressure, and respiration are also known to occur in response to nociceptive input (62, 64, 65) [See Nansel and Slazack for a recent review which discusses the topic of suprasegmental responses (66)]. Nociceptive induced stimulation of neuroendocrine centers of the hypothalamus can result in the release of catecholamines and catabolic hormones such as cortisol, which can lead to a catabolic state with a negative nitrogen balance (62). It should be clear that pain is only one potential outcome of nociceptive input; and thus, the commonly used term "pain receptor" does not accurately or effectively describe the nature or function of a nociceptor.

Clearly, the clinical significance of the extraordinary abundance of nociceptors and their subsequent activation should not be taken lightly by chiropractors. It is quite possible that nociceptive input is responsible for the generation of most of the symptoms which respond to chiropractic care. Despite the fact that physiological evidence supports this contention, only a handful of authors present evidence which suggests that the chiropractic adjustment reduces nociception (22, 23, 25,33,

Journal of Manipulative and Physiological Therapeutics 283
Volume 20 • Number 4 • May, 1997
Commentary

34, 37,67-70). Indeed, except for the work of a handful of authors, nociception is rarely, if ever, a topic of focus in chiropractic literature or the chiropractic research setting.

Mechanoreceptors. An examination of Table 1 reveals that mechanoreceptors are found in the skin and in various musculoskeletal structures. Most texts tell us that different mechanoreceptors encode different types of stimuli. For example, Pacinian corpuscles most effectively encode vibratory stimuli, whereas Meissner's corpuscles most effectively encode pressure (9, 10). Typically, we are not given any indication as to whether mechanoreceptors in different structures have additional functions. Herein lies the source of much confusion. Save for proprioception, it should be understood that the additional functions of mechanoreceptor activation are not well known by most students and practitioners. As mentioned earlier in this paper, the activation of mechanoreceptors can inhibit nociception (22-24), modulate somatomotor output (25-27), modulate segmental sympathetic output (26, 28), and modulate suprasegmental motor control (29).

Clearly, this information about mechanoreceptors has significant clinical and research significance for the chiropractic profession because, as mentioned earlier, numerous authors suggest that spinal adjustments activate mechanoreceptors (12, 22, 23, 25, 33-36, 68-70). However, a review of chiropractic literature demonstrates that mechanoreceptors, like nociceptors, are very rarely a focus of attention.

Conclusion

Understanding the location and distribution and function of spinal nociceptors and mechanoreceptors is critical for the chiropractic profession because these are the neurological structures by which we influence the nervous system. Without detailed knowledge about the properties of these receptors, it will be impossible to ever truly appreciate the important role chiropractors can and should play in the health care field. I would recommend that the nociceptor-mechanoreceptor classification system replace the obsolete and inaccurate interoceptor-exteroceptor-proprioceptor classification system. I would also suggest that the chiropractic departments, basic/core science departments, and research departments at our chiropractic colleges make an effort to make spinal nociceptors and mechanoreceptors a topic of focus so that students and doctors can develop a well-rounded understanding of the neurological structures so intimately related to chiropractic care.

David Seaman, D.C.
1871 Hendersonville Road, #302
Asheville, NC 28803

REFERENCES

1. Berne R, Levy M. Physiology. 3rd ed. St Louis: Mosby-Year Book, 1993:110.
2. Cramer G, Darby S, eds. Basic and clinical anatomy of the spine, spinal cord and ANS. St. Louis: Mosby-Year Book, 1995:251-4, 355-72.
3. Daube J, Reagan T, Sandok B, Westmoreland B. Medical neurosciences. 2nd ed. Boston: Little, Brown, 1986:115-8.
4. Kapit W, Macey R, Meisami E. The physiology coloring book. Philadelphia: Harper Collins, 1987:83-5.
5. Light A, Perl E. Peripheral sensory systems. In: Dyck P, Thomas P, Griffin J, Low P, Poduslo J, eds. Peripheral neuropathy. 3rd ed. Philadelphia: WB Saunders, 1993:149-65.
6. Martin J. Coding and processing of sensory information. In: Kandel E, Schwartz J, Jessell T, eds. Principles of neural science. 3rd ed. New York: Elsevier, 1991:329-40.
7. Shepard G. Neurobiology. 2nd ed. New York: Oxford University Press, 1988:205-11.
8. Williams P, Warwick R, eds. Gray's Anatomy. 36th ed. WB Saunders: Philadelphia, 1980: 851.
9. Martin J, Jessell T. Modality coding in the somatic sensory system. In: Kandel E, Schwartz J, Jessell T, eds. Principles of neural science. 3rd ed. New York: Elsevier, 1991:341-52.
10. Willis W, Coggeshall R. Sensory mechanisms of the spinal cord. 2nd ed. New York: Plenum Press, 1991:13-45.
11. Maciewicz R. Organization of pain pathways. In: Ashbury A, McKhann G, McDonald W, eds. Diseases of the nervous system: clinical neurobiology. Vol 2. 2nd ed. Philadelphia: WB Saunders, 1992:849-57.
12. Bergmann T, Peterson D, Lawrence D. Chiropractic technique. New York: Churchill Livingstone, 1993.
13. Cox J. Low back pain. 5th ed. Baltimore: Williams & Wilkins, 1990.
14. Eder M, Tilscher H, Gengenbach M. Chiropractic therapy: diagnosis and treatment. Rockville, MD: Aspen Publishers, 1990.
15. Gatterman M. ed. Foundations of chiropractic: subluxation. St Louis: Mosby, 1995.
16. Haldeman S, ed. Principles and practice of chiropractic. 2nd ed. Norwalk, CT: Appleton & Lange, 1992.
17. Leach R. The chiropractic theories: principles and clinical applications. 3rd ed. Baltimore: Williams & Wilkins, 1994.
18. Fitz-Ritson D. Neuroanatomy and neurophysiology of the upper cervical spine. In: Vernon H, ed. Upper cervical syndrome: chiropractic diagnosis and treatment. Baltimore: Williams & Wilkins, 1988:48-85.
19. Sherrington C. The integrative action of the nervous system. New York: Charles Scribner's Sons, 1906.
20. Propropception. Taber's Cyclopedic Medical Dictionary. Thomas C, ed. 16th ed. Philadelphia: FA Davis, 1989:638,930,1495.
21. Fisher A. Vestibular-proprioceptive processing and bilateral integration and sequencing deficits. In: Fisher A, Murray E, Bundy C, eds. Sensory integration: theory and practice. Philadelphia: FA Davis, 1991: 71-107.
22. Wyke B. Articular neurology and manipulative therapy. In: Glasgow E, Twomey L, Scull E, et al. eds. Aspects of manipulative therapy. 2nd ed. New York: Churchill Livingstone, 1985:72-7.
23. Gillette R. Potential antinociceptive effects of high level somatic stimulation: chiropractic manipulation therapy may coactivate both tonic and phasic analgesic system—some recent evidence. Trans Pacific Consortium Res. 1986; 1(A4): 1-9.
24. Woolf C. Segmental afferent fibre-mediated analgesia: transcutaneous electrical nerve stimulation (TENS) and vibration. In Wall P, Melzack R, eds. Textbook of pain. 2nd ed. New York: Churchill Livingstone, 1989:884-96.
25. Dvorak J, Dvorak V. Manual medicine: diagnostics. 2nd ed. New York: Thieme Med Pub, 1990:35-45.
26. Hooshmand H. Chronic pain: reflex sympathetic dystrophy, prevention and management. Boca Raton, FL: CRC Press, 1993: 33-56.
27. Gordon J. Spinal mechanisms of motor coordination. In: Kandel E, Schwartz J, Jessell T, eds. Principles of neural science. 3rd ed. New York: Elsevier, 1991:581-95.
28. Levine J, Coderre T, Basbaum A. The peripheral nervous system

and the inflammatory process. In: Dubner R, Gebhart G, Bond M, eds. Proceedings of the 5th World Congress on Pain. New York: Elsevier, 1987:33-43.

29. Masdeu J, Brazis P. The anatomic localization of lesions in the thalamus. In: Brazis P, Masdeu J, Biller J. eds. Localization in clinical neurology. 2nd ed. Boston: Little, Brown & Co, 1990: 319-43.

30. Price D. Psychological and neural mechanisms of pain, New York: Raven Press, 1988:86

31. Schmidt R, Schaible H, Mefslinger K, et al. Silent and active nociceptors: Structure, functions, and clinical implications. In: Gebhart G, Hammond D, Jensen T. eds. Proceedings of the 7th World Congress on Pain , Seattle: IASP Press, 1994:213-50.

32. Willis W. Central plastic responses to pain. In: Gebhart G, Hammond D, Jensen T. eds. Proceedings of the 7th World Congress on Pain , Seattle: IASP Press, 1994:301-24.

33. Ferezy J. Sensory innervation of the spinal joint and effects of manipulation, (Appendix 5-B). In: Ferezy, J. ed. The chiropractic neurological examination Gathersburg, MD: Aspen Publishers, 1992: 71-3.

34. Sandoz R. Some reflex phenomena associated with spinal derangements and adjustments. Ann Swiss Chiropr Assoc. 1981; 7:45-65.

35. Slosberg M. Effects of altered afferent input on sensation, proprioception, muscle tone and sympathetic reflex response, J Manipulative Physiol Ther. 1988; 11:400-8.

36. Suter E, Herzog W, Conway PJ, Zhang YT. Reflex response associated with manipulative treatment of the thoracic spine. JNMS: J Neuro Sys 1995;2(3):124-30.

37. Gillette R. A speculative argument for the coactivation of diverse somatic receptor populations by forceful chiropractic adjustments. Manual Med 1987; 3:1-14.

38. Sato A. Spinal reflex physiology. In: Haldeman, S. ed. Principles and practice of chiropractic. 2nd ed. Norwalk, CT: Appleton & Lange, 1992: 87-103.

39. Brass A, Netter F. The Ciba collection of medical illustrations, nervous system (volume I-part I), anatomy and physiology. West Caldwell, New Jersey: CIBA, 1986:164-5,185.

40. Burt A. Textbook of neuroanatomy. Philadelphia: WB Saunders, 1993:198-201, 308-10.

41. Dvorak J, Dvorak V. Manual medicine: diagnostics. New York: Thieme-Stratton, 1984:21-26.

42. Guyton A. Basic neuroscience. 2nd ed. Philadelphia: WB Saunders, 1991:103.

43. Martin J. Somatic sensory system I: receptor physiology and submodality coding. In: Kandel E, Schwartz J, eds. Principles of neural science. 1st ed. New York: Elsevier, 1981:157-69.

44. Martin J. Receptor physiology and submodality coding in the somatic sensory system. In: Kandel E, Schwartz J, eds. Principles of neural science. 2nd ed. New York: Elsevier, 1985:287-300.

45. Nicholls J, Martin A, Wallace B. From neuron to brain. 3rd ed. Sunderland, MA: Sinauer Associates, 1992:467-97.

46. Snell R. Clinical neuroanatomy for medical students. 3rd ed. Boston: Little, Brown and Company, 1992:123.

47. Williams P, Warwick R, Dyson M, Bannister L, eds. Gray's Anatomy. 37th ed. Edinburgh: Churchill Livingstone, 1989: 908.

48. Barr M, Kiernan J. The human nervous system: an anatomical viewpoint. 5th ed. Philadelphia: JB Lippincott, 1993:33-42.

49. Barr M, Kiernan J. The human nervous system: an anatomical viewpoint. 6th ed. Philadelphia: JB Lippincott, 1993:36-44.

50. Nolte J. The human brain. 2nd ed. St Louis: Mosby-Year Book, 1988:96.

51. Nolte J. The human brain. 3rd ed. St Louis: Mosby-Year Book, 1993:101.

52. Hnik P, Soukup T, Vejsada R, Zelena J. Mechanoreceptors: development, structure and function. New York: Plenum Press, 1988.

53. Bogduk N. Innervation, pain patterns, and mechanisms of pain production. In Twomey L, Taylor J, eds. Physical therapy of the low lack. 2nd ed. New York: Churchill Livingstone, 1994:93-109.

54. Grieve G. Common vertebral joint problems. 2nd ed. New York: Churchill Livingstone, 1988:51-2.

55. Haldeman S. The neurophysiology of spinal pain. In: Haldeman S. ed. Principles and practice of chiropractic. 2nd ed. Norwalk, CT: Appleton & Lange, 1992:165-84.

56. Wyke B. The neurological basis of thoracic pain. Physiotherapy. 1970; 10:356-67

57. Charman R. Pain and nociception: mechanisms and modulation in sensory context. In: Boyling J, Palastanga N. eds. Grieve's modern manual therapy. 2nd ed. New York: Churchill Livingstone, 1994: 253-70.

58. Zimmerman M. Neurophysiology of nociception, pain and pain therapy. In Bonica J, Ventafridda V, eds. Advances in pain research and therapy, Vol 2. New York: Raven Press, 1979:13-29.

59. Fields H. Pain. New York: McGraw Hill, 1987: 16.

60. Bonica J. Anatomic and physiologic basis of nociception and pain. In: Bonica J, ed. The management of pain. 2nd ed. Philadelphia: Lea & Febiger, 1990: 28-94.

61. Hooshmand H. Chronic Pain: Reflex sympathetic dystrophy, prevention, and management. Boca Raton, FL: CRC Press, 1993: 33-5.

62. Bonica J. Clinical importance of hyperalgesia. In: Willis W, ed. Hyperalgesia and allodynia. New York: Raven Press, 1992: 17-43.

63. Feinstein B. Experiments on pain referred from deep somatic tissues, J Bone Joint Surg 1954; 36-A(5):981-97.

64. Cramer G, Darby S. Anatomy related to the spinal subluxation. In: Gatterman M, ed. Foundations of chiropractic: subluxation. St. Louis: Mosby, 1995:18-34.

65. Sato Y, Schaible H, Schmidt R. Reactions of cardiac postganglionic sympathetic neurons to movements of normal and inflammed knee joints. J Autonomic Nerv Sys 1985; 12:1-13.

66. Nansel D, Szlazak M. Somatic dysfunction and the phenomenon of visceral disease simulation: A probable explanation for the apparent effectiveness of somatic therapy in patients presumed to be suffering from true visceral disease. J Manipulstive Physiol Therap 1995; 18(6):379-97.

67. Patterson M. The spinal cord: Participant in disorder. Spinal Manipulation. 1993: 9(3):2-11.

68. Will T. The biochemical basis of manipulative therapeutics: hypothetical considerations. J Manip Physiol Therap 1978; 1(3):153-6.

69. Terrett A, Vernon H. Manipulation and pain tolerance. A controlled study of the effect of spinal manipulation on paraspinal cutaneous pain tolerance levels. Am J Phys Med 1984; 63:217-25.

70. Vernon H, Dhami M, Howley T, Annett R. Spinal manipulation and beta-endorphin: A controlled study of the effect of a spinal manipulation on plasma beta-endorphin levels in normal males. J Manip Physiol Therap 1986; 9:115-23.

634 Journal of Manipulative and Physiological Therapeutics
Volume 20 • Number 9 • November/December, 1997
Commentary

COMMENTARY

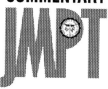

Joint Complex Dysfunction, A Novel Term to Replace Subluxation/Subluxation Complex: Etiological and Treatment Considerations

SUBLUXATION–A HISTORY OF CONFUSION

Gatterman has determined that over 100 synonyms for subluxation have been used over the years:

> The word subluxation has been daubed in a kaleidoscope of colors and embedded with a multitude of meanings by chiropractors during the past 100 years. To some it has become a holy word; to others, an albatross to be discarded. Currently subluxation is the most loved and hated, hotly debated, and consecrated term used by chiropractors.(1)

Clearly, "subluxation" is an emotional topic. Dictionaries provide several definitions for the word 'emotional.' *The Random House Dictionary of the English Language* defines 'emotional' as "actuated, effected, or determined by emotion rather than reason; An emotional decision is often a wrong decision." (2) Based on this definition, does it make sense for the chiropractic profession to continue using the word "subluxation?" This question, which simply seeks to determine the utility, necessity, and appropriateness of the word "subluxation," most likely ignites the passions of many chiropractors, because it is held that, "the concept of vertebral subluxation is central to chiropractic." (1) Indeed, many in the chiropractic profession feel that "subluxation" is an unique chiropractic word. Even though such feelings exist, it is important to ascertain if this feeling about subluxation is actually consistent with reality.

Practice Guidelines for Straight Chiropractic defines subluxation as

> a misalignment of one or more articulations of the spinal column or its immediate weight-bearing articulations, to a degree less than a luxation, which by inference causes alteration of nerve function and interference to the transmission of mental impulses, resulting in a lessening of the body's innate ability to express its maximum potential (3).

This text credits D. D. and B. J. Palmer for generating this definition of subluxation; however, a review of relevant dictionaries demonstrates that only the hypothetical nerve function component of this definition is unique to chiropractic.

In 1828, almost 70 yr before D. D. Palmer delivered the first chiropractic adjustment, Noah Webster published his first edition of the *American Dictionary of the English Language*, in which subluxation was defined as "in surgery, a violent sprain; also, an incomplete dislocation." (4) Today, standard dictionaries continue to define subluxation as "a partial dislocation, as of a joint; sprain." (2) Medical dictionaries (5, 6) and textbooks on biomechanics (7) also define subluxation as "an

incomplete or partial dislocation." Based on this information, it seems that subluxation is a medical word, and not a word with a unique chiropractic heritage.

Clearly, both medical doctors and many chiropractors generally agree on the definition of subluxation; however, treatment approaches differ widely. Chiropractors use the manual adjustment or manipulation to reduce a subluxation. Such an adjustment is most commonly characterized as a high velocity, low amplitude thrust into the subluxated joint. The medical approach to treating subluxation is very different. White and Panjabi indicate that upper cervical subluxations should be reduced by skeletal traction and then cervical fusion (7). Regarding the treatment of subluxations, Bland indicates that "manipulation is dangerous"; instead, treatment should involve immobilization and fusion (8). These conflicting treatments demand that the following question be asked. How could a subluxation at C1-C2 approach the level of a medical/surgical emergency for one professional and, for another professional, an upper cervical subluxation is viewed as a spinal lesion in need of a high velocity adjustment? Obviously, the two so-called subluxations are very different, despite the fact that, for many years, they were defined in exactly the same fashion.

Efforts to define more accurately the chiropractic variety of subluxation have been made by a small handful of authors (9-14). As a result of this effort, the term "subluxation complex" emerged. "Subluxation complex" refers to pathological or degenerative changes that occur in the structures that make up the joint complex such as the joint capsule, spinal ligaments, disc, tendons, muscles, and blood vessels.

Despite the advent of a revised, contemporary definition of subluxation, it is still unlikely that non-chiropractors will appreciate the "new" chiropractic variety of subluxation or its relationship to the nervous system. The term "subluxation complex" will necessarily connote a complex of problems that occur in response to a partial dislocation. In short, it will be impossible for a small, disorganized and somewhat marginal profession such as chiropractic to redefine a word and expect it to be understood and appreciated by allopaths, scientists, attorneys, legislators, and laymen. For at least 170 yr, both medical and nonmedical dictionaries have defined subluxation as a "partial dislocation," and it is very likely that this definition will live on forever.

It is time that the chiropractors accept the fact that "subluxation" and "subluxation complex" have outlived their usefulness. Neither "subluxation" or "subluxation complex" effectively or accurately conveys the nature of the joint problem that

Journal of Manipulative and Physiological Therapeutics **635**
Volume 20 • Number 9 • November/December, 1997
Commentary

chiropractors treat. History demonstrates that (a) "subluxation" is not a chiropractic word (4); (b) there is considerable confusion regarding the word "subluxation" (1, 15) and (c) efforts by the chiropractic profession to define and redefine the word "subluxation" have not been effective (15, 16). Furthermore, because "subluxation" is poorly defined, it is not possible to effectively study the pathogenesis of the condition or develop a rational treatment approach. Thus, it seems that it is time to replace "subluxation" with a more contemporary, accurate and physiological term. For these reasons, I propose that the term "joint complex dysfunction" replace "subluxation/subluxation complex."

There is no doubt that objections will arise regarding the addition of another term to the list of over 100 names that already exist to describe the chiropractic lesion; however, this proposal offers an important distinction to consider. The purpose of this commentary is to propose a name for the spinal lesion that chiropractors treat, discuss likely pathogenic factors, examine possible pathophysiological factors that are involved in symptom generation and offer appropriate methods of treatment. At the present time, no text or paper has yet to take such an approach. Keating indicates that, "the subluxation concept itself has remained more metaphor than a scientific, operationally defined phenomenon." (15) Indeed, a functional definition of subluxation was not provided by texts devoted to chiropractic practice guidelines (3 ,17) or a recent text devoted to the topic of subluxation itself (1).

It should be mentioned that, like the chiropractic profession, the medical profession has yet to put forth a reasonable name to describe the lesion responsible for spine pain. Indeed, regarding the majority of neck and back pains, Wall states that, "we are faced with a crisis epidemic of painful states where no peripheral pathology has been discovered" (18).

Consider the irony of this situation. The medical profession has determined that no overt pathology, such as a partial dislocation (subluxation), exists in the great majority of patients with spinal pain. Meanwhile, in the eyes of the medical and scientific community, the chiropractic profession continues to promote the notion that the purpose of chiropractic care is to remove partial dislocations from patients with pain and without pain. This situation exists in spite of the fact that the majority chiropractors know that partial dislocations rarely occur in their patient population.

In summary, the professions of chiropractic, physical therapy and medicine have yet to come up with a reasonable name for the musculoskeletal lesion of the spine that all three professions attempt to treat when patients present with spinal pain and related symptoms. Clearly, new terminology is needed. To fill this need, the name "joint complex dysfunction" is proposed.

JOINT COMPLEX DYSFUNCTION

The word "complex" is used to describe something that is composed of many interconnected parts (2). Any discussion about joints necessarily involves all of the specific joint structures, as well as muscles, ligaments, and blood supply and

Table 1. *Negative effects of immobilization (reprinted with permission from Liebenson C. Pathogenesis of chronic back pain. J Manipulative Physiol Ther 1992; 15:299-308).*

Joints
  Shrinks joint capsules
  Increases compressive loading
  Leads to joint contracture
  Increases synthesis rate of glycosaminoglycans
  Increase in periarticular fibrosis
  Irreversible changes post-8-wk immobilization
Ligament
  Lowers failure or yield point
  Decreased thickness of collagen fibers
Disc biochemistry
  Decreased oxygen
  Decreased glucose
  Decreased sulfate
  Increase lactate concentration
  Decreased proteoglycan content
Bone
  Decreases bone density
  Eburnation
Muscle
  Decreased thickening of collagen fibers
  Decreased oxidative potential
  Decreased muscle mass
  Decreased saromeres
  Decreased cross-sectional area
  Decreased mitochondrial content
  Type 1 muscular atrophy
  Type 2 muscular atrophy
  20% loss of muscle strength per week
Cardiopulmonary
  Increased maximal heart rate
  Decreased VO2 maximum
  Decreased plasma volume

nerve supply (19). The term "joint complex" is used here to collectively describe all of these structures. Thus, the term "joint complex dysfunction" refers to dysfunction of joint complex structures.

Although the term joint complex dysfunction is new, dysfunction of joint complex structures has been described in the literature by chiropractors (14, 20, 21), physical therapists (22, 23) and medical doctors (24-26). All agree that reduced mobility promotes pathological changes in the structures that make up the joint complex, and that pain, inflammation and stiffness are common manifestations of the lesion. Restoring mobility is often a primary objective of treatment for this very common type of musculoskeletal lesion. Table 1 outlines the pathological changes that occur in joint complex structures due to immobilization.

In addition to the pathological changes that occur in the muscular system because of immobilization, axial and appendicular muscle undergo functional imbalances such as muscle tightening or shortening, and also develop myofascial trigger points. It appears that both muscle imbalances and trigger points are intimately associated with joint hypomobility/immobility; thus, both varieties of muscle dysfunction are considered to be a component joint complex dysfunction.

Janda states that, "the tendency for some muscles to develop weakness or tightness does not occur randomly; rather, typical 'muscle imbalance patterns' can be described" (27). Janda indicates that muscle imbalance develops mainly between mus-

636 Journal of Manipulative and Physiological Therapeutics
Volume 20 • Number 9 • November/December, 1997
Commentary

cles prone to develop tightness, such as the hamstrings and erector spinae muscles, and muscles prone to develop inhibition, such as the gluteal and abdominal muscles (27). It seems that this variety of muscle dysfunction, which promotes faulty movement patterns, is an essential component of joint complex dysfunction (20, 27, 27).

Myofascial trigger points were first described in an organized fashion by Travell and Rinzler in 1952 (29). In this landmark paper, the location and zones of pain referral were illustrated for trigger points in both spinal and extremity muscles. Trigger points were defined as "small hypersensitive region[s] from which impulses bombard the central nervous system and give rise to referred pain" (29). It is generally held that trigger points most commonly develop in response to muscle macro/microtrauma. There may also be a relationship between joint hypomobility and the development of trigger points. Simons states that, "articular dysfunction is marked by a loss of normal joint 'play' or mobility" and further explains that "joint dysfunction can be a potent perpetuator of myofascial trigger points, if not the origin of a myofascial pain syndrome" (30). For the details on biochemical and pathophysiological mechanisms that have been implicated in the development of trigger points, see Travell and Simons (31), Simons (30), Sola and Bonica (32), Yunus (33), Rachlin (34) and Sandman (35).

Simons and Travell state that, "myofascial trigger points are among the most common, yet poorly recognized and inadequately-managed, causes of musculoskeletal pain seen in medical practice." (36) Sola and Bonica indicate that patients are often unaware that they have a muscle problem, "and might complain instead of headache, neck pain, joint pain, backache, or sciatica-like pain in the buttocks or lower extremities" (32). A clinical study performed in a comprehensive pain center demonstrated that myofascial trigger points were the primary cause of pain in 85% of 283 consecutive admissions (30). In another study, trigger points in the upper trapezius, sternocleidomastoid, splenii, and suboccipital muscles were found to be the most common cause of head pain in a group of patients with chronic headache (31). According to Davidoff, a great number of migraine episodes are initiated by trigger points, yet a surprising number of clinicians overlook this common phenomenon; treating triggers points may be the only way to offer relief to those who suffer with migraines (37). Davidoff also states that it is worthwhile to check for trigger points in patients whose history demonstrates macro/microtraumatic injury (37).

In summary, it should be clear that the word "subluxation" (i.e., a partial dislocation) cannot not be used to describe the negative effects of immobilization, imbalances in muscle function and myofascial trigger points. Terms such as joint restriction, joint fixation, hypomobility, somatic dysfunction and joint blockage are also inappropriate because they merely refer to reduced joint mobility and not to the negative effects of immobilization, imbalances in muscle function, and myofascial trigger points.

It should be mentioned that Mayer and Gatchel put forth the term "deconditioning syndrome" to describe patients with (a) the degeneration and atrophy that occurs in hypomobile spinal tissues (referred to in the present commentary as joint complex dysfunction), (b) a reduction in cardiovascular fitness and (c) pain (24). It should be clear that the deconditioning syndrome is not a synonym for joint complex dysfunction; rather, joint complex dysfunction is a component of the deconditioning syndrome.

Pathogenesis of joint complex dysfunction. It is likely that joint complex dysfunction develops before pain is generated. It is known that the muscle pathology (i.e., degeneration and atrophy, and connective tissue pathology can exist in asymptomatic subjects. Parkkola and Kormano have demonstrated that lumbar intervertebral discs and muscles degenerate without any symptoms in apparently healthy volunteers ranging in age from 19 to 74 years (38). The asymptomatic disc degeneration is characterized by reduced discal height, loss of water content, and, sometimes protrusion and prolapse. The asymptomatic muscle degeneration is characterized by atrophied muscles and enhanced fat deposition within the muscles (38). Such muscle degeneration is of special concern because researchers have concluded that the lumbar paravertebral musculature plays a role in stabilizing the spinal column and that muscle weakness can predispose the spine to injury (39).

It appears that there are two main promoters of spinal muscle degeneration, a sedentary lifestyle and repetitive strain/microtrauma. Parkkola and Kormano determined that the degeneration of the discs and muscles was found to increase as people age. Thus,

> degeneration of both the discs and the muscles of the lumbar spine might be considered a normal consequence of aging. However, aging cannot explain the early degeneration of discs detected in persons under 20 years of age (38).

Indeed, investigators have concluded that "modern sedentary man does not expose his back to work loads sufficient for Type 2 muscle fibers to retain their "normal" size" (40). Liebenson indicates that, repetitive microtrauma from prolonged overuse of muscles, joints and ligaments and/or constrained postures can lead to a gradual weakening and atrophy of the strained musculoskeletal structures, such that painful injury can occur without obvious trauma, or noticeable inflammation or swelling (20). Based on this information, it is reasonable to suggest that the great majority of individuals suffer from asymptomatic joint complex dysfunction before spinal tissue injury generates pain. Once tissue injury occurs, an entirely new set of dynamics come into play, including inflammation, nociception and pain, all of which promote joint immobility and further development of joint complex dysfunction.

Inflammation, a promoter of joint complex dysfunction. It is a well-accepted fact that tissue injury results in the generation of the inflammatory process (41). The inflammatory process consists of three phases, including the acute inflammatory phase, which lasts from 0-72 hr, the repair phase, which lasts from 48 hr to 6 wk, and the remodeling phase, which lasts from 3 wk to 1 yr or more (23, 42).

The acute inflammatory phase is characterized by the release of such chemical mediators as bradykinin, serotonin, histamine

Journal of Manipulative and Physiological Therapeutics **637**
Volume 20 • Number 9 • November/December, 1997
Commentary

and prostaglandins from injured tissues. These and other chemical mediators are responsible for driving both the vascular and cellular components of the acute inflammatory phase (41, 42). The repair phase of the inflammatory process is characterized by the random deposition of fibrous tissue such as collagen and proteoglycans. The purpose of the remodeling phase is to organize and realign the randomly deposited fibrous tissue. Effective remodeling is dependent on tissue mobility (20, 23, 42). Unfortunately, it is thought that fibrous scar tissue proliferation is seen in virtually all soft tissue injuries (43). Two main factors are thought to drive such fibrous tissue production: the release of the inflammatory chemical mediators (43, 44), and reduced mobility (26, 45, 46). Such fibrous tissue deposition will reduce mobility and further promote joint complex dysfunction.

Nociception, a promoter of joint complex dysfunction. Nociceptors are the bare, or unmyelinated, beginnings of C fibers and A-delta fibers. They are thought to have a 'chicken wire' appearance and weave throughout the tissues in which they are found (47).

Nociceptors are located in virtually every tissue of the joint complex (47-54). Not only is nociceptor innervation nearly ubiquitous, recent research suggests that nociceptors may be the predominant receptor type found in joint structures. A recent paper explained that the majority of afferent fibers innervating the knee joint of the cat are those which are most commonly associated with nociception, namely A-delta and C fibers (55). In the medial articular nerve, 21% were found to be A-delta fibers and 70% were C fibers. In the posterior articular nerve, 14% were found to be A-delta fibers and 60% were C fibers. Other authors have commented on the abundance of nociceptive fibers. Zimmerman has estimated that about half of the afferent fibers entering the spinal cord via the dorsal roots are nociceptive (56). Fields presents evidence which indicates that approximately 55% of afferents in typical cutaneous nerve are nociceptive C fibers (57). Charman maintains that C fibers form about 70% of all dorsal root afferents (47).

Under normal biomechanical and physiological conditions, nociceptors are not stimulated because their thresholds of activation are too high (54, 58). It is known nociceptors respond to noxious stimuli, such as tissue injury/damage, or to stimuli that is potentially tissue damaging (58, 59). As mentioned in the section on inflammation, tissue injury releases chemical mediators which drive the inflammatory process. These same chemical mediators also activate nociceptors (57, 60-62).

Nociceptor activity can be dramatically enhanced via a sensitization process in which nociceptors acquire abnormally low thresholds of activation (63). Sensitization is promoted by many of the same chemical mediators which initially activate nociceptors (57, 60, 63). In addition, the nociceptor itself can play a role in promoting inflammation and the sensitization process. Fields states that, "it is not generally appreciated that substances contributing to nociception are present in the terminals of primary afferent nociceptors and that they can be released by those terminals when the nociceptor is active" (57).

Examples include substance P and calcitonin gene-related peptide, both of which cause vasodilation (64). Levine et al. explain that introducing synthetic substance P into peripheral tissues causes vasodilation, increased vascular permeability, pavementing of leukocytes in venules, stimulation of phagocytosis by polymorphonuclear leukocytes, and mast degranulation which involves the release of histamine, serotonin and leukotrienes (65). Fields indicates that substance P release from nociceptors causes histamine release from mast cells, serotonin release from platelets, and the accumulation of bradykinin (57). The term "neurogenic inflammation" is used to describe the vasodilation, edema, and the nociceptor sensitization which are promoted by the many actions of substance P (64).

As mentioned earlier, sensitized nociceptors have abnormally low thresholds. In this state they are capable of being stimulated by innocuous input such as that associated with light touch and normal body movement (66, 67). Research has demonstrated that the resting discharge of the medial articular nerve of the cat knee joint consists of some 1,800 impulses per 30-sec intervals. During inflammation, the resting discharge increases to 11,000 impulses. During normal movement without inflammation, some 4,400 impulses are generated per 30-sec interval, whereas during inflammation the same movement generated some 30,900 impulses, reflecting a sevenfold difference (60). When "individual afferents have been studied under normal and inflamed conditions, the afferent discharge sometimes increased more than 100-fold."(60)

As a consequence of the sensitization that occurs in tissue nociceptors, referred to as peripheral sensitization, the increased nociceptive input promotes a phenomenon known as central sensitization (68). "Intense nociceptive barrage produces stimulation and sensitization of neurons in the dorsal horn, interneurons, and neurons located in the anterior and anterolateral cord" (66). The outcome of this activity can have dramatic effects on the muscular component of the joint complex. "Stimulation and sensitization of somatomotor neurons result in skeletal muscle spasm.... which through positive feed back loops generate and sustain nociceptive impulses from the muscles and thus aggravate pain and discomfort" (66). It should be understood that central sensitization and the subsequent reflex muscle spasm are not merely segmental phenomena.

> Based on both experimental and clinical evidence, the sensitization spreads not only in the those segments that receive input from affected nociceptive fibers, but with time it causes changes of neurons in adjacent spinal segments that become involved in the expansion of the area of hyperalgesia, allodynia, reflex muscle spasm, and other segmental responses (69).

It is generally agreed that the purpose of muscles spasm is to reduce mobility of the injured tissue (69-71). Thus, it is reasonable to conclude that nociceptive-induced muscle spasm can reduce mobility and further promote joint complex dysfunction.

As mentioned above, nociceptive input also activates seg-

638 Journal of Manipulative and Physiological Therapeutics
Volume 20 • Number 9 • November/December, 1997
Commentary

Appendix B: Reprinted Articles   p. 251

mental preganglionic sympathetic neurons. Since at least the 1960s, it has been known that such a relationship exists between nociceptive afferents and sympathetic postganglionic fibers (65). There are several ways in which nociceptive-induced segmental sympathetic hyperactivity may actually help to promote inflammation and nociception and thus help to promote the development of joint complex dysfunction. First, it is known that sympathetic hyperactivity contributes to the development of inflammation, which is referred to as "neurogenic inflammation." Research has demonstrated that sympathetic nerve stimulation causes an increase in vascular permeability, and chemical sympathectomy potently inhibits the plasma extravasation induce by the injection of histamine and serotonin (65). Second, it has been shown that the interaction between sympathetic efferents and nociceptors can increase local tissue production of prostaglandins (65). Third, it is known that norepinephrine release into injured tissues from sympathetic terminals can contribute to nociception. It is thought that norepinephrine may play a role in nociceptor sensitization by up-regulating the production of alpha-1-adrenergic receptors on the nociceptor membrane (72, 73). Experimental evidence has demonstrated that norepinephrine injection into the skin of normal patients does not cause pain, whereas it can cause pain in pain patients who have been rendered pain-free with sympathetic blockade (73).

In addition to enhancing inflammation and nociception, it is possible that sympathetic fibers may play a more direct role in promoting joint complex dysfunction. It is known that muscle spindles are innervated by sympathetic efferent fibers (74, 75), which suggests that sympathetic hyperactivity may promote muscle spasm (75).

Pain, a promoter of joint complex dysfunction. Pain is very different than inflammation or nociceptive-induced muscle spasm. Inflammation, nociception and muscle spasm are physiological processes and do not require the involvement of our brain in a conscious fashion. In other words, when joint hypomobility is induced by inflammation and nociceptive-induced muscle spasm, it is done physiologically and without a patient's conscious participation. However, pain is a psychological state that does involve the conscious participation of the patient.

It is known that the experience of pain drives a patient to consciously immobilize an injured area in a position of comfort for the purpose of reducing pain (22). Norkin and Levangie state that "if the joint is immobilized for a few weeks in the position of comfort, contractures will develop in the surrounding soft tissues and as a consequence, a normal range of joint motion will be impossible" (22) and thus further promote joint complex dysfunction.

It should be mentioned that peripheral and central nociceptive sensitization can cause allodynia and hyperalgesia to develop. Allodynia is defined as pain produced by innocuous stimuli and hyperalgesia is defined as abnormally intense pain produced by noxious stimuli (59, 63). In clinical practice it is common to find patients who complain that normal movements are very painful. It is also common to find patients who are abnormally sensitive to normal and deep palpation, particularly

in the cervical spine. It is likely that these patients, who manifest signs of allodynia and hyperalgesia, would be particularly devoted in their efforts to consciously immobilize their injured joint complex structures.

SYMPTOM GENERATION FROM JOINT COMPLEX DYSFUNCTION

Two main theories have been put forth to explain how symptom generation occurs with spinal joint dysfunction. Chiropractors put forth a nerve interference model of subluxation. The Osteropaths maintained that osteopathic lesion was associated with irritated sensory receptors, particularly proprioceptors, which caused segmental spinal cord activity to become hyperexcitable (referred to as segmental facilitation) and capable of promoting various symptoms and disease states via the enhancement of segmental somatomotor and sympathetic output. It will be demonstrated shortly that neither of these models sufficiently describe a mechanism by which various symptoms may develop; for this reason; a dysafferentation model of symptom-generation is proposed.

Nerve interference model of symptom generation. Classical chiropractic theory maintains that subluxations cause nerve interference. The precise nature of this interference has yet to be precisely described. For example, *Practice Guidelines for Straight Chiropractic* states that a subluxation "by inference causes alteration of nerve function and interference to the transmission of impulses, resulting in a lessening of the body's innate ability to express its maximum potential" (3). The word "interference" is used in a fashion which suggests that subluxations interrupt mental/nerve impulse generation and this may result in the development of symptoms wherever the body is unable to express itself maximally. In reality, classic chiropractic theorists and their modern day proponents offer nothing more than an esoteric description of nerve root compression and the associated "conduction block" that occurs in compromised fibers. Because it is well-known that nerve compression is an uncommon occurrence in clinical practice (48, 50, 76-78), I recommend that chiropractors use the term "nerve interference" only for the rare patient that demonstrates signs and symptoms of nerve compression.

Proprioceptor model of symptom generation. Although the shortcomings of the nerve interference model are very obvious, the inadequacies of the so-called proprioceptor model are not so clear. The proprioceptor model of symptom generation suggests that spinal joint dysfunction can abnormally excite resident tissue proprioceptors which bombard the spinal cord to create a facilitated segment (i.e., central sensitization), which, in turn, can promote segmental sympathetic hyperactivity and create the symptoms of visceral disease. Irvin Korr has been credited for developing this model (79), which has gained favor in the chiropractic profession (82, 81). It should be mentioned that Korr's work was based, in part, upon the earlier work of Denslow and colleagues (82-84).

There are two primary problems with the proprioceptor model. First, both Denslow (82) and Korr (85, 86) incorrectly focused on the notion that dysfunctional proprioceptors were the source of exaggerated afferent input that created central

p. 252   *Clinical Nutrition for pain, inflammation & tissue healing*

Journal of Manipulative and Physiological Therapeutics 639
Volume 20 • Number 9 • November/December, 1997
Commentary

sensitization, rather than nociceptors. The focus that Denslow and Korr placed on so-called proprioceptors is surprising. Perl indicates that in 1926, "Adrian noted that noxious mechanical stimulation of the skin provoked no greater frequency of activity from low-threshold cutaneous sense organs than innocuous mechanical stimuli" (87). In other words, research in 1926 suggested that the so-called proprioceptors do not fire excessively in the presence of a noxious stimulus. More recently, researchers have indicated that the so-called proprioceptors are incapable of being irritated or abnormally excited by noxious stimuli (55, 88, 89). In fact, some may actually reduce their firing in the presence of a noxious stimulus (89). Schaible and Grubb indicated that group II afferents from joints, which are the afferents associated with so-called proprioceptors, do not increase their activity in the presence of inflammation (90).

The second problem with the proprioceptor model is notion that segmental sympathetic hyperactivity can create symptoms of visceral disease. A recent paper demonstrated that there is very little evidence to suggest that the segmental sympathetic hyperactivity, induced by nociceptive input from joint complex dysfunction, will commonly damage segmentally innervated organs and create symptoms (79).

Based on this information, it is no longer reasonable to support the theory that a proprioceptive-driven, facilitated spinal cord can promote segmental sympathetic hyperactivity and create the symptoms of visceral disease. It is time for chiropractors to officially abandon the so-called proprioceptive insult hypothesis. My recent paper even suggested that "proprioceptor" should no longer be used because it is an inaccurate word and one that creates confusion (91).

Despite the inaccuracies in the proprioceptor model, it should be mentioned that the thinking of Denslow and Korr was far ahead of their time. They realized the fact that spinal cord neurons become hyperexcitable or sensitized in the presence of a noxious stimulus. Unfortunately, their pioneering efforts have not been recognized by modern researchers. According to Dubner (92), it was not until the work of Woolf in 1983 that the scientific community began to embrace and focus on the existence of spinal cord hyperexcitability. Woolf stated that, "electrophysiological analysis of the injury-induced increase in excitability of the flexion reflex shows that it in part arises from changes in the activity of the spinal cord," (93) which is nearly the same conclusion made some 40 years earlier by Denslow and Korr.

Dysafferentation model of symptom generation. Joint complex structures are innervated by two main types of sensory receptors, nociceptors and mechanoreceptors (85, 86). As discussed earlier, nociceptors are depolarized by noxious mechanical stimuli and the chemical mediators released in response to tissue injury. Mechanoreceptors are very different from nociceptors in their morphology and method of activation.

The family of mechanoreceptors consists of muscle spindles and golgi tendon organs which are innervated by A-alpha fibers, and many additional receptors which are found in the skin, muscle and joint structures, such as Pacinian corpuscles,

Meissner's corpuscles, Ruffini corpuscles and Merkel's receptors which are all innervated by A-beta fibers (94). Mechanoreceptors only respond to innocuous mechanical stimuli such as that associated with touch and normal body movements (55, 90, 91).

Based on this information, it is reasonable to suggest that joint complex dysfunction would influence the function of both types of receptors, leading to excitation of the nociceptive system and reduced activity in the mechanoreceptive system. Indeed, Hooshmand illustrates how restricted joint mobility causes an increase firing of nociceptive axons (A-delta and C fibers) and a decreased firing of large diameter mechanoreceptor axons (A-beta fibers) (95).

In the biomedical literature, the prefix "dys" is used to describe activity that is abnormal, bad, difficult or disordered (6). It is proposed here that the chiropractic profession adopts the word "dysafferentation" to describe the increased nociceptive input and reduced mechanoreceptive input which are associated with joint complex dysfunction. Research suggests that dysafferent input can produce numerous symptoms that one would not normally ascribe to altered joint complex function.

In addition to causing pain, allodynia, and hyperalgesia, nociceptive input can also excite the hypothalamus and medulla centers (66), which results in the generation symptoms that are usually associated with visceral disease. In a recent review, Nansel and Szlazak explained that nociceptive input from joint complex structures can cause symptoms such as sweating, pallor, nausea, vomiting, abdominal pain, sinus congestion, dyspnea, cardiac palpitations, and chest pain that mimics heart disease (79).

As with enhanced activity in the nociceptive system, reduced activity in the mechanoreceptive can also promote a variety of symptoms. First, it should be mentioned that an important function of mechanoreceptive input is to inhibit nociception at the level of the spinal cord (96-98). Thus, it is likely that reduced mechanoreception may magnify the symptoms generated by nociceptive input. Reduced mechanoreception can also promote symptoms which are independent from the nociceptive system. It is known that mechanoreceptor afferents directly or indirectly end in nuclei of the spinal cord, brainstem, cerebellum, thalamus and cerebral cortex (99-101), and subsequently play a major role in equilibrium (102), proprioception (98, 103) and suprasegmental motor control (104). Based on this information, the reduced joint mobility associated with joint complex dysfunction might reduce mechanoreceptor activation and create symptoms such as dysequilibrium, vertigo and faulty motor control. In fact, many researchers have discussed such relationships (105-115).

As described above, the dysafferentation created by joint complex dysfunction has the potential for creating a wide variety of symptoms. It should be understood, however, that not all patients will develop similar symptoms. As an example, it has been known for more than 40yr that noxious irritation of spinal tissues does not affect each individual in the same fashion. Feinstein et al. were the first to clearly describe visceral symptoms associated with noxious irritation of spinal

640 Journal of Manipulative and Physiological Therapeutics
Volume 20 • Number 9 • November/December, 1997
Commentary

tissues. Hypertonic saline was injected into interspinous tissues and paraspinal muscles of normal volunteers for the purpose of characterizing local and referred pain patterns that might develop. What they discovered was surprising:

> The pain elicited from muscles was accompanied by a characteristic group of phenomena which indicated involvement of other than segmental somatic mechanisms...The manifestations were pallor, sweating bradycardia, fall in blood pressure, subjective "faintness," and nausea, but vomiting was not observed. Syncope occurred in two early procedures in the series of paravertebral injections and was subsequently avoided by quickly depressing the subjects head or by having him lie down at the first sign of faintness. These features were not proportional to the severity of or to the extent of radiation; on the contrary, they seemed to dominate the experience of subjects who complained of little pain, but who were overwhelmed by this distressing complex of symptoms (116).

Feinstein et al. referred to these symptoms as "autonomic concomitants." Commenting on their findings, they indicated that "this is an example of the ability of deep noxious stimulation to activate generalized autonomic responses independently of the relay of pain to conscious levels." In other words, pain may not be the symptomatic outcome of nociceptive stimulation of spinal structures. Such a conclusion has profound implications for the chiropractic profession. Clearly, patients do not need to be in pain to be candidates for spinal adjustments and moreover, non-pain patients with joint complex dysfunction and dysafferentation will not necessarily present with the same combination of symptoms.

TREATMENT OF JOINT COMPLEX DYSFUNCTION

Based upon the pathophysiological nature of joint complex dysfunction, a logical treatment approach would necessarily involve restoring joint motion, lengthening shortened/tightened muscles, trigger point therapy, rehabilitating deconditioned tissues, and reducing chemical mediator release. At the present time, neither the chiropractors or medical doctors recognize the importance of treating patients in such an integrated fashion.

Restoration of joint motion. The main treatment focus of the chiropractor is the restoration of joint motion via the chiropractic adjustment (1, 10, 20). Patterson states that adjustments can reduce motion restrictions, increase proper fluid in fusion and reduce nociceptive inputs to the spinal cord (117). Research also suggests that the adjustment can restore mechanoreceptive input to the central nervous system (54, 69, 96).

Although the adjustment provides benefits beyond the biomechanical effect or restoring joint complex motion, it is clear that the adjustment as a single therapy is incapable of resolving joint complex dysfunction. First, the adjustment cannot lengthen muscles that are chronically shortened. Second, the adjustment cannot eliminate trigger points. Third, the adjustment cannot rehabilitate degenerated and deconditioned tissues. Fourth, a biomechanical therapy such as the adjustment cannot directly influence the production of chemical mediators of inflammation and nociception.

Lengthening of shortened/tightened muscles. Shortened muscles and their fascia can be lengthened by manual techniques,

referred to by Liebenson as manual resistance techniques or MRT (118). A typical technique requires the doctor or therapist to actively stretch a shortened muscle after the muscle has been engaged in an isometric effort [see Liebenson for details (118)].

As mentioned earlier in this paper, it is thought that muscle imbalances are extremely common, which suggests that all patients should be screened [see Janda (27), Liebenson (118), and Liebenson and Oslance (119) for details]. Indeed, a recent case study by Graber demonstrated that MRT was required to achieve a more permanent resolution of back pain (120).

The importance of MRT in patient care should not be underemphasized. If shortened/tight muscles are not lengthened/stretched, it will be difficult to perform rehabilitation exercises to strengthen and promote the healing of joint complex structures. For this reason, Liebenson states that "MRT should be used at the beginning of any rehabilitation program before initiating a strengthening program" (123).

Trigger point therapy. There are many available methods that help to reduce trigger points, such as injection therapy (121), electrical modalities (122), stretch-and-spray with flourimethane (30), and manual pressure (123). Although chiropractors use electrical modalities and stretch-and-spray, the most common technique is direct manual pressure upon the trigger point. Chiropractors refer to this manual method as receptor-tonus technique, which was developed by Ray Nimmo, D.C., during the 1950s (123).

Rehabilitation of deconditioned tissues. Numerous authors have discussed the benefit of rehabilitation exercise in improving muscle strength and reducing spinal pain (24, 124-131). Liebenson clearly describes the need to include rehabilitation exercise in clinical practice. "Chiropractors or myofascial specialists who concentrate exclusively on passive intervention (i.e., spinal adjustments, trigger point therapy) to treat a specific pain generator (joint or soft tissue) are placing patients at risk for deconditioning" (20). McCune and Sprague explain that passive manual techniques such as the chiropractic are most effective for restoration of segmental mobility; however, exercises are essential for retaining this mobility and for restoring strength and health to deconditioned tissues (124). In a recent paper, Twomey and Taylor discuss the effectiveness of spinal manipulation in the treatment of low back pain; however, they focus on the emerging evidence which demonstrates that rehabilitation exercises are required if a patient wishes to approach full recovery (136). Manniche et al. state that on theoretical grounds, rehabilitation exercises should probably be considered a lifelong activity for those with low back pain (128).

Physical therapy modalities should also be considered for the treatment of joint complex dysfunction. Several texts outline the utility of electrical stimulation and ultrasound for reducing pain and inflammation and helping in the rehabilitation process (132-134).

Reduction of the chemical mediators of inflammation and nociception. One way to reduce the production of biochemical mediators is via pharmacologic therapy, specifically through the use of

Journal of Manipulative and Physiological Therapeutics 641
Volume 20 • Number 9 • November/December, 1997
Commentary

non-steroidal anti-inflammatory drugs (NSAIDs). It is known that NSAIDs inhibit the synthesis of prostaglandins and thromboxanes, interfere with bradykinin synthesis and also decrease the generation of free radials (135). In the clinical setting, it is known that NSAIDs can reduce objective muscle spasm, tenderness and increase spinal motion; however, research suggests that the combination of a muscle relaxant and an NSAID is more effective than NSAIDs alone (136). Unfortunately, NSAID use can have serious side effects, including gastrointestinal ulceration (137), increase gut permeability (138), and a reduction in articular cartilage and bone repair (139, 140). To circumvent these problems, nutritional methods can be used instead.

Research indicates that both dietary factors and nutritional supplements should be used to help reduce inflammation and nociception. For example, Kjeldsen-Kragh et al. demonstrated that dietary modification can dramatically reduce the pain and inflammation associated with rheumatoid arthritis (141). The findings of this research suggest that consuming large quantities of fruits and vegetables can have an anti-inflammatory effect. Unfortunately, it is known that in the United States, the population's intake of these foods is remote from recommended levels (142). Block states that, "it is likely that substantial public health benefits and disease reduction could be achieved if consumption of fruits and vegetables were greatly increased over the low levels seen in the United States and other industrialized nations (142)."

Nutritional supplements can be used to support an anti-inflammatory diet. Many supplements have demonstrated an anti-nociceptive and/or anti-inflammatory effect such as ginger (143), omega-3 fatty acids (144,145), magnesium (146, 147), bioflavonoids (148, 149), and glucosamine and chondroitin sulfate (148). See Bucci for examples of supplement programs that have been proposed to help treat tissue injury and inflammation (148).

CONCLUSION

In a recent paper, Gelardi discussed the division between the so-called straight and mixer varieties of chiropractor and stated that, "the locus of the chiropractic profession's division is clearly the matter of definition, i.e., who are we and what do we strive to do?" (150). This statement implies that we already have sufficient data to define ourselves, and we simply disagree on the definitive definition of chiropractic. Such an assumption is unwarranted. It is much more likely that the chiropractic profession at large has been unaware of available data about joint complex function, and/or ignored pertinent information and, consequently, we have been unable develop a functional definition for the spinal lesion that chiropractors treat, and equally unable to develop a sound philosophical foundation by which to practice chiropractic.

A review of what appears to be the available research suggests that (a) joint complex structures undergo pathological changes before and after spinal injury, (b) inflammation, nociception and pain serve to promote joint hypomobility/immobility, (c) axial and appendicular muscles undergo functional changes

such as muscle tightening or shortening, (d) trigger points commonly develop in conjunction with joint hypomobility, and (e) symptom generation develops as a consequence of dysafferent input. Based on this information, it is clear that terms such as subluxation, subluxation complex, joint blockage, joint restriction, joint dysfunction and joint hypomobility do not adequately convey the complex nature of the spinal lesion that is most commonly treated by chiropractors. For this reason, it is proposed here that the chiropractors (a) adopt the term "joint complex dysfunction" and (b) accept the evidence which demonstrates that the pathophysiological nature of this variety of spinal lesion requires a five-fold approach to care involving joint adjusting, muscle lengthening/stretching, trigger point therapy, rehabilitation exercises and a variety of nutritional interventions.

David R. Seaman, D.C.
1871 Hendersonville Rd, Ste 302
Asheville, NC 28803

REFERENCES

1. Gatterman M. What's in a word? In: Gatterman M, editor. Foundations of chiropractic: subluxation. St. Louis: Mosby; 1995. p.5-17.
2. The Random House Dictionary of the English Language. 2nd ed. New York: Random House; 1987. Emotional, p.637; Subluxation; p. 1894.
3. Boone W, Brotman D, Brown M, et al., moderators, Practice guidelines for straight chiropractic. Chandler (AZ): World Chiropractic Alliance; 1993. p.29, 98.
4. Webster N. American dictionary of the English Language. New York: S. Converse; 1828
5. Dorland's illustrated medical dictionary. 25th ed. Philadelphia: W.B. Saunders; 1974. Subluxation p.1488.
6. Encyclopedia and dictionary of medicine, nursing, and allied health. 4th ed. Philadelphia: W.B. Saunders; 1987: Dys-, p. 383-8; Subluxation, p.1185.
7. White A, Panjabi M. Clinical biomechanics of the spine. 2nd ed. Philadelphia: Lippincott; 1990. p.683.
8. Bland J. Differential diagnosis and specific treatment. In: Bland J, editor. Disorders of the cervical spine. 2nd ed. Philadelphia: WB Saunders; 1994. p. 223-70.
9. Faye L. The subluxation complex (class notes). Huntington Beach (CA): Motion Palpation Institute; 1986.
10. Schafer R, Faye L. Motion palpation and chiropractic technique. 2nd ed. Huntington Beach (CA): Motion Palpation Institute; 1990.
11. Dishman R. Review of the literature supporting a scientific basis for the chiropractic subluxation complex. J Manipulative Physiol Ther 1985; 8:163-74.
12. Dishman R. Static and dynamic components of the chiropractic subluxation complex: A literature review. J Manipulative Physiol Ther 1988; 11:98-107.
13. Lantz C. The vertebral subluxation complex. ICA Rev 1989; 45(5):37-61
14. Lantz C. The vertebral subluxation complex. In Gatterman M. editor. Foundations of chiropractic: subluxation. St. Louis: Mosby, 1995. p. 149-74.
15. Keating J. Toward a philosophy of the science of chiropractic: a primer for clinicians. Stockton (CA): Stockton Foundation for Chiropractic Research; 1992

642 Journal of Manipulative and Physiological Therapeutics
Volume 20 • Number 9 • November/December, 1997
Commentary

16. Wardwell W. Chiropractic: history and evolution of a new profession. St. Louis: Mosby Year Book; 1992.
17. Haldeman S, Chapman-Smith D, Petersen D. editors. Guidelines for chiropractic quality assurance and practice parameters. Gaithersburg (MD): Aspen Publishers; 1993.
18. Wall P. Introduction to the edition after this one. In: Wall P, Melzack R, editors. Textbook of pain. 3rd ed. New York: Churchill Livingstone; 1994 p. 1-7.
19. Williams P, Warwick R. Gray's Anatomy. 36th ed. New York: Churchill Livingstone; 1980 p. 419-503.
20. Liebenson C. Integrating rehabilitation into chiropractic practice (blending active and passive care). In: Liebenson C, editor. Rehabilitation of the spine: a practitioner's manual. Baltimore: Williams & Wilkins, 1996. p. 13-43.
21. Liebenson C. Pathogenesis of chronic back pain. J Manipulative Physiol Ther 1992; 15:299-308.
22. Norkin C, Levangie P. Joint Structure and Function: a comprehensive analysis. 2nd ed. Philadelphia: F.A. Davis; 1992 p. 87,88,120.
23. Engles M. Tissue response. In: Donatelli R, Wooden M. editors. Orthopaedic physical therapy. 2nd ed. New York: Churchill Livingstone, 1994 p. 1-31.
24. Mayer T, Gatchel R. Functional restoration for spinal disorders: the sports medicine approach. Philadelphia: Lea & Febiger; 1988.
25. Salter R. Continuous passive motion: a biological concept for the healing, and regeneration of articular cartilage, ligaments, and tendons— from its origination to research to clinical applications. Baltimore: Williams & Wilkins; 1993.
26. Kirkaldy-Willis W. Pathology and pathogenesis of low back pain. In: Kirkaldy-Willis W, Burton C. editors. Managing low back pain. 3rd ed. New York: Churchill Livingstone; 1992. p. 49-79.
27. Janda V. Evaluation of muscular imbalance. In: Liebenson C, editor. Rehabilitation of the spine: a practitioner's manual. Baltimore: Williams & Wilkins; 1996. p. 97-112.
28. Janda V. Muscles and motor control in cervicogenic disorders: assessment and management. In: Grant R, editor. Physical therapy of the cervical and thoracic spine. 2nd ed. New York: Churchill Livingstone, 1994. p. 195-216.
29. Travell J, Rinzler S. The myofascial genesis of pain. Postgrad Med J 1952; 11:425-34.
30. Simons D. Myofascial pain syndromes of head, neck and low back. In: Dubner R, Geghart G, Bond M, editors. Proceedings of the 5th World Congress on Pain, 1987, Hamburg, Germany. New York: Elsevier; 1988. p. 186-200.
31. Travell J, Simons D. Myofacial pain and dysfunction: the trigger point manual. Baltimore: Williams & Wilkins; 1983.
32. Sola A, Bonica J. Myofascial pain syndromes. In: Bonica J. editor. The management of pain. 2nd ed. Philadelphia: Lea & Febiger; 1990. p. 352-67.
33. Yunus M. Fibromyalgia syndrome and myofascial pain syndrome: clinical features, laboratory tests, diagnosis, and pathophysiologic mechanism. In: Rachlin E, editor. Myofascial pain and fibromyalgia: trigger point management. St. Louis: Mosby; 1994. p. 3-29.
34. Rachlin E. Trigger points. In: Rachlin E. editor. Myofascial pain and fibromyalgia: trigger point managment. St. Louis: Mosby; 1994. p. 145-57.
35. Sandman K. Myofascial pain syndromes: their mechanisms, diagnosis and treatment. J Manipulative Physiol Ther 1981; 4:135-40.
36. Simons D, Travell J. Myofascial pain syndromes. In: Wall P, Melzack R, editors. Textbook of Pain. 2nd ed. New York: Churchill Livingstone; 1989. p. 263-76.
37. Davidoff R. Migraine: manifestations, pathogenesis, and management. Philadelphia: F A Davis; 1995. p. 38-9.
38. Parkkola R, Kormano M. Lumbar disc and back muscle degeneration on MRI: Correlation to age and body mass. J Spinal Disord 1992; 5(1):86-92.
39. Hayashi N, Tamaki T, Yamada H. Experimental study of denervated muscle atrophy following severance of posterior rami of lumbar spinal nerves. Spine 1992; 17:1361-67.
40. Rantanen J, Hurme M, Falck B et al. The lumbar multifidus muscle five years after surgery for a lumbar intervertebral disc herniation. Spine 1993; 18:568-74.
41. Cotran R, Kumar V, Robbins S, editors. Robbins pathologic basis of disease. 5th ed. Philadelphia: W.B. Saunders; 1994. p. 51-92.
42. Kellett J. Acute soft tissue injuries: a review of the literature. Med Sci Sports Exer 1986; 18:489-500.
43. Foreman S, Croft A. Whiplash injuries. Baltimore: Williams & Wilkins, 1988. p. 301.
44. Chamberlain G. Cyriax's friction massage: a review. J Orthop Sports Phys Ther 1982; 4(1):16-22.
45. Hammer W. Friction massage. In: Hammer W, editor. Functional soft tissue examination by manual methods. Gaithersburg (MD): Aspen Publishers; 1991. p. 235-49.
46. Kottke F. Therapeutic exercise to maintain mobility. In: Kottke F, Lehmann J, editors. Kruzen's handbook of physical medicine and rehabilitation. 4th ed. Philadelphia: W.B. Saunders; 1990. p. 436-51.
47. Charman R. Pain and nociception: mechanisms and modulation in sensory context. In: Boyling J, Palastanga N, editors. Grieve's modern manual therapy. 2nd ed. New York: Churchill Livingstone; 1994. p. 253-70.
48. Bogduk N. Innervation patterns of the cervical spine. In: Grant R, editor. Physical therapy of the cervical and thoracic spine. 2nd ed. New York: Churchill Livingstone; 1994. p. 65-76.
49. Bogduk N, Valencia F. Innervation patterns of the thoracic spine. In: Grant R, editor. Physical therapy of the cervical and thoracic spine. 2nd ed. New York: Churchill Livingstone; 1994. p. 77-87.
50. Bogduk N. Innervation, pain patterns, and mechanisms of pain production. In: Twomey L, Taylor J, editors. Physical therapy of the low back. 2ndd ed. New York: Churchill Livingstone; 1994. p. 93-109.
51. Grieve G. Common vertebral joint problems. 2nd ed. New York: Churchill Livingstone. 1988. p. 51-52.
52. Haldeman S. The neurophysiology of pain. In; Haldeman S, editor. Principles and practice of chiropractic. 2nd ed. East Norwalk (CT): Appleton-Century-Crofts; 1992. p. 165-84.
53. Wyke B. The neurological basis of thoracic pain. Rheumatol Phys Med 1970; 10(7):356-67
54. Wyke B. Neurological aspects of pain therapy. In: Swerdlow M, editor. The therapy of pain. Philadelphia: Lippincott; 1980. p. 1-30.
55. Schmidt R, Schaible H, Mefslinger K, et al. Silent and active nociceptors: Structure, functions, and clinical implications. In: Gebhart G, Hammond D, Jensen T. editors. Proceedings of the 7th World Congress on Pain, 1993, Paris, France. Seattle: IASP Press; 1994. p. 213-50.
56. Zimmerman M. Neurophysiology of nociception, pain and pain therapy. In: Bonica J, Ventafridda V. editors. Advances in pain research and therapy, vol 2. New York: Raven Press; 1979. p. 13-29.
57. Fields H. Pain. New York: McGraw-Hill; 1987. p.13-40.
58. Meyer R, Campbell J, Raja S. Peripheral neural mechanisms of nociception. In: Wall P, Melzack R, editors. Textbook of pain. 3rd ed. New York: Churchill Livingstone; 1994. p. 13-44.
59. Portenoy R, Kanner R. Definition and assessment of pain. In: Portenoy R, Kanner R, editors. Pain managment: theory and practice. Philadelphia: F.A. Davis; 1996. p. 3-18.
60. Hanesch U, Hepplemann B, Messlinger K, Schmidt R. Noci-

ception in normal and arthritic joints: structural and functional aspects. In: Willis W. editor. Hyperalgesia and Allodynia. New York: Raven Press; 1992. p. 81-106.

61. Portenoy R. Basic mechanisms. In: Portenoy R, Kanner R, editors. Pain managment: theory and practice. Philadelphia: F. A. Davis; 1996. p. 19-39.

62. Bonica J. Anatomic and physiologic basis of nociception and pain. In: Bonica J, Editor. The management of pain. 2nd ed. Philadelphia: Lea & Febiger; 1990. p. 28-94.

63. Casey K. Nociceptors and their sensitization: overview. In: Willis W, editor. Hyperalgesia and allodynia. New York: Raven Press; 1992. p. 13-5.

64. Fields H. Introduction. In: Fields H, editor. Pain syndromes in neurology. Boston: Butterworth-Heinemann; 1991. p. 1-18.

65. Levine J, Coderre T, Bausbaum A. The peripheral nervous system and the inflammatory process. In: Dubner R, Gebhart G, Bond M, editorss. Proceedings of the 5th World Congress on Pain. New York: Elsevier; 1988. p. 33-43.

66. Bonica J. Clinical importance of hyperalgesia. In: Willis W, Editor. Hyperalgesia and allodynia. New York: Raven Press; 1992. p. 17-43.

67. Light A. The initial processing of pain and its descending control: spinal and trigeminal systems. New York: Karger; 1992. p. 28.

68. Woolf C. Generation of acute pain: central mechanisms. Br Med Bull 1991;47:523-33.

69. Peterson D. Principles of adjustive technique. In: Bergmann T, Peterson D, Lawrence D, editors. Chiropractic technique: principles and procedures. New York: Churchill Livingstone, 1993. p. 123-95.

70. Zohn D. Musculoskeletal pain: diagnosis and physical treatment. 2nd ed. Boston: Little, Brown and Co., 1988. p. 76.

71. Muhlemann D, Cimino J. Therapeutic muscle stretching. In: Hammer W, editor. Functional soft tissue examination and treatment by manual methods: the extremities. Gaithersburg (MD): Aspen Publishers; 1991. p. 251-75.

72. Campbell J, Raja S, Belzberg A, Meyer R. Hyperalgesia and the sympathetic nervous system. In Boivie J, Hansson P, Lindblom U. eds, Touch, temperature, and pain in health and disease: mechanisms and assessments—progress in pain research and management, vol 3. Seattle: IASP Press, 1994. p. 249-65.

73. Campbell J, Meyer R, Davis K, Raja S. Sympathetically maintained pain: a unifying hypothesis. In: Willis W, editor. Hyperalgesia and allodynia. New York: Raven Press; 1992. p. 141-49.

74. Fitz-Ritson D. The anatomy and physiology of the muscle spindle, and its role in posture and movement. JCCA 1982; 26:144-50.

75. Hubbard D, Berkoff G. Myofascial trigger points show spontaneous needle EMG activity. Spine 1993; 18:1803-07.

76. Peterson D, Bergmann T. Joint assessment principles and procedures. In: Bergmann T, Peterson D, Lawrence D, editors. Chiropractic technique: principles and procedures. New York: Churchill Livingstone; 1993. p. 51-121.

77. Jull G. Headaches of cervical origin. In: Grant R, editor. Physical therapy of the cervical and thoracic spine. 2nd ed. New York: Churchill Livingstone, 1994. p. 261-285.

78. Bogduk N, Twomey L. Clinical anatomy of the lumbar spine. 2nd ed. New York: Churchill Livingstone; 1991. p. 151-59.

79. Nansel D, Szlazak M. Somatic dysfunction and the phenomenon of visceral disease simulation: a probable explanation for the apparent effectiveness of somatic therapy in patients presumed to be suffering from true visceral disease. J Manipulative Physiol Ther 1995; 18:379-97.

80. Haldeman S. The pathophysiology of the spinal subluxation. JCCA 1975; 5-11.

81. Mootz R. Theoretic models of chiropractic subluxation. In:

Gatterman M, editor. Foundations of chiropractic: subluxation. St. Louis: Mosby; 1995. p. 175-89.

82. Denslow J, Clough G. Reflex activity in the spinal extensors. J Neurophysiol 1941; 4:430-37.

83. Denslow J, Hassett C. The central excitatory state associated with postural abnormalities. J Neurophysiol 1942; 5:393-402.

84. Denslow J, Hassett C. Spontaneous and induced muscle spasm in structural abnormalities. J Am Osteo Assoc 1943; 42:207-12.

85. Korr I. The neural basis of the osteopathic lesion. J Am Osteopath Assoc 1947; 47:191-98.

86. Korr I. Proprioceptors and somatic dysfunction. J Am Osteopath Assoc 1975; 74:638-50.

87. Perl E. Pain and nociception. In: Darian-Smith I, editor. Handbook of physiology - the nervous system III. Bethesda (MD): American Physiology Society; 1984. p. 915-75.

88. Willis W. Central plastic responses to pain. In: Gebhart G, Hammond D, Jensen T, editors. Proceedings of the 7th World Congress on Pain, 1993 Paris, France. Seattle: IASP Press; 1994. p. 301-24.

89. Price D. Psychological and Neural Mechanisms of Pain. New York: Raven Press; 1988. p. 86.

90. Schaible H, Grubb B. Afferent and spinal mechanisms of joint pain. Pain 1993; 55:5-54.

91. Seaman D. Proprioceptor: an obsolete, inaccurate word. J Manipulative Physiol Ther 1997; 20:279-84.

92. Dubner R, Basbaum A. Spinal dorsal horn plasticity following tissue or nerve injury. In: Wall P, Melzack R, editors. Textbook of pain. 3rd ed. New York: Churchill Livingstone; 1994. p. 225-41.

93. Woolf C. Evidence for a central component of post-injury pain hypersensitivity. Nature 1983; 306:686-688.

94. Martin J, Jessell T. Modality coding in the somatic sensory system. In: Kandel E, Schwartz J, Jessell T, editors. Principles of Neural Science. 3rd ed. New York: Elsevier, 1991. p. 341-52.

95. Hooshmand H. Chronic pain: reflex sympathetic dystrophy, prevention and management. Boca Raton(FL): CRC Press; 1993. p. 33-55.

96. Gillette R. A speculative argument for the coactivation of diverse somatic receptor populations by forceful chiropractic adjustments. Manual Med 1987; 3:1-14.

97. Woolf C. Segmental afferent fibre-mediated analgesia: transcutaneous electrical nerve stimulation (TENS) and vibration. In: Wall P, Melzack R. editors. Textbook of pain. 2nd ed. New York: Churchill Livingstone; 1989. p. 884-96.

98. Wyke B. Articular neurology and manipulative therapy. In: Glasgow E, Twomey L, Scull E, et al. editors. Aspects of manipulative therapy. 2nd ed. New York: Churchill Livingstone; 1985. p. 72-77.

99. Brodal A. Neurological anatomy. 3rd ed. New York: Oxford University Press; 1981.

100. Carpenter M. Core text of neuroanatomy. 4th ed. Baltimore: Williams & Wilkins; 1991. p. 234-49.

101. Nolte J. The human brain. 3rd ed. St. Louis: Mosby; 1993.

102. Guyton A. Basic neuroscience. 2nd ed. Philadelphia: W.B. Saunders, 1991. p. 221.

103. Willis W, Coggeshall R. Sensory mechanisms of the spinal cord. 2nd ed. New York: Plenum Press; 1991. p. 428-30.

104. Masdeu J, Brazis P. The anatomic localization of lesions in the thalamus. In: Brazis P, Masdeu J, Biller J, editors. Localization in clinical neurology. 2nd ed. Boston: Little, Brown; 1990. p. 319-43.

105. Weeks V, Travell J. Postural vertigo due to trigger areas in the sternocleidomastoid muscle. J Pediatr 195; 47:315-27.

106. Gray L. Extra labyrinthine vertigo due to cervical muscle lesions. J Laryngol Otol 1956; 70:352-61.

644   Journal of Manipulative and Physiological Therapeutics
Volume 20 • Number 9 • November/December, 1997
Commentary

107. Wing L, Hargrave-Wilson. Cervical vertigo. Aust NZ J Surg 1974; 44:275-7.

108. Fitz-Ritson D. Cervicogenic vertigo. J Manipulative Physiol Ther 1991; 14:193-98.

109. Lewit K. Manipulative therapy in rehabilitation of the locomotor system. 2nd ed. Boston: Butterworth Heinemann, 1991. p.18.

110. Caranasos G, Israel R. Gait disorders in the elderly. Hosp Pract 1991; (26):67-94.

111. Revel M, Andre-Deshays C, Minguet M. Cervicocephalic kinesthetic sensibility in patients with cervical pain. Arch Phys Med Rehabil 1991;72:288-91.

112. Revel M, Minguet M, Gergoy P, Vaillant J, Manuel J. Changes in cervicocephalic kinesthesia after a proprioceptive rehabilitation program of in patients with neck pain: a randomized controlled study. Arch Phys Med Rehabil 1994;75:895-9.

113. Hulse M. Disequilibrium, caused by a functional disturbance in the upper cervical spine: clinical aspects and differential diagnosis. Man Med 1983; 1:18-22.

114. Hinoki M, Ushio N. Lumbomuscular proprioceptive reflexes in body equilibrium. Acta Otolaryngol Suppl (Stockh) 1975; 330: 197-210.

115. Hildingsson C, Wenngren B, Toolanen G. Eye motility after soft-tissue injury of the cervical spine: A controlled, prospective study of 38 patients. Acta Orthop Scand 1993; 64:129-32.

116. Feinstein B, Langton J, Jameson R, Schiller F. Experiments on pain referred from deep somatic tissues, J Bone Joint Surg Am 1954; 36-A:981-97.

117. Patterson M. The spinal cord: participant in disorder. Spinal Manipulation 1993; 9(3):2-11.

118. Liebenson C. Manual resistance techniques and self-stretches for improving flexibility/mobility. In: Liebenson C. editor. Rehabilitation of the spine: a practioner's manual. Baltimore: Williams & Wilkins; 1996. p. 253-92.

119. Liebenson C, Oslance J. Outcomes assessment in the small private practice. In: Liebenson C, editor. Rehabilitation of the spine: a practioner's manual. Baltimore: Williams & Wilkins; 1996. p. 73-95.

120. Graber D. Muscle dysfunction as a contributor to low back pain: A case study. J Sports Chiropr Rehabil 1997; 11:21-27.

121. Rachlin E. Injection of specific trigger points. In: Rachlin E, editor. Myofascial pain and fibromyalgia: trigger point management. St. Louis: Mosby; 1994. p. 197-360.

122. Kahn J. Electrical modalities in the treatment of myofascial conditions. In: Rachlin E, editor. Myofascial pain and fibromyalgia: trigger point management. St. Louis: Mosby; 1994. p. 473-85.

123. Cohen J, Schneider M. Receptor-tonus technique: an overview. Chiropr Technique 1990; 2:13-16.

124. McCune D, Sprague R. Exercise for low back pain. In: Basmajian J, Wolf S, editors. Therapeutic exercise. 5th ed. Baltimore: Williams & Wilkins, 1990. p. 299-321.

125. Liebenson C. editor. Rehabilitation of the spine: a practioner's manual. Baltimore: Williams & Wilkins; 1996.

126. Tietz C, Cook D. Rehabilitation of neck and low back injuries. Clin Sports Med 1985; 4:455-76.

127. Manniche C, Bentzen L, Hesselsoe G, Christensen I, Lundberg E. Clinical trial of intensive muscle training for chronic low back pain. Lancet 1988; 2:1473-6.

128. Manniche C, Lundberg E, Christensen I, Bentzen L, Hesselsoe G. Intesive dynamic back exercises for chronic low back pain: a clinical trial. Pain 1991; 47:53-63.

129. Moffroid M, Haugh L, Haig A, Henry S, Pope M. Endurance training of trunk extensor muscles. Phys Ther 1993; 73(1):3-10.

130. Risch S, Norvell N, Pollock M et al. Lumbar strengthening in chronic low back pain patients: physiologic and psychological benefits. Spine 1993; 18:232-38.

131. Twomey L, Taylor J. Exercise and spinal manipulation in the treatment of low back pain. Spine 1995; 20(5):615-19.

132. Kahn J. Principles and Practice of Electrotherapy. 3rd ed. New York: Churchill Livingstone; 1994.

133. Nelson R, Currier D. Clinical electrotherapy. 2nd ed. East Norwalk (CT): Appleton & Lange; 1991.

134. Prentice W, editor. Therapeutic modalities in sports medicine. St Louis: Times Mirror/Mosby; 1990.

135. Shearn M. Nonsteroidal anti-inflammatory agents; nonopiate analgesics; drugs used in gout. In: Katzung B, editor. Basic and clinical pharmacology. 3rd ed. East Norwalk (CT): Appleton & Lange; 1987. p. 396-413.

136. Borenstein D. Medical therapy of low back pain. Drug Therapy 1992; 22(10):93-102.

137. Arthritis unyielding to drugs. Med Advertis News 1991; 26-7.

138. Bjarnason I, So A, Levi A et al. Intestinal permeability and inflammation in rheumatoid arthritis: effects of nonsteroidal anti-inflammatory drugs. Lancet 1984; 2:1171-4.

139. David M, Vignon E, Peschard M, Broquet P, Louisot P, Richard M. Effect of non-steroidal anti-inflammatory drugs (NSAIDS) on glycosyltransferase activity from human osteoarthritic cartilage. Br J Rheumatol 1992; 31Suppl 1:13-7.

140. Newman N, Ling R. Acetabular bone destruction related to non-steroidal anti-inflammatory drugs. Lancet 1985; 2:11-3.

141. Kjeldsen-Kragh J, Haugen M, Borchgrevink C, et al. Controlled trial of fasting and one-year vegetarian diet in rheumatoid arthritis. Lancet 1991; 338:899-902.

142. Block G. Dietary guidelines and the results of food consumption surveys. Am J Clin Nutr 1991; 53 Suppl 1:356S-7S.

143. Srivistava K, Mustafa T. Ginger (*Zingiber officinale*) in rheumatism and musculoskeletal disorders. Med Hypothesis 1992; 39:342-8.

144. Kremer J. Clinical studies of omega-3 fatty acid supplementation in patients who have rheumatoid arthritis. Rheum Dis Clin N Am 1991; 17(2)391-402

145. Nettleton J. Omega-3 fatty acids and health. New York: Chapman & Hall, 1995. p. 207-209.

146. Dreosti I. Magnesium status and health. Nutr Rev 1995; 53: S23-S7.

147. Elin R. Magnesium: the fifth but forgotten electrolyte. Am J Clin Pathol 1994; 102:616-22.

148. Bucci L. Nutrition applied to injury rehabilitation and sports Medicine. Boca Raton (FL): CRC Press; 1995. p. 205-8.

149. Macheix J, Fleuriet A, Billot J. Fruit phenolics. Boca Raton (FL): CRC Press, 1990. p. 272-3.

150. Gelardi T. The science of identifying professions as applied to chiropractic. J Chiropr Human 1997; 6(1):11-7.

Reprinted by permission of the Journal of Manipulative and
Physiological Therapeutics

Journal of Manipulative and Physiological Therapeutics   267
Volume 21 • Number 4 • May, 1998
0161-4754/98/2104-0267 $4.00/0 ©1998 JMPT

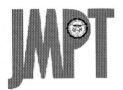

Dysafferentation: a Novel Term to Describe the Neuropathophysiological Effects of Joint Complex Dysfunction. A Look at Likely Mechanisms of Symptom Generation

David R. Seaman, D.C.[1] and James F. Winterstein, D.C[2]

ABSTRACT

Background and Objectives: Since the founding of the chiropractic profession, very few efforts have been made to thoroughly explain the mechanism(s) by which joint complex dysfunction generates symptoms. Save for a few papers, only vague and physiologically inconsistent descriptions have been offered. The purpose of this paper is to propose a precise and physiologically sound mechanism by which symptoms may be generated by joint complex dysfunction.

Data Sources: The data was accumulated over a period of years by reviewing contemporary articles and books, and subsequently retrieving relevant papers. Articles were also selected from volumes 1-4 of the Chiropractic Research Archives Collection. *The Nexus,* published by the David D. Palmer Health Sciences Library, and *In Touch,* published by Logan College of Chiropractic Library, were reviewed and relevant articles were retrieved. Medline searches were found to be ineffective because appropriate key indexing terms were difficult to identify.

Data Synthesis: The symptoms generated by joint complex dysfunction, such as pain, nausea and vertigo, are probably caused by increased nociceptive input and/or reduced mechanoreceptive input.

Conclusions: Joint complex dysfunction should be included in the differential diagnosis of pain and visceral symptoms because joint complex dysfunction can often generate symptoms which are similar to those produced by true visceral disease. (J Manipulative Physool Ther 1998; 21:267-80).

Key Indexing Terms: Allodynia; Central Sensitization; Dysafferentation; Joint Complex Dysfunction; Mechanoreception; Nociception; Nociceptor Sensitization

INTRODUCTION

In a recent paper, the term *joint complex dysfunction* was suggested as a replacement subluxation/subluxation complex (1). Joint complex dysfunction refers to pathological and functional changes which occur in joint complex structures including (a) the negative effects of hypomobility/immobility, (b) functional imbalances such as muscle tightening or shortening and (c) myofascial trigger points. In short, the article demonstrated how the term joint complex dysfunction allows for a more descriptive and pathophysiologically precise discussion of spinal dysfunction compared to the term subluxation/subluxation complex. The author also proposed that the chiropractic profession adopt the term "dysafferentation" to describe the neuropathophysiological effects of joint complex dysfunction which act to generate symptoms (1).

The topic of symptom generation has remained a source for debate within the chiropractic profession. For example, B. J. Palmer, who was often referred to as the "developer" of chiropractic maintained "a peculiar belief in the perfection of the incoming (afferent) sensory system." (2) In his writings Palmer indicated that subluxations only affected efferent pathways and not the afferent system (2). Many modern-day chiropractors still promote this notion. It is believed that subluxations impinge upon spinal nerves at the level of the intervertebral foramina and

> interfere with the conduction of impulses innately generated within the brain and which subsequently pass through neural tissue, with the result that tissue supplied by the affected nerves could suffer some form of functional insult" (3).

Another popular notion is that upper cervical subluxations or misalignments can somehow impinge upon the medulla and interfere with the transmission of "the mental impulse life force" (4).

To our knowledge, at the present time, there is no evidence to support these opinions about such a relationship between joint complex dysfunction and efferent nerve function. However, as will be discussed in this paper, a great deal of information suggests that joint complex dysfunction affects the afferent system by altering the function of nociceptors and mechanoreceptors found within the structures of the joint complex.

The purpose of this paper is to describe the sensory receptors and their relationship to afferent input and describe possible symptoms that can develop in response to enhanced nociceptor input and reduced mechanoreceptor input, which

[1] Research and Development, NutrAnalysis, Inc., Hendersonville, North Carolina
[2] President, National College of Chiropractic, Lombard, Illinois.
Submit requests for reprints to: Dr. David Seaman, P.O. Box 9, Lake Lure, NC.
Paper submittes July 11, 1997

268 Journal of Manipulative and Physiological Therapeutics
Volume 21 • Number 4 • May, 1998
Dysafferentation • *Seaman and Winterstein*

has been referred to previously as dysafferentation (1). We should mention that much confusion exists regarding sensory receptor terminology (5). Consequently, a discussion about receptors and their function can lead to unnecessary arguments (6, 7). For this reason and for the sake of clarity in general, pertinent terminology will be discussed in appropriate sections of this article.

DISCUSSION

Afferentation and Deafferentation

Afferentation refers to the transmission of afferent nerve impulses; deafferentation is defined as the elimination or interruption of afferent nerve impulses, as by destruction of the afferent pathway (8). In the neurological literature, the word "deafferentation" is typically reserved for conditions in which peripheral nerves are either damaged, completely severed or avulsed (9-11). Because joint complex dysfunction is very rarely associated with peripheral nerve injury, it is not appropriate to use the word deafferentation.

Dysafferentation

Dysafferentation refers to an imbalance in afferent input such that there is an increase in nociceptor input and a reduction in mechanoreceptor input (1). Notice that proprioceptors are not mentioned; this is because contemporary texts do not consider proprioceptors a category of receptor. A recent article explained why proprioceptor is actually an obsolete, inaccurate word (5).

According to standard texts in neurology, there are two categories of somatic receptors: nociceptors and mechanoreceptors (5, 12-14). At the present time, an emerging body of research indicates that abnormal joint complex function can alter the activity of nociceptors (15-19) and mechanoreceptors (20-23), such that nociceptive activity increases and mechanoreceptive activity decreases. Many authors and researchers involved in joint adjusting and manipulation realize this fact, and use the terms "altered afferent input," "abnormal afferent input," or similar terms when discussing the neuropathophysiological component of joint complex dysfunction (24-32). For example, Peterson states that, "somatic dysfunction and/or joint dysfunction induce persistent nociceptive input and altered proprioceptive input" (26). Peterson and Bergmann describe "vertebral joint dysfunctions—and their associated mechanical alterations, pain, and potential local inflammation—as lesions capable of inducing chronically altered nociceptive and proprioceptive input" (27). Hooshmand illustrated how restricted joint mobility results in a decreased firing of large diameter mechanoreceptor axons (A-beta fibers) and increased firing of nociceptive axons (A-delta and C fibers) (20). Henderson uses the term "altered somatic afferent input theory" to classify a neurophysiologic theory of the chiropractic subluxation (28). He proposes that a chiropractic adjustment may normalize articular afferent input to the nervous system which reestablishes normal nociceptive and kinesthetic reflex thresholds.

The information in the previous paragraph demonstrates that researchers in different professions have acknowledged the fact that compromised joint function will alter afferent input, such that nociception is enhanced and mechanoreception is reduced. In the biomedical literature, the prefix "dys" is used to describe activity that is abnormal, bad, difficult or disordered (33). For this reason, we propose that the chiropractic profession adopt the word 'dysafferentation' to describe the abnormal afferent input associated with joint complex dysfunction (1).

The remainder of this paper will discuss potential symptoms which may develop as a consequence of dysafferent input (i.e., increased nociception and reduced mechanoreception). To accomplish this task, both the neuroanatomy and physiology related to nociceptors and mechanoreceptors will be discussed and then related to symptom generation.

Nociceptors

Neuroanatomy. It is thought that spinal tissue nociceptors can be found in

• skin,
• subcutaneous and adipose tissue,
• fibrous capsules of apophyseal and sacroiliac joints,
• spinal ligaments,
• periosteum covering vertebral bodies and arches (and attached fascia, tendons and aponeurosis),
• dura mater and epidural fibro-adipose tissue,
• the walls of blood vessels supplying the spinal joints, sacroiliac joints, and the vertebral cancellous bone,
• the walls of epidural and paravertebral veins and
• the walls of intramuscular arteries at the outer third of the annulus fibrosis (34-41).

Wyke provides the most vivid anatomical description of the nociceptive receptor system (41). He described interstitial nociceptors as "a continuous tridimensional plexus of unmyelinated nerve fibers that weaves (like chicken-wire) in all directions throughout the tissue." A similar plexus of unmyelinated nerve fibers is embedded in the adventitial sheath and encircles each blood vessel. Commenting on nociceptive C fiber innervation, Charman states that the "network of each C fibre innervates a three-dimensional receptive field of between 6 and 15 mm in diameter and of variable depth with extensive field overlapping between adjacent C-fibres" (37). Thus, we can envision the presence of an almost unending meshwork of nociceptors within the various tissues described earlier.

Nociceptors are classified as mechanical nociceptors, mechanothermal nociceptors and polymodal nociceptors, depending on the type of energy used to activate them in the nociceptive range. Polymodal nociceptors are activated by noxious mechanical and thermal stimulation, as well as by chemical mediators released from the injured tissues (42).

Recent research has demonstrated the presence of articular nociceptors with thresholds so high that they cannot be excited by acute noxious stimulation, for example mechanical injury to the joint (17-19, 43). Thus, these nociceptors are normally mechano-*insensitive* and have been characterized as solely chemosensitive (43). This special category of nociceptors is called silent or sleeping nociceptors. Sleeping nociceptors are thought to awaken in the presence of chemical mediators

Journal of Manipulative and Physiological Therapeutics   269
Volume 21 • Number 4 • May, 1998
Dysafferentation • *Seaman and Winterstein*

released from injured tissues (17, 18, 43), upon which they become mechanosensitive. It is thought that the activation of these afferents may not only represent an extra source of nociceptive input, but may also be important in promoting central sensitization (43).

Generally speaking, mechanical and mechanothermal nociceptors are innervated by A-delta axons, whereas polymodal and silent nociceptors receive their innervation from C fibers. Within the spinal cord, nociceptive afferents send collaterals to supra- and infra-adjacent segments. For example, A-delta fibers spread collaterals three to six segments rostrally and an equal number caudally, whereas C fibers spread two to three (or possibly more) segments above and below the level of entry (44).

A recent review by Charman provides a vivid description of the central connections of nociceptive afferents (37). Nociceptive afferents travel up the anterolateral system and ultimately terminate in the spinal cord, a variety of brainstem nuclei, the limbic system, frontal lobes, parietal lobes, insula cortex and temporal lobes.

Peripheral nociceptive sensitization. Nociceptors have high thresholds of activation, meaning that, under normal circumstances, only stimuli which are either potentially or overtly tissue-damaging can depolarize a nociceptor (45, 46). Normally, light touch and normal joint motion cannot depolarize a nociceptor (5).

Although nociceptors normally have high thresholds, certain physiologic environments can result in the lowering of nociceptive thresholds, such that light touch and normal movement patterns can cause nociceptor depolarization and excitation of nociceptive afferent pathways. Peripheral sensitization is the term used to describe the process by which nociceptor thresholds are lowered (47), which enhances the transmission of nociceptive impulses into the spinal cord. The driving force behind the sensitization process appears to be the chemical mediators released after tissue injury. Prostaglandin E-2, leukotriene B-4, bradykinin, histamine, and 5-hydroxytryptamine are thought to be the main chemical mediators which can sensitize nociceptors (10, 47). Local tissue acidity is also thought to be capable of participating in the sensitization process (47-49).

Recent research suggests that norepinephrine release from sympathetic terminals into the area of tissue injury, can also sensitize nociceptors (47, 51-52). The exact mechanism by which this occurs is not well understood. It is possible that norepinephrine released from sympathetic terminals activates alpha-1-adrenergic receptors found on the nociceptor membrane (50). It is also possible that sympathetic discharge into the area of tissue injury promotes the release of prostaglandins (53).

It is not clear whether substance P is directly involved in the sensitization process (10, 47, 54). We known that substance P is produced in the dorsal root ganglion cells and then transmitted to the spinal cord and to the nociceptor. Substance P is released from nociceptors after they are activated by noxious input. The activity of substance P in this local environment can cause further accumulation of bradykinin and the release of histamine

from mast cells and 5-hydroxytryptamine from platelets, all of which can promote the sensitization of local nociceptors (10).

It is thought that chemical mediators depolarize and/or sensitize a nociceptor through their interaction with chemosensitive receptors on the membrane of the nociceptor, which influences the flow of sodium, calcium and potassium ions. Some of the chemical mediators have receptors linked directly to ion channels, whereas the receptors for other mediators are linked to second messenger systems which modulate ion channels. For more details see Rang et al. (53).

It is important to consider the degree to which nociceptor sensitization can influence the activity of the associated afferent fibers and the spinal cord. Hanesch et al. provide a vivid example of afferent fiber function after nociceptor sensitization (17). They studied the medial articular nerve in cats and discovered that, in normal joints, the afferent volley during a simple flexion movement comprises approximately 4,400 impulses per 30 seconds, including resting discharges. During inflammation, which promotes nociceptor sensitization, the afferent volley comprises some 30,900 impulses per 30 seconds, which represents about a seven-fold increase compared to normal conditions. They indicate that, "in individual afferents that have been studied consecutively under both normal and inflamed conditions, the afferent discharges sometimes increased more than 100-fold."

It is thought that an increased nociceptive barrage caused by sensitized nociceptors play a role in the development of central nociceptive sensitization. Researchers have yet to discover all of the details about central sensitization. Nonetheless, we will attempt to provide the most relevant data in the next section.

Central nociceptive sensitization. After tissue injury, nociceptors exhibit spontaneous activity, lowered thresholds and increased responsiveness to noxious stimuli, which leads to hyperexcitability and altered neuronal processing in the spinal cord and brain (55). The term 'central sensitization' refers to this increased excitability of nociceptive neurons in the central nervous system (CNS) (56). Of importance to the chiropractic profession is the fact that joint nociceptors, as with nociceptors in other tissues, can be sensitized (57). In addition, joint and muscle nociceptors are much more capable of producing central nociceptive sensitization than cutaneous nociceptors (58).

In 1942, Denslow and Hassett reviewed the literature and demonstrated that the concept of spinal cord hyperexcitability had been around since at least the 1930s (30). At that time, the term central excitatory state was used to describe central sensitization. Denslow and Hassett were the first to suggest and demonstrate that spinal dysfunction, (i.e. joint complex dysfunction) was associated with central sensitization. They credited Charles Sherrington for developing the concept of the central excitatory state. They state that

the evocation of additional activity by a stimulus which, in the normal would be ineffective, is explained by Sherrington's concept of a motoneuron pool in which there is an enduring subliminal central excitatory state (CES) created by subthreshold stimuli" (30).

In 1947, Denslow et al. used the terms facilitation and central facilitation in an effort to describe what is now referred to as central sensitization (59). Recently, Patterson indicated that Irvin Korr is credited for coining the term facilitated segment (60) about which Korr wrote numerous papers (61-67).

In 1983, and apparently without knowledge of the work by Denslow et al., Woolf hypothesized and then experimentally demonstrated the presence of a hyperexcitable central component in post-injury pain hypersensitivity (68). In 1987, Woolf provided a clear explanation of central sensitization; "C fiber input to the spinal cord, in addition to producing an input concerning the onset, location and duration of the peripheral noxious stimuli, also produces a prolonged increase in the excitability of the spinal cord" (58). Research demonstrated that brief conditioning stimuli of nociceptive C fibers (up to 20 sec) at low frequencies (1 Hz) can produce a prolonged excitation (up to 90 minutes) of the spinal cord. Additionally, it was shown that C fibers innervating deep structures, such as joints or muscles, can more readily produce central facilitation than can cutaneous C fibers (58). The activation of nociceptive C afferents can also produce profound changes in the receptive field properties of dorsal horn neurons, such as an expansion of the receptive field size, increases in spontaneous activity, and increases in response to innocuous stimuli (58).

Since Woolf's initial paper in 1983, a great deal of research has been devoted to understanding the process of central sensitization (55, 56, 69-81). Most authors now agree that central sensitization manifests in CNS neurons as increased spontaneous activity, reduced thresholds or increased responsivity to afferent inputs, which are prolonged after discharge to repeated stimulation, and expanded receptive fields of dorsal horn neurons (56). It is thought that these CNS changes are caused by an increase in excitatory inputs and/or a loss of inhibitory inputs, which results in a net excitation of the dorsal horn (69).

At the present time, an emerging impression is that spinal cord plasticity is responsible for the development of central sensitization (55, 55, 69-71, 82). In general, plasticity refers to an adaptation of the nervous system in response to changes in the associated internal or external environment (83). Kandel states that plasticity is a "change in the effectiveness of specific synaptic connections." (85) Research suggests that the physiological basis of plasticity involves an increase in gene expression, particular intermediate-early genes such as *c-fos* and *c-jun* (71, 86). With respect to central sensitization, plastic changes begin after the release of various excitatory transmitter substances from nociceptive afferents, such as substance P, calcitonin gene-related peptide, aspartate and glutamate, and their subsequent action at N-methyl-D-asparte receptor sites. Dubner and Ruda provide a review of this proposed mechanism (70).

It is thought that central sensitization extends to neurons in the dorsal and anterior horns of the spinal cord, the thalamus and even higher centers (57,87,88). In other words, noxious input leads to the hyperexcitability of alpha-motoneurons, preganglionic sympathetic neurons, spinal cord nociceptive projection neurons, thalamic projection neurons and other neurons in the brain. A variety of symptoms and conditions can develop in response to these changes. For example, it is known that nociceptor sensitization and central nociceptive sensitization of projection neurons causes increased pain (55). From a clinical perspective, chiropractors routinely encounter pain associated with a sensitized nociceptive system. It is common to discover that gentle or normal palpation of spinal tissues results in the experience of pain. The word allodynia is used to describe this state in which normally painless stimuli results in pain (47).

Considering the fact that the nociceptive input reaches subcortical areas such as the brainstem hypothalamus (37), it is also likely that a wide variety of neuroendocrine responses and seemingly unrelated symptoms could develop in response to a sensitized nociceptive system. The following two sections discuss these relationships in some detail.

Neuroendocrine responses caused by nociceptive input to subcortical centers. We know that nociceptive afferent input travels up the anterolateral pathway, which contains the spinoreticular and spinothalamic tracts. Bonica provides a succinct explanation of the neuroendocrine responses associated with such activity (87):

> Suprasegmental reflex responses result from nociceptive-induced stimulation of medullary centers of ventilation and circulation, hypothalamic (predominantly sympathetic) centers of neuroendocrine function, and some limbic structures. These responses consist of hyperventilation, increased hypothalamic neural sympathetic tone, and increased secretion of catecholamines and other catabolic hormones. The increased neural sympathetic tone and catecholamine secretion add to the effects of spinal reflexes and further increase cardiac output, peripheral resistance, blood pressure, cardiac workload and myocardial oxygen consumption. In addition to catecholamine release, there is an increased secretion of cortisol, adrenocorticotrophic hormone, glucagon, cyclic AMP, antidiuretic hormone, growth hormone, renin and other catabolically acting hormones, with a concomitant decrease in the anabolically acting hormones insulin and testosterone.... Cortical responses, in addition to and including the perception of pain as an unpleasant sensation and negative emotion, initiate the psychodynamic mechanisms of anxiety, apprehension and fear. These in turn produce cortically mediated increases in blood viscosity, clotting time, fibrinolysis and platelet aggregation. Indeed, cortisol and catecholamine responses to anxiety usually exceed the hypothalamic response that is provoked directly by nociceptive impulses reaching the hypothalamus.

Bonica demonstrates the degree to which nociceptive input can metabolically compromise the host. As implied above, subcortical responses can occur with or without the experience of pain. Perhaps such asymptomatic neuroendocrine responses, induced by nociceptive input, play a role in the pathogenesis of degenerative diseases such as cardiovascular disease, cancer, diabetes, arthritis, and Alzheimer's disease. We need more research in this area, which becomes more obvious when the devastating effects of hypercortisolemia considered.

Cortisol levels are increased by nociception, pain, inflammation, trauma, anxiety, fear, apprehension, prolonged and

p. 262   *Clinical Nutrition for pain, inflammation & tissue healing*

Journal of Manipulative and Physiological Therapeutics   271
Volume 21 • Number 4 • May, 1998
Dysafferentation • *Seaman and Winterstein*

strenuous exercise and hypoglycemia (87, 88). When stressors are present for protracted periods of time, feedback suppressibility of cortisol can be impaired (88).

The damaging effects of excess endogenous cortisol are as jeopardizing as those associated with exogenous intake in the form of medication. Such a relationship can be better appreciated when we understand that cortisol secretion can rise 20-fold when the adrenal gland is chronically stimulated (88).

Excess cortisol produces a continuous drain on body protein stores, most notably in muscle, bone, connective tissue and skin. Hypercortisolemia causes a variety of tissue-specific changes, including a reduction in rapid-eye-movement sleep; a reduction of cell-mediated immunity by inhibiting the production of interleukin-1, interleukin-2 and gamma interferon; a decrease in the proliferation of osteoblasts; and a reduction in collagen synthesis. We know cortisol antagonizes the action of insulin, which results in decreased glucose use. Cortisol stimulates lipogenesis in specific body locations, including the abdomen, trunk and face (88).

Chronic hypercortisolemia may play a role in spinal muscle degeneration. We known that cortisol preferentially reduces the ratio of slow oxidative type I muscle fibers to fast glycolytic type II-B fibers (88). This may enhance the deconditioning of spinal muscles that occurs as a consequence of sedentary living and aging and promote spinal injury and chronic joint complex dysfunction.

There are also a number of diseases that are driven by hypercortisolemia. Dilman and Dean actually characterizes hypercortisolemia as a disease (89). They coined the term hyperadaptosis which is characterized in its latent stage by an excessive and prolonged elevation of cortisol levels in response to stressors, and in the overt state by an elevation of basal cortisol levels in the absence of apparent stressors. Several conditions are known to develop as a consequence of hypercortisolemia including heart disease, various cancers, hypertension, depression, obesity and diabetes (89).

Symptoms caused by nociceptive input to subcortical centers. Feinstein et al. was the first to clearly describe some symptoms associated with noxious irritation of spinal tissues (90). They injected hypertonic saline into interspinous tissues and paraspinal muscles of normal volunteers for the purpose of characterizing local and referred pain patterns that might develop. What he discovered was surprising:

> The pain elicited from muscles was accompanied by a characteristic group of phenomena which indicated involvement of other than segmental somatic mechanisms…The manifestations were pallor, sweating bradycardia, fall in blood pressure, subjective "faintness," and nausea, but vomiting was not observed. Syncope occurred in two early procedures in the series of paravertebral injections and was subsequently avoided by quickly depressing the subject's head or by having him lie down at the first sign of faintness. These features were not proportional to the severity of or to the extent of radiation; on the contrary, they seemed to dominate the experience of subjects who complained of little pain, but who were overwhelmed by this distressing complex of symptoms.

Feinstein et al. referred to these symptoms as autonomic concomitants (90). It is likely that these autonomic concomitants were caused by nociceptive stimulation of autonomic centers in the brainstem, particularly the medulla (87). Feinstein et al. indicates that "this is an example of the ability of deep noxious stimulation to activate generalized autonomic responses independently of the relay of pain to conscious levels" (90). In other words, pain may not be the symptomatic outcome of nociceptive stimulation of spinal structures. Such a conclusion has profound implications for the chiropractic profession. Clearly, patients do not need to be in pain to be candidates for spinal adjustments.

Nansel and Szlazak published the most recent paper devoted to autonomic concomitants associated with nociceptive input (91). They explain that it is now well-established that nociceptive input from somatic and visceral structures "converge on common pools of interneurons within the spinal cord and brainstem." As a consequence, nociceptive input from somatic structures can "create complex patterns of signs and symptoms that can often be virtually identical to and, therefore, easily mistaken for those induced by primary visceral disease." The authors have collected over 200 scientific articles that deal with various somatic visceral disease mimicry syndromes.

In summary, there are many neuroendocrine and symptomatic presentations that can occur in response to nociceptive input. It is very likely that no two patients will present in the exact same fashion even if joint complex dysfunction exists in the same spinal location. The symptomatic picture can become even more complex when the consequences of reduce mechanoreception are considered.

Mechanoreceptors

Mechanoreceptors are located in the skin, muscles, joint structures and the intervertebral disc (13, 14, 92). Examples of mechanoreceptors include muscle spindles, golgi tendon organs (GTOs) and a variety of corpuscular mechanoreceptors such as Ruffini endings, Merkel cell complexes, Meissner's corpuscles, Pacinian corpuscles and many others (14).

Many believe that, as a group, mechanoreceptors respond only to weak mechanical stimuli, such as touch and joint movement, and not to nociceptive stimuli with higher frequencies (18, 19, 42, 94). As would be expected, several authors suggest that reduced joint movement results in less mechanoreceptor activation (20-23); however, the degree to which mechanoreceptor input would be compromised by joint hypomobility is unknown at the present time. Although it may be difficult to quantify such mechanoreceptor deficits in the laboratory, research suggests that a reduction in mechanoreceptor afferent input can result in the development of symptoms that can be identified in the clinical setting. For example, de Jong et al. injected human subjects with lidocaine into the area halfway between the mastoid process and carotid tubercle at the level of the second and third cervical vertebrae (94). Injections were made unilaterally. Immediately after injection, symptoms of dysequilibrium began to appear. Symptoms included ataxia, hypotonia of the ipsilateral arm and leg and a strong sensation

272   Journal of Manipulative and Physiological Therapeutics
Volume 21 • Number 4 • May, 1998
Dysafferentation • *Seaman and Winterstein*

of ipsilateral falling or tilting. The symptoms were more pronounced on the side of injection and lasted for about an hour. The authors suggest that the injection of local anesthetics "interrupted the flow of afferent information from neck and muscle receptors," which can affect vestibular nuclei function and promote a variety of vestibular symptoms (94). Presumably, the receptor types to which the authors refer include corpuscular mechanoreceptors, muscle spindles and GTOs.

A brief review of mechanoreceptor subtypes, their basic functions, and the neuroanatomical pathways associated with mechanoreceptors will help to outline potential symptoms that may develop due to joint complex dysfunction.

Corpuscular mechanoreceptors. Corpuscular mechanoreceptors are found in the skin, joint structures and muscles (14, 21, 95). It is generally held that corpuscular mechanoreceptors are associated with A-beta fibers (12, 13).

Mechanoreceptor afferents (A-beta fibers) influence the nervous system in many ways. For example, at the spinal cord level, mechanoreceptor input can inhibit nociception (14, 20, 96-99). Thus, it is very likely that reduced mechanoreceptive activity will enhance the nociceptive input associated with joint complex dysfunction. Also, mechanoreceptor afferents can reduce sympathetic hyperactivity (20, 99, 100). Thus, it is reasonable to suggest that reduced mechanoreception will enhance segmental sympathetic hyperactivity and somatomotor output.

Clearly, mechanoreceptor afferents have important functions in the CNS. It appears that it would be ideal to have an abundance of mechanoreceptors functioning at an optimal level at all times. Unfortunately, it appears that there are relatively few corpuscular mechanoreceptors compared to nociceptors.

The precise concentration of corpuscular mechanoreceptors in somatic tissues is unknown. Recent research suggests that the concentration of nociceptors far exceeds that of corpuscular mechanoreceptors. Schmidt et al. discuss the percentage of fiber types in the medial articular nerve and posterior articular nerve of the cat (19). Only 9% of the fibers in the medial articular nerve and 26% in the posterior articular nerve were mechanoreceptive (19). Such a low percentage of mechanoreceptive afferents suggests that maintaining proper joint mobility is very important.

Muscle spindles. Muscle spindles are classically described as receptors which send information into the CNS about muscle length or the rate of change of muscle length. It is generally held that muscle spindles lie parallel to extrafusal fibers in the belly of a muscle. Muscle spindles have primary endings associated with a group Ia afferent fiber, and secondary endings associated with a group II afferent fiber. Both group Ia and II fibers are thought to have numerous connections within the spinal cord.

Group Ia afferents are involved in several cord reflexes that modulate extrafusal muscle function, such as the stretch reflex, recurrent inhibition, reciprocal inhibition and the cross extensor reflex (101). All of these reflexes are very important for promoting smooth and controlled movements. Group II afferents are not as well described as Ia afferents. It is generally

believed that group II afferents primarily affect the static component of the stretch reflex.

In general, the greatest concentration of muscle spindles are located in muscles involved in fine movements and posture, whereas the lowest concentration is found in muscles involved in gross movement (102). Research has demonstrated that the digits and neck contain the greatest density of muscle spindles. Indeed, it has been stated that the neck muscles contain a "bewildering number of muscle spindles" (103). Dvorak and Dvorak indicate that, per gram of muscle tissue, the rectus femoris contains 50 muscle spindles, whereas the suboccipital muscles contain approximately 150-200 muscle spindles and the intertransverse muscles in the cervical spine contain between 200-500 muscle spindles (99). It has been suggested that the intertransverse muscles of the neck and low back, may actually function as mechanoreceptors and not as muscles (104).

The distribution of muscle spindles within muscles is far more varied and complex than the classical description. Richmond et al. indicate that muscle spindles can be associated with one another in several ways including

> (a) paired associations in which two or more spindles lie side-by-side, (b) parallel associations, in which two or more intrafusal fiber bundles are contained within a common capsule for some part of their length and (c) tandem associations, in which two or more spindle units are linked in series by a common intrafusal fiber that runs through each spindle unit in succession."

It is not uncommon to find muscle spindles linked in complex arrays that span the length of an intervertebral muscle. Some spindles are also found in close contact with Paciniform corpuscles and GTOs (103).

GTOs. GTOs are usually described as muscle tension receptors. Many believe that GTOs lie in series with extrafusal fibers. In other words, GTOs are found at the junction of a muscle and its tendon.

GTOs are stimulated when muscle contraction generates tension in a muscle. The frequency of firings increase in proportion to the increasing muscle tension (103). GTOs are innervated by a group Ib afferent fiber. The Ib afferent enters the cord and excites an interneuron located in the intermediate region of spinal cord gray matter. This so-called Ib inhibitory interneuron serves to inhibit the alpha-motoneuron that innervates the same muscle that was contracted and created the tension. It should be mentioned that the Ib inhibitory interneuron receives convergent input from Ia afferents from muscle spindles and A-beta afferents from cutaneous and joint receptors (100, 105).

GTOs are highly concentrated in neck muscles. Their distribution tends to be nonuniform. They are found along internal aponeurosis and where muscles attach to vertebral process. In both the deep and more superficial neck muscles spindles and GTOS are often clustered in complex receptor arrays (103).

In recent years, it has been shown the GTOs have a dynamic sensitivity and are more suited to signaling rapidly changing

Journal of Manipulative and Physiological Therapeutics   273
Volume 21 • Number 4 • May, 1998
Dysafferentation • *Seaman and Winterstein*

tensions rather than static levels of tension. Research has shown GTOs respond to forces as low as 4 mg.

Supraspinal connections. We know that afferent input from corpuscular mechanoreceptors, muscles spindles and GTOs can influence brain function. Researchers have stated that mechanoreceptive input is partially responsible for proprioception (14, 96) and suprasegmental motor control (106). Indeed, it appears that many supraspinal centers depend on afferent input, including the cerebellum and cerebral cortex. For example, Carpenter states that afferent fiber input to the cerebellum exceeds efferent fibers by a ratio of approximately 40:1, which demonstrates the degree to which afferent input is needed by the CNS (107). With this information in mind, it is important to consider the probability that joint complex dysfunction is associated with the degeneration, atrophy and deconditioning of mechanoreceptor rich tissues, such as muscles and joint structures (1,107-109).

The following sections describe the main afferent and subsequent efferent connections of the cerebellum and cerebral cortex. Based on these connections and related research findings, a variety of potential symptoms that may manifest in response to the reduced mechanoreceptive input associated with joint complex dysfunction.

Cerebellum. Brodal provides a detailed description of mechanoreceptive input to the cerebellum (95). Afferents enter the cerebellum through all three cerebellar peduncles. Whereas the superior peduncle contains mostly efferent fibers and some afferent fibers, the middle peduncle contains only afferent fibers and the inferior peduncle contains mostly afferent fibers and some efferent fibers. The discussion which follows focuses on afferent information that travels through the middle and inferior peduncles.

Afferents entering the middle cerebellar peduncle come from the cerebral cortex via the corticopontocerebellar tract, which contains some 20 million fibers (95). The majority of these fibers project to the lateral cortex of the cerebellum, which is involved in the coordination and regulation of sequential and volitional motor activities initiated by the cerebral cortex (95, 110). Clearly, without afferent input, the lateral cortex could not properly modulate motor control.

The lateral cortex is often called the cerebrocerebellum because it receives input exclusively from the cerebral cortex by way of the pontine nuclei (111). The heaviest projections come from the primary motor area (Brodmann area 4), the primary sensory area (Brodmann area 3, 1, and 2), a somatosensory association area (Brodmann area 5) and from parts of the visual areas related to the peripheral visual field (95). Areas 3, 1, and 2, the primary sensory area, each receive afferents from specific receptors (95). Group Ia muscle spindle afferents project to area 3a. Cutaneous afferents project to area 3b. Joint afferents project to area 2. Area 1 receives input from both cutaneous and deep tissue receptors. This information makes it is clear that a significant level of mechanoreceptor afferent input indirectly reaches the cerebellum by way of the cerebral cortex.

The inferior peduncle contains some 0.5 millions fibers (95), most of which originate from receptors in axial and appendicular structures. Afferents from spinal structures end in the cerebellar vermis, whereas afferents from the extremities end in the intermediate cortex which is also referred to as the paravermal region. Of importance to note is that this input is somatotopically organized. Nolte indicates that the principle sources of afferent input to the vermis and intermediate cortex comes, via the spinal cord, from mechanoreceptors in the skin, muscle and joints (110). For this reason, the vermis and intermediate cortex are often referred to as the spinocerebellum. It should be mentioned that the both the vermis and intermediate cortex also receive afferent input from the motor cortex, by way of the corticopontocerebellar tract. This input is somatotopically organized so that the cortical fibers end in the same pattern as those from mechanoreceptor afferents (110).

As far back as 1960, it was determined that the dorsal spinocerebellar tract conveys information to the vermis and intermediate cortex from muscle spindles, GTOs and corpuscular mechanoreceptors in the skin. Later, it was determined that the dorsal spinocerebellar tract also conveys information from joint receptors (95). It is known that the dorsal spinocerebellar tract conveys mechanoreceptive information from the lower half of the body and the cuneocerebellar tract relays mechanoreceptor afferent input from the upper half (95,107). The importance of the spinocerebellar pathways is demonstrated by the conduction velocity of its component fibers. We is known that impulses are transmitted at velocities up to 120 m/sec for the purpose of instantaneously apprising the cerebellum about peripheral movements (12). Additional afferents that travel through the inferior cerebellar pedumcle to end in the spinocerebellum arise from the inferior olive and central-cervival nucleus.

The inferior olive also provides input to the cerebellum from mechanoreceptor afferents, which end somatotopically in the olive (95). Carpenter (107) indicates that afferents from cutaneous receptors and Ib afferents from GTOs contribute to the spino-olivary tract. Proske indicates that the principal supraspinal site of termination for GTO afferents is the cerebellum (105). The major projection is from the spinocerebellar tracts and the secondary projection comes from the inferior olive via the spino-olivary tract (105). If the spino-olivary tract is consistent with other ascending mechanoreceptive tracts, it is likely that all types of mechanoreceptor afferents project to the inferior olive. Brodal states that, "the quantitatively most important contingents of afferents mediate spinal impulses." (95)

The inferior olive is a very important structure and far too complex to discuss in this paper. In brief, we know that the inferior olive projects to all parts of the cerebellar cortex and all deep cerebellar nuclei (i.e, the dentate, globose, emboliform, (nucleus interpositus) and fastigial). There are even reciprocal connections between each cerebellar nucleus and the olive. In addition to mechanoreceptor afferents, the inferior olive also receives input from the cerebral cortex (chiefly the motor cortex), red nucleus, mesencephalic reticular formation, superior colliculus and pretectum (115). The symptoms associated with experimental oblation of the inferior olive are similar to

274   Journal of Manipulative and Physiological Therapeutics
Volume 21 • Number 4 • May, 1998
Dysafferentation • *Seaman and Winterstein*

those associated with destruction of the entire contralateral cerebellum (110).

The central cervical nucleus (CCN), located in lamina VII of the first four cervical segments, projects to the cerebellar vermis (95). Originally, the CCN was thought to receive only upper cervical mechanoreceptor afferents (95, 121). Recent research suggests that the CCN may receive mechanoreceptor afferents from as low as the lumbar spine (113). However, there is evidence to suggest that the CCN is most powerfully influence by receptors in deep neck muscles (114).

The vermis functions to control equilibrium, posture, muscle tone and locomotion (12, 95, 107). Ghez states that the vermis is involved in axial and proximal motor control (111). It must be remembered that, without proper afferent input, these functions would be compromised.

Assuming that the vermis receives sufficient mechanoreceptive input, it will modulate motor function by projecting to a variety of nuclei. The vermis projects somatotopically organized information to the fastigial nucleus, which then projects bilaterally to the lateral vestibular nucleus and reticular formation nuclei (111), particularly the nucleus reticularis pontis caudalis and the nucleus reticularis gigantocellularis (95). The tracts associated with these nuclei include the lateral vestibulospinal tract, the medial reticulospinal tract, and the lateral reticulospinal tract, respectively. It is known the fastigial nucleus also projects to the thalamus, and ultimately, to the motor cortex (95, 111).

The intermediate cortex mainly coordinates the actions of the distal extremities (95, 107, 111). It accomplishes this task by projecting to nucleus interpositus, which projects mainly to the red nucleus and motor cortex, affecting the rubrospinal tract and corticospinal tract, respectively. It is thought that the intermediate cortex compares commands emanating from the motor cortex with the actual position and velocity of the moving part (it receives this information from mechanoreceptors); then, by way of the nucleus interpositus, the intermediate cortex issues correcting signals (110). Without adequate mechanoreceptor input, the ability of the intermediate cortex to modulate motor control would be compromised.

Thus far, both the cerebrocerebellum and spinocerebellum have been discussed. The third division of the cerebellum is known as the vestibulocerebellum, so named because it receives afferent input from the vestibular nerve and vestibular nuclei. The flocculonodular lobe is the specific area of the cerebellum referred to as the vestibulocerebellum. Afferents to vestibulocerebellum also travel through the inferior cerebellar peduncle.

Most texts indicate that only vestibular afferents end in the flocculonodular lobe (11, 110, 111); however, this is not the case. Guyton alludes to the fact that mechanoreceptor afferents from the neck, also gain access to the flocculonodular lobe (12). He explains that mechanoreceptors from the neck and body transmit information directly into the vestibular nuclei and indirectly, by way of the cerebellum, into the flocculonodular lobe. Apparently, mechanoreceptor input from the neck transmit signals that oppose the signals from the vestibular appa-

ratus, which prevents a person from developing dysequilibrium when the head is laterally flexed or rotated. Guyton further stated that, "by far the most important proprioceptive information needed for the maintenance of equilibrium is that derived from the joint receptors of the neck." (12) Although not described by Guyton, several other authors describe a specific relay nucleus by which mechanoreceptor afferents gain access to the vestibulocerebellum (95, 113, 114).

Brodal states that mechanoreceptor afferents project to the flocculonodular lobe via the group X nucleus located in the region of the vestibular nuclei (95). Bakker and Abrahams explain that the neurons of group X appear to serve as a primary relay for cervical mechanoreceptor afferent input to the cerebellum (114). Research also suggests that thoracic and lumbar mechanoreceptor afferents project to group X (113).

In summary, the flocculonodular lobe receives input from the vestibular apparatus in the inner ear and mechanoreceptor afferents, and then projects ipsilaterally to the middle, superior and inferior vestibular nuclei. Relatively few fibers project to the lateral vestibular nucleus (95).

Most authors agree that the medial vestibulospinal tract originates in the medial vestibular nucleus and descends bilaterally into the cervical and perhaps upper thoracic cord (95, 110, 111). Ghez state that, "this tract participates in the reflex control of neck movements so that the position of the head can be maintained accurately and is correlated with eye movements" (111).

The medial longitudinal fasciculus (MLF) is believed to originate in the superior and medial vestibular nuclei. Fibers in the MLF project to abducens, trochlear and oculomotor nuclei, which allows a person's gaze to stay fixed on an object while the head is moving (110). This is known as the vestibulo-ocular reflex; Maeda has demonstrated that the cervical spine mechanoreceptors participate in this reflex by projecting to the group X nucleus (115).

The MLF also projects to the interstitial nucleus of Cajal (128). It is thought that this nucleus probably plays an important role in mediating effects on the neck and body musculature in response to optic and vestibular impulses and may also influence certain central effects on the autonomic system (125).

The vestibular nuclei also project to the cerebral cortex via both direct and indirect pathways. Animal experiments have revealed that within the facial region of the primary sensory area, there is a marked convergence of vestibular and somatosensory impulses arising from muscle spindles and from mechanoreceptors in skin and joints (95). These connections may exist in humans; Nolte indicates that each superior vestibular nucleus sends projections bilaterally to the facial region of the primary sensory area (110). Through these connections it is likely that the vestibular nuclei play a role in the conscious appreciation of body position (95, 110).

The vestibular nuclei also have extensive reciprocal connections with the reticular formation. "The vestibuloreticular connections are presumably involved in vomiting and cardiovascular reactions observed on vestibular irritation" (95).

In a classical sense, the vestibulocerebellum is primarily

p. 266   *Clinical Nutrition for pain, inflammation & tissue healing*

Journal of Manipulative and Physiological Therapeutics 275
Volume 21 • Number 4 • May, 1998
Dysafferentation • *Seaman and Winterstein*

thought to play a role in equilibrium. This is because lesions to the flocculonodular lobe can result in general dysequilibrium and vertigo (110). However, the vestibular nuclei have widespread connections; therfore, lesions within the vestibulocerebellum may also result in conditions such as nystagmus and a variety of autonomic concomitants (95). It is quite possible that similar symptoms can develop when adequate mechanoreceptive input does not reach the vestibular nuclei and flocculonodular lobe.

Cerebral cortex. As mentioned in the cerebellum section, each area in the primary somatosensory region receives afferents from specific receptors (107). Group Ia muscle spindle afferents project to area 3a. Cutaneous afferents project to area 3b. Joint afferents project to area 2. Area 1 receives input from both cutaneous and deep tissue receptors. It is well-known that the dorsal columns and medial lemniscus carry this mechanoreceptive information. The importance of such mechanoreceptor afferent input to the cerebral cortex is described by many neuroanatomists.

Carpenter states that

> although impulses generated in neurons in the primary motor area (M I), the premotor area, and in the supplementary motor area (M II) are responsible for movement, motor control, changes in muscle tone and maintenance of posture, these motor activities are initiated by inputs that arise from the thalamus, other cortical areas and peripheral receptors (119).

According to Masdeu and Brazis, sensorimotor control is carried out by various thalamic nuclei, such as the ventrolateral nucleus, which predominantly coordinate the finer distal motor movements (106): "The ventrolateral nucleus integrates input from the cerebellum, basal ganglia and mechanoreceptors from the musculoskeletal system; it projects to the precentral cortex or primary motor cortex (area 4)." Wyke maintains that Type I joint receptors, which are similar to Ruffini spray endings, excite the paracentral and parietal regions of the cerebral cortex and make a significant contribution to the perceptual experiences of postural sensation and kinesthesis (96). Clearly, appropriate mechanoreceptor afferent input is required by the cerebral cortex to perform a host of conscious and subconscious motor functions.

Other authors indicate that afferent input plays a role that extends beyond that of motor control. Both Guyton (12) and Nolte (110) indicate that if afferent signals are eliminated, the cerebrum would be incapable of functioning in a conscious manner and would actually approach a permanent state of coma.

A more precise anatomical look at the cerebral cortex reveals that somatosensory input plays an additional role in human function, such that mechanoreceptor input is actually needed to help us function as humans. The human neocortex accounts for more than 90% of our total cortical area (110) and is divided into six separate layers (107). Layer I, the molecular layer is the most external. Layer II is the external granular layer. Layer III is the external pyramidal layer. Layer IV is the internal granular layer. Layer V is the internal pyramidal layer. Layer VI is the deepest and is known as the multiform layer.

Generally speaking, layers II and IV receive afferent input and layers III and V mainly receive efferent (112). Layer II receives cortical afferents and, depending on the location in the neocortex, layer IV receives afferents from somatosensory receptors, the medial geniculate body for audition and the lateral geniculate body for vision (see discussion below on primary sensory areas). Layer III projects ipsilaterally and contralaterally to other areas of the cerebral cortex via association fibers and commissural fibers. Layer V gives rise to corticostriate fibers, corticopontine fibers, corticobulbar fibers and corticospinal fibers (c107). Layer VI is also thought to be largely efferent and mainly project fibers to the thalamus. Cortical interneurons allow the various layers in a specific area to communicate with one another (112).

The term 'great sensory pathways" has classically been used to describe the somatosensory, optic and acoustic systems (95). Each has an individual primary sensory area in the cerebral cortex. Area 17 in the occipital lobe is for vision. Area 41 in the temporal lobe is for audition, and areas 3,1 and 2 in the parietal lobe are for somatosensory input. Once afferent input is received in a specific primary sensory area, the information is integrated and then communicated to other parts of the brain via commissural and association fibers. The great majority of commissural fibers travel in the corpus callosum, which is thought to contain about 180 million fibers. The projections between homotopic regions are thought to very precise. For example, the commissural connections of the primary and secondary sensory areas seem to be extremely specific (95).

Association fibers are ipsilateral, and four main fiber pathways are typically described. One passes through the cingulate gyrus and is known as the cingulum. The superior longitudinal fasciculus connects the frontal lobe to the occipital lobe. The inferior longitudinal fasciculus connects the occipital lobe to the temporal lobe. The uncinate fasciculus passes from the temporal lobe to the frontal lobe (95, 110). It should be understood that none of the association pathways are discrete, point-to-point pathways. Fibers freely enter and leave along the course the pathways (110). Thus, the association pathways allow for an almost unimaginable number of connections. We know that the primary sensory areas (for somatosensory input, vision and audition) all communicate in various association areas, such as the parieto-occipito-temporal association area and the prefrontal association area, via the commissural and association pathways (95, 112).

The prefrontal association area also receives input from the limbic system; thus, this association area receives information about all modalities as well as information regarding motivational and emotional state (112). All of this input is integrated, which allows one to appropriately engage a given environmental situation. A reduction in limbic input, visual input, auditory input or somatosensory input would necessarily compromise one's ability to function.

Janse provided a most elegant commentary on the importance of mechanoreceptor afferent input (116). "Numerically, the somatic sensory factors comprise by far the major activating vehicle of the nervous system and the overtones of the

276   Journal of Manipulative and Physiological Therapeutics
Volume 21 • Number 4 • May, 1998
Dysafferentation • *Seaman and Winterstein*

body's conduct are significantly conditioned and controlled by their input." Regarding the total sensorial experience of humans, which includes mechanoreceptive, nociceptive and special senses, Janse stated that humans are provided "with sentiencies [sic] of emotional, mental and spiritual affectivities that defy total comprehension." Janse suggested that an divergence in the totality of sensory input could ultimately result in pathology, or symptoms of pathology, in seemingly unrelated tissues and organs (116).

Symptoms associated with reduced mechanoreceptor input. Mechanoreceptive information reaches numerous centers in the CNS. Consequently, a reduction in mechanoreceptor input, due to joint complex dysfunction has the potential to promote numerous symptoms which could mimic lesions of the vestibular nuclei, cerebellum, cerebral cortex and basal ganglia. Although much more research is still needed in this area, evidence exists to support this contention. For example, as early as 1845, "Longet reported that surgical damage of neck muscles in a wide range of species led to generalized but transient motor disturbances characterized by an ataxia similar to that which followed cerebellectomy." (103) More recently, a study of patients with soft tissue injuries in the neck lead the authors to conclude that oculomotor abnormalities may be due to abnormal mechanoreceptor input (117).

Fitz-Ritson found that 112 out of 235 patients with cervical spinal trauma experienced cervical vertigo (118). The definition of vertigo used in this study can be either "a subjective vertigo, i.e., the patient feels that he/she is rotating, [and] objective vertigo, i.e., the feeling that the room or environment is rotating." After 18 treatments, which involved chiropractic adjustments to restore mobility to restricted joints, 101 of the 112 patients (90.2 %) were symptom free. This finding is consistent with the findings of Lewit who states that manipulation is very effective for reducing vertigo and dizziness (119).

It seems that symptoms of enhanced nociception often accompany those associated with reduced mechanoreception. For example, Weeks and Travell demonstrated that a clinical syndrome characterized by postural vertigo or dizziness, imbalance, and usually headache may be caused by dysfunction of the sternocleidomastoid muscle (120). Gray reported on a series of case histories that described how injured cervical muscles can play a role in the production of vertigo, pain, nausea and tinnitus (121).

In a paper entitled *Cervical Vertigo*, Wing and Hargrave-Wilson described 80 patients, all of whom had some form of vertigo, which varied from the severe rotary type to generalized unsteadiness (122). All patients had a thorough examination of the ears, nose and throat, and the results were normal in 96% of the cases. Electronystagmographic abnormalities were found in all patients. Some 69% of the patients also had either occipital headaches or cervical pain. All patients had "tender muscle guarding" in the upper cervical region which was thought to exist due to "partial fixation of the involved vertebra." The authors state that manipulation was a "bastion" of treatment. After treatment, electronystagmographic recordings were significantly improved in 73% of the patients. A total

of 53% of patients had complete relief of symptoms, and 36% had significant improvement to the point where they required no medication and could return to normal activities.

Several additional authors have discussed the relationship between a dysfunctional cervical spine and symptoms of pain, vertigo and dizziness (123-126). Research also suggests that joint complex dysfunction in the lumbar spine can affect equilibrium (127).

Reduced mechanoreception may also impact the nonmotor functions of the cerebellum. In 1978, Watson explained how traditional concepts of cerebellar physiology emphasize motor control functions; he also points out that an emerging body of literature demonstrates a relationship between the cerebellum and psychological processes (128).

Specifically , data have suggested that this brain structure may participate in sensory integration activities, motor skills learning, visual and auditory discrimination performance, emotion and motivation control, and reinforcement processes.

Many articles have discussed the cerebellum's participation in emotional expression (128-132). The most dramatic work was completed by Heath during the 1970s (132).

Through experimentation, Heath demonstrated that brain sites for emotional expression are anatomically connected and functionally related to sensory relay nuclei for all modalities and also to sites involved in facial expression and motor coordination (132). His research demonstrated that efferent pathways from the vermis/fastigial nucleus could stimulate pleasure centers located in the septal nuclei of the hypothalamus and corticomedial amygdala, and simultaneously inhibit adversive emotion centers located in the hippocampus and dorsolateral amygdala. Heath applied electrical stimulation to vermis to activate this pathway in the treatment of psychiatric patients. To access the cerebellum, suboccipital craniotomy was performed and 2.0 mm electrodes were implanted subtentorially over the rostral vermal and paravermal regions of the cerebellum. A pace-making device delivered a stimulus at selected time intervals. Heath applied this method to 11 patients with intractable psychiatric illness, all of whom were pronounced incurable by at least two physicians. The length of illness varied from 6 to 23 yr. Of the 11 patients, four had uncontrollable violence-aggression (two with no demonstrable organic brain disease and two with brain pathology), five were schizophrenics, and two had lifetime patterns of severe neurosis. After treatment, ten of the eleven patients were out of the hospital and functioning without medications or other treatment [except for cerebellar stimulation]. Some were symptom free and others demonstrated significant improvements. The one patient who failed to respond had an adhesion between the tentorium and the rostral vermis, that extended 2.5 cm to either side of midline, which apparently damaged the targeted cerebellar neurons.

Heath's work is important for chiropractors because the rostral vermal and paravermal neurons of the cerebellum receive axial and appendicular mechanoreceptor input from all levels of the spinal cord (see earlier discussion on the cerebellum). Although this does not prove that dysafferentation

p. 268 *Clinical Nutrition for pain, inflammation & tissue healing*

Journal of Manipulative and Physiological Therapeutics 277
Volume 21 • Number 4 • May, 1998
Dysafferentation • *Seaman and Winterstein*

due to joint complex dysfunction is a cause of psychiatric illness, it is clear that interesting implications do exist and should be investigated.

CONCLUSION

The information presented in this article demonstrated that the CNS is greatly influenced by somatosensory input. Numerous, seemingly unrelated symptoms can be generated when nociceptive input is enhanced and mechanoreceptive input is reduced. Research evidence leads us to believe that such dysafferent input is associated with joint complex dysfunction, which explains why so many seemingly bizarre symptoms respond to chiropractic care.

As stated earlier, according to classical neuroanatomy, the great sensory systems include the visual system, the auditory system and the somatosensory system. At the present time, there are specialists devoted to the visual and auditory systems. As of yet, no profession has effectively stepped forward to specialize in treating somatosensory system dysfunction (i.e., dysafferentation induced by joint complex dysfunction). That chiropractic has not assumed such a role is surprising. Indeed, it seems that Janse envisioned that chiropractors filling this role (116).

Apparently, Janse was so convinced that the chiropractic profession would pursue research in the field of somatosensory neurology that he wrote, "let us be a trifle bold and quite foolish; let us try to imagine what a symposium on Principles of Sensory Communication might be like in 10 or 15 years hence." (134) Janse went on to discuss numerous aspects of somatosensory function which could have served as research topics for chiropractors. Unfortunately, save for a few scattered articles, the idea that chiropractors should be the doctors or care takers of one of the great sensory systems has not been pursued. Janse warned future generations of chiropractors about neglecting the somatosensory system. He stated

it is not to be forgotten that essentially man is a sensorial organism. He functions by virtue of the inputs he experiences via the cutaneum, the subdermal, the myofascial planes, the diarthrodial complexes of the musculoskeletal system, especially the spine; the related proprioceptive phenomena (116).

Suggestions for Chiropractic Education

At the present time, the basic sciences in most chiropractic colleges are taught in the same fashion as in medical school. Students are taught to view anatomy, physiology and diagnosis based solely on a pathology model. In other words, a differential diagnosis involves ruling out pathological changes in anatomical structures and metabolic pathways. This approach should not be abandoned; however, joint complex dysfunction and dysafferentation must be included in every differential diagnosis whenever it is determined that nociceptive and mechanoreceptive input can directly or indirectly influence the structures from which the symptoms are generated. This demands that students and practitioners be well versed in the details of the central connections of the many neuroanatomical pathways related to nociceptive and mechanoreceptive input.

Without this knowledge it will be impossible for students and doctors to understand and explain how joint complex dysfunction can affect the many conditions which afflict the human body.

At the present time, only a few articles explain how to include joint complex dysfunction in the differential diagnosis, all of which focus on the topic of dizziness and vertigo (99, 118, 133, 134). This must change if chiropractic is to ever become a truly mainstream profession that reaches a majority of the population.

REFERENCES

1. Seaman D. Joint complex dysfunction: A novel term to replace subluxation/subluxation complex. Etiological and treatment considerations. J Manipulative Physiol Ther 1997; 20:634-44.
2. Waagen G, Strang V. Origin and development of traditional chiropractic philosophy. In Haldeman S. editor. Principles and Practice of Chiropractic. 2nd ed. Norwalk: Appleton &Lange; 1992. p. 29-43.
3. Practice guidelines for straight chiropractic. Proceedings of the International Straight Chiropractic Consensus Conference. Chandler, (AZ): World Chiropractic Alliance, 1992. p. 98.
4. Kale Clinic & Research Center. Houston Control (patient pamphlet). Spartanburg: South Carolina; 1993.
5. Seaman D. Proprioceptor: An obsolete, inaccurate word. J Manip Physiol Ther1997; 20(4):279-84.
6. Seaman D. Letter to Editor. Top Clin Chiropr 1997; 4(1):vi-viii.
7. Cramer G, Darby S. Letter to Editor. Top Clin Chiro 1997; 4(1):viii-xi.
8. Deafferentation Dorland's Medical Dictionary. 25th ed. Philadelphia: W.B. Saunders, 1974. p. 409.
9. Burchiel K. Deafferentation syndromes and dorsal root entry zone lesions. In: Fields H, editor. Pain syndromes in neurology. Boston: Butterworth-Heinemann, 1990. p. 201-22.
10. Fields H. Pain. New York: McGraw-Hill, 1987.
11. Tasker R. Management of nociceptive, deafferentation and central pain by surgical intervention. In: Fields H, editor. Pain syndromes in neurology. Boston: Butterworth-Heinemann, 1990. p. 143-200.
12. Guyton A. Basic neuroscience. 2nd ed. Philadelphia: WB Saunders, 1991.
13. Martin J, Jessell T. Modality coding in the somatic sensory system. In Kandel E, Schwartz J, Jessell T, eds. Principles of neural science. 3rd ed. New York: Elsevier, 1991. p. 341-52.
14. Willis W, Coggeshall R. Sensory mechanisms of the spinal cord. 2nd ed. New York: Plenum Press, 1991.
15. Schaible H, Schmidt R. Direct observation of the sensitization of articular afferents during an experimental arthritis. In: Dubner R, Gebhart G, Bond M, editors. Proceedings of the 5th World Congress on Pain; 1987 Aug 2-7; Hamburg, Germany. New York: Elsevier, 1988. p. 44-50.
16. Guilbaud G. Peripheral and central electrophysiological mechanisms of joint muscle pain. . In: Dubner R, Gebhart G, Bond M, editors. Proceedings of the 5th World Congress on Pain. 1987 Aug 2-7; Hamburg, Germany. New York: Elsevier, 1988. p. 201-15.
17. Hanesch U, Heppelmann B, Messlinger K, Schmidt R. Nociception in normal and arthritic joints: Structural and functional aspects. In: Willis W, editor. Hyperalgesia and allodynia. New York: Raven Press, 1992. p. 81-106.
18. Schaible H, Grubb B. Afferent and spinal mechanisms of joint pain. Pain 1993; 55:5-54.
19. Schmidt R, Schaible H, Messlinger K, Heppelmann B, Hanesch

278 Journal of Manipulative and Physiological Therapeutics
Volume 21 • Number 4 • May, 1998
Dysafferentation • *Seaman and Winterstein*

U, Pawlak M. Silent and active nociceptors: structure, functions, and clinical implications. In: Gebhart G, Hammond T, Jensen T, editors. Proceedings of the 7th World Congress on Pain, Progress in Pain Research and Management; 1993; Paris, France. Seattle: IASP Press, 1994. p. 213-50.

20. Hooshmand H. Chronic pain: reflex sympathetic dystrophy, prevention and management. Boca Raton(FL): CRC Press; 1993. p. 33-55.

21. Jozsa L, Balint J, Kannus P, Jarvinen M, Lehto M. Mechano-receptors in human myotendinous junction. Muscle & Nerve 1993; 16. p. 453-7.

22. Lephart S. Reestablishing proprioception, kinesthesia, joint position sense, and neuromuscular control in rehabilitation. In: Prentice, W ed. Rehabilitation techniques in sports medicine. 2nd ed. St. Louis: Mosby, 1994. p. 118-37.

23. Parkhurst T, Burnett C. Injury and proprioception in the lower back. J Orthop Sports Phys Ther 1994; 19:282-95.

24. Slosberg M. Effects of altered afferent input on sensation, proprioception, muscle tone and sympathetic reflex response. J Manipulative Physiol Ther 1988; 11:400-8.

25. Jones M, Christensen N, Carr J. Clinical reasoning in orthopedic manual therapy. In: Grant R, editor. Physical therapy of cervical and thoracic spine. 2nd ed. New York: Churchill-Livingstone, 1994. p. 89-108.

26. Peterson D. Principles of adjustive technique. In: Bergmann T, Peterson D, Lawrence D, editors. Chiropractic technique. New York: Churchill-Livingstone, 1993. p. 123-95.

27. Peterson D, Bergmann T. Joint assessment principles and procedures. In: Bergmann T, Peterson D, Lawrence D, editors. Chiropractic technique. New York: Churchill-Livingstone; 1993. p. 51-121.

28. Henderson C. Three neurophysiologic theories on the chiropractic subluxation. In: Gatterman M, editor. Foundations of chiropractic - subluxation, St. Louis: Mosby, 1995. p. 225-33.

29. Murphy D. The locomotor system: Korr's "primary machinery of life" J Manipulative Physiol Ther 1994; 17:562-4.

30. Denslow J, Hassett C. The central excitatory state associated with postural abnormalities. J Neurophysiol 1942; 5:393-402.

31. Korr I. The neural basis of the osteopathic lesion. J Am Osteopath Assoc 1947; 47:191-7.

32. Patterson, M. A model mechanism for spinal segmental facilitation. J Am Osteopath Assoc 1976; 76:62-72.

33. Miller B, Keane C, editors. Encyclopedia and dictionary of medicine, nursing and allied Health. Philadelphia: WB Saunders; 1987. p. 383-8.

34. Bogduk N. Innervation patterns of the cervical spine. In: Grant R, editor. Physical therapy of the cervical and thoracic spine. 2nd ed. New York: Churchill-Livingstone, 1994. p. 65-76.

35. Bogduk N, Valencia F. Innervation patterns of the thoracic spine. In: Grant R, editor. Physical therapy of the cervical and thoracic spine. 2nd ed. New York: Churchill-Livingstone, 1994. p. 77-87.

36. Bogduk N. Innervation, pain patterns, and mechanisms of pain production. In: Twomey L, Taylor J, editors. Physical therapy of the low back. 2nd ed. New York: Churchill-Livingstone, 1994, p, 93-109.

37. Charman R. Pain and nociception: mechanisms and modulation in sensory context. In: Boyling J, Palastanga N, editors. Grieve's modern manual therapy: the vertebral column. 2nd ed. New York: Churchill-Livingstone, 1994. p. 253-70.

38. Grieve G. Common vertebral joint problems. 2nd ed. New York: Churchill-Livingstone; 1988. p. 51-2.

39. Haldeman S. The neurophysiology of pain. In: Haldeman S, editor. Principles and practice of chiropractic. 2nd ed. Norwalk (CT): Appleton-Century-Crofts; 1992. p. 165-84.

40. Wyke B. The neurological basis of thoracic pain. Rheumatol Phys Med 1970; 10:356-67.

41. Wyke B. Neurological aspects of pain therapy. In: Swerdlow M, editor. The therapy of pain. Philadelphia: JB Lippincott; 1980. p. 1-30.

42. Price D. Psychological and neural mechanisms of pain. New York: Raven Press; 1988. p. 76-99.

43. McMahon S, Koltzenburg M. Novel classes of nociceptors: beyond Sherrington. Trends Neurosci 1990; 13:199-201.

44. Bonica J. Anatomic and physiologic basis of nociception and pain. In: Bonica J, editor. Management of pain. 2nd ed. Philadelphia: Lea & Febiger, 1990. p. 28-94.

45. Bonica J. Definitions and taxonomy of pain. In: Bonica J. editor The management of pain. 2nd ed. Philadelphia: Lea & Febiger; 1990. p. 18-27.

46. Maciewicz R. Organization of pain pathways. In: Ashbury A, McKhann G, McDonald W, eds. Diseases of the nervous system: clinical neurobiology. Philadelphia: WB Saunders; 1992. p. 849-57.

47. Casey K. Nociceptors and their sensitization: overview. In: Willis W, editor Hyperalgesia and allodynia. New York: Raven Press; 1992. p. 13-5.

48. Handwerker H, Reeh P. Nociceptors: chemosensitivity and sensitization by chemical agents. In: Willis W, editor. Hyperalgesia and allodynia. New York: Raven Press, 1992. p. 107-15.

49. Steen KH, Reeh PW, Anton F, Handwerker HO. Protons selectively induce long lasting excitation and sensitization to mechanical stimulation of nociceptors in rat skin, *in vitro*. J Neurosci 1992; 12:86-95.

50. Campbell J, Meyer R, Davis K, Raja S. Sympathetically maintained pain: A unifying hypothesis. In: Willis W, editor Hyperalgesia and allodynia. New York: Raven Press, 1992. p. 141-9.

51. Levine J, Coderre T, Basbaum A. The peripheral nervous system and the inflammatory process. In: Dubner R, Gebhart G, Bond M, editors. Proceedings of the Fifth World Congress on Pain; 1987 Aug 2-7; Hamburg, Germany. New York: Elsevier; 1987. p. 33-43.

52. Levine J, Taiwo Y, Heller P. Hyperalgesic pain: inflammatory and neuropathic. In: Willis W, editor Hyperalgesia and allodynia. New York: Raven Press, 1992. p. 117-23.

53. Rang H, Bevan S, Dray A. Chemical activation of nociceptive peripheral neurones. Br Med Bull 1991;47:534-48.

54. Reeh P. Chemical excitation and sensitization of nociceptors: In Urban L, editor. Cellular mechanisms of sensory processing. Berlin: Springer-Verlag, 1994. p. 119-31.

55. Dubner R. Spinal cord neuronal plasticity: mechanisms of persistent pain following tissue damage and nerve injury. In: Vecchiet D, Albe-Fessard D, Lindblom U, Giamberardino M, editors. New trends in referred pain and hyperalgesia. New York: Elsevier Sci Pub, 1993. p. 109-17.

56. Coderre T, Katz J, Vaccarino A, Melzack R. Contribution of central neuroplasticity to pathological pain: review of clinical and experimental evidence. Pain 1993; 52:259-85.

57. Light A. The initial processing of pain and its descending control: spinal and trigeminal systems. New York: Karger, 1992:28

58. Woolf C. Physiological, inflammatory and neuropathic pain. Adv Tech Standards Neurosurg 1987; 15:39-62.

59. Denslow J, Korr I, Krems A. Quantitative studies of chronic facilitation in human motoneurons. Am J Physiol 1947; 150: 229-38.

60. Patterson M. The spinal cord: participant in disorder. Spinal Manipulation 1993; 9(3):2-11.

61. Korr I. Symposium on the functional implications of segmental facilitation: A research report. J Am Osteopath Assoc 1955; 54:265-82.

62. Korr I. The facilitated segment: A factor in injury to the body framework. Osteopathic Annals 1973; 1:10-12,17-18.

63. Korr I. Andrew Taylor Still memorial lecture: Research and

Journal of Manipulative and Physiological Therapeutics 279
Volume 21 • Number 4 • May, 1998
Dysafferentation • *Seaman and Winterstein*

practice — a century later. J Am Osteopath Assoc 1974; 73:362-70.

64. Korr I. Proprioceptors and somatic dysfunction. J Am Osteopath Assoc 1975; 74:638-50.

65. Korr I. Sustained sympathicotonia as a factor in disease. In: Korr I, editor. The neurobiologic mechanisms in manipulative therapy. New York: Plenum Press, 1978. p. 229-68.

66. Korr I. Somatic dysfunction, osteopathic manipulative treatment, and the nervous system: A few facts, some theories, many questions. J Am Osteopath Assoc 1986; 86:109-14.

67. Korr I. Osteopathic research: the needed paradigm shift. J Am Osteopath Assoc 1991; 91:156-71.

68. Woolf C. Evidence for a central component of post-injury pain hypersensitivity. Nature 1983; 306:686-8.

69. Dubner R. Neuronal Plasticity in the spinal and medullary dorsal horns: A possible role in central pain mechanisms. In: Casey K. Pain and central nervous system disease: the central pain syndromes. New York: Raven Press; 1991. p. 143-55.

70. Dubner R, Ruda M. Activity-dependent neuronal plasticity following tissue injury and inflammation. Trends Neurosci 1992; 15(3):96-103.

71. Dubner R, Basbaum A. Spinal cord plasticity following tissue or nerve injury. In: Wall R, Melzack R. editors. Textbook of pain. 3rd ed. New York: Churchill-Livingstone; 1994. p. 225-41.

72. Hoheisel U, Mense S. Long-term changes in discharge behavior of cat dorsal horn neurones following noxious stimulation of deep tissues. Pain 1989; 36:239-47.

73. Ren K, Hylden J, Williams G, Ruda M, Dubner R. The effects of a non-competitive NMDA receptor antagonist, MK-801, on behavioral hyperalgesia and dorsal horn neuronal activity in rats with unilateral inflammation. Pain 1992; 50:331-44.

74. Richmond C, Bromley L, Woolf C. Preoperative morphine pre-empts postoperative pain. Lancet 1993; 342:73-5.

75. Roberts W. A hypothesis on the physiological basis for causalgia and related pains. Pain 1986; 24:297-311.

76. Wall, P, Woolf C. Muscle but not cutaneous C-afferent input produces prolonged increases in the excitability of the flexion reflex in the rat. J Physiol 1984; 356:443-58.

77. Woolf C. Long term alterations in the excitability of the flexion reflex produced by peripheral tissue injury in the chronic decerebrate rat. Pain 1984; 18:325-43.

78. Woolf C. Generation of acute pain: Central mechanisms. Br Med Bull 1991; 47:523-33.

79. Woolf C, Excitability changes in central neurons following peripheral damage: Role of central sensitization in the pathogenesis of pain. In: Willis W, editor. Hyperalgesia and allodynia. New York: Raven Press; 1992. p. 221-43.

80. Woolf C. The dorsal horn: state-dependent sensory processing and the generation of pain. In: Wall P, Melzack R, editors. The textbook of pain. 3rd ed. New York: Churchill-Livingstone; 1994. p. 101-12.

81. Simone D. Neural mechanisms of hyperalgesia. Curr Opin Neurobiol 1992; 2:479-83.

82. Gillette R. Spinal cord mechanisms of referred pain and related neuroplasticity. In: Gatterman M, ed. Foundations of chiropractic: subluxation. St. Louis: Mosby, 1995. p. 279-301.

83. Huttenlocher P. Neural plasticity. In: Asbury A, McKhann G, McDonald W. eds. Diseases of the nervous system: clinical neurobiology. Philadelphia: W B Saunders, 1992. p. 63-71.

84. Kandel E. Cellular mechanisms of learning and the biological basis of individuality. In: Kandel E, Schwartz J, Jessell T, editors. Principles of neural science. 3rd ed. New York: Elsevier; 1991. p. 1009-31.

85. Teyler T, Grover L. Forms of long-term potentiation induced by NMDA and non-NMDA receptor activation. In: Baudry M, Thompson R, Davis J. editors Synaptic plasticity: molecular, cellular aspects. Cambridge, (MA): MIT Press, 1993. p. 73-86.

86. Bonica J. Introduction: semantic, epidemiologic, and educational issues.In: Casey, K, editor. Pain and central nervous system disease: the central pain syndromes. New York: Raven Press; 1991. p. 13-29.

87. Bonica J. Clinical importance of hyperalgesia. In: Willis W, editor. Hyperalgesia and allodynia. New York: Raven Press; 1992. p. 17-43.

88. Berne R, Matthew L. Physiology. 3rd ed. St. Louis: Mosby Year Book, 1993. p. 949-79.

89. Dilman V, Dean W. The neuroendocrine theory of aging and degenerative disease. Pensacola: The Center for Bio-Gerontology; 1992. p. 23-30.

90. Feinstein B, Langton J, Jameson R, Schiller F. Experiments on pain referred from deep somatic tissues, J Bone Joint Surg Am 1954; 36:981-97.

91. Nansel D, Szlazak M. Somatic dysfunction and the phenomenon of visceral disease simulation: A probable explanation for the apparent effectiveness of somatic therapy in patients presumed to be suffering from true visceral disease. J Manipulative Physiol Ther 1995; 18:379-97.

92. Mendel T, Wink C, Zimny M. Neural elements in human cervical intervertebral discs. Spine 1992; 17(2):132-5.

93. Willis W. Central plastic responses to pain. In: Gebhart G, Hammond D, Jensen T, editors. Proceedings of the 7th World Congress on Pain: 1993; Paris, France. Seattle: IASP Press; 1994. p. 301-24.

94. De Jong P, de Jong J, Cohen B, Jongkees L. Ataxia and nystagmus induced by injection of local anesthetics in the neck. Ann Neurol 1977; 1:240-46.

95. Brodal A. Neurological Anatomy. 3rd ed. New York: Oxford Univ Press, 1981.

96. Wyke B. Articular neurology and manipulative therapy. In: Glasgow E, Twomey L, Scull E, Kleynhans A, Idczak R,. editors. Aspects of manipulative therapy. 2nd ed. New York: Churchill-Livingstone, 1985. p. 72-7.

97. Gillette R. Potential antinociceptive effects of high level somatic stimulation—Chiropractic manipulation therapy may coactivate both tonic and phasic analgesic systems. Some recent evidence. Trans Pacific Consortium Res. 1986; 1:A4(1)-A4(9).

98. Woolf C. Segmental afferent fibre-mediated analgesia: transcutaneous electrical nerve stimulation (TENS) and vibration. In: Wall P, Melzack R, editors. Textbook of pain. 2nd ed. New York: Churchill-Livingstone; 1989. p. 884-96.

99. Dvorak J, Dvorak V. Manual medicine: diagnostics. 2nd ed. New York: Thieme Med Pub; 1990. p. 35-45.

100. Gordon J. Spinal mechanisms of motor coordination. In: Kandel E, Schwartz J, Jessell T, editors. Principles of neural science. 3rd ed. New York: Elsevier, 1991. p. 581-95.

101. Sato A. Spinal reflex physiology. In: Haldeman S, editor. Principles and practice of chiropractic. 2nd edition. Norwalk (CT): Appleton & Lange; 1992. p. 87-103.

102. Fitz-Ritson D. The anatomy and physiology of the muscle spindle, and its role in posture and movement: Review. JCCA 1982; 26:144-50.

103. Richmond F, Bakker D, Stacey M. The sensorium: receptors of neck muscles and joints. In: Peterson B, Richmond F, editors. Control of head movement. New York: Oxford University Press; 1988. p. 49-62.

104. Bogduk N, Twomey L. Clinical Anatomy of the Lumbar spine. 2nd ed. New York: Churchill-Livingstone; 1991. p. 86.

105. Proske U. The golgi tendon organ. In: Dyck P, Thomas P, Griffin J, Low P, Podusko J, editors. Peripheral neuropathy. 3rd ed. Philadelphia: WB Saunders; 1993. p. 141-8.

106. Masdeu J, Brazis P. The anatomic localization of lesions in the thalamus. In: Brazis P, Masdeu J, Biller J, editors. Localization in clinical neurology. 2nd ed. Boston: Little, Brown and Company; 1990. p. 319-43.

280 Journal of Manipulative and Physiological Therapeutics
Volume 21 • Number 4 • May, 1998
Dysafferentation • *Seaman and Winterstein*

107. Carpenter M. Core Text of Neuroanatomy. 4th ed. Baltimore: Williams & Wilkins; 1991. p. 224-49.

108. Lantz C. The vertebral subluxation complex. ICA Rev Chiropr 1989:37-61.

109. Lantz C. The vertebral subluxation complex. In: Gatterman M, editor. Foundations of chiropractic: subluxation. St. Louis: Mosby, 1995. p. 149-74.

110. Nolte J. The human brain. 3rd ed. St. Louis: Mosby; 1993. p. 337-59.

111. Ghez C. The cerebellum. In: Kandel E, Schwartz J, Jessell T, editors. Principles of neural science. 3rd ed. New York: Elsevier; 1991. p. 626-46.

112. Brodal P. The Central Nervous System: Structure and Function. New York: Oxford University Press; 1992

113. Fitz-Ritson D. Neuroanatomy and neurophysiology of the upper cervical spine. In: Vernon H, editor. Upper cervical spine: chiropractic diagnosis and treatment. Baltimore: Williams & Wilkins; 1988. p. 48-85.

114. Bakker D, Abrahams V. Central projections from nuchal afferent systems. In: Peterson B, Richmond F, editors. Control of head movement. New York: Oxford University Press; 1988. p. 63-89.

115. Maeda M. Neck influences on the vestibulo-ocular reflex arc and the vestibulocerebellum. Prog Brain Res 1979; 50:551-9.

116. Janse J. The integrative purpose and function of the nervous system: A review of classical literature. J Manipulative Physiol Ther 1978; 1:182-91.

117. Hildingsson C, Wenngren B, Toolanen G. Eye motility after soft-tissue injury of the cervical spine: a controlled, prospective study of 38 patients. Acta Orthop Scand 1993; 64:129-32.

118. Fitz-Ritson D. Cervicogenic vertigo. J Manipulative Physiol Ther 1991; 14:193-8.

119. Lewit K. Manipulative therapy in rehabilitation of the locomotor system. 2nd edition. Boston: Butterworth Heinemann, 1991:18

120. Weeks V, Travell J. Postural vertigo due to trigger areas in the sternocleidomastoid muscle. J Pediatr 195; 47:315-27.

121. Gray L. Extra labyrinthine vertigo due to cervical muscle lesions. J Laryngol Otol 1956; 70:352-61.

122. Wing L, Hargrave-Wilson. Cervical Vertigo. Aust NZ J Surg 1974; 44(3):275-77.

123. Caranasos G, Israel R. Gait disorders in the elderly. Hosp Pract 1991:67-94.

124. Revel M, Andre-Deshays C, Minguet M. Cervicocephalic kinesthetic sensibility in patients with cervical pain. Arch Phys Med Rehabil 1991;72:288-91.

125. Revel M, Minguet M, Gergoy P, Vaillant J, Manuel J. Changes in cervicocephalic kinesthesia after a proprioceptive rehabilitation program of in patients with neck pain: A randomized controlled study. Arch Phys Med Rehabil 1994;75:895-9.

126. Hulse M. Disequilibrium, caused by a functional disturbance in the upper cervical spine: clinical aspects and differential diagnosis. Man Med 1983; 1:18-22.

127. Hinoki M, Ushio N. Lumbomuscular proprioceptive reflexes in body equilibrium. Acta Otolaryngol Suppl (Stockh) 1975; 330: 197-210.

128. Watson P. Nonmotor functions of the cerebellum. Psychol Rev 1978; 85:944-67.

129. Courchesne E, Yeung-Courchesne R, Press G, Hesselink J, Jernigan T. Hypoplasia of cerebellar vermal lobules VI and VII in autism. New Eng J Med 1988; 318:1349-54.

130. Gutzmann H, Kuhl K. Emotion control and cerebellar atrophy in senile dementia Arch Gerontal Geriatr 1987; 6:61-71.

131. Lalonde R, Botez M. The cerebellum and learning processes in animals. Brain Res Rev 1990; 15:325-32.

132. Heath R. Modulation of emotion with a brain pacemaker J Nerv Ment Dis 1977; 165(5):300-17.

133. Douglas F. The dizzy patient: strategic approach to history, examination, diagnosis, and treatment. Chiropr Technique 1993; 5:5-14.

134. Schimp D. A diagnostic algorithm for the dizzy patient. Chiropr Technique 1994; 6:123-37.

Appendix C - The RDA Nutrients

Nutrient	RDA 1968	RDA 1989 [481]	DRI 1997-98**	Machlin [278]	Linder [275]
Protein	65 g	.75 g/kg body weight/day			
Calories		Approx. 2,200 ♀ cal (p.33) Approx. 2,900 ♂ cal			
Vitamin C	60 mg	60 mg (p.118) 1 g or more is non toxic (p121)	Scheduled to be updated in 1999	60 mg (p.221) Low toxicity	60 mg (p.144) Toxicity very low
Biotin	300 mcg	30-100 mcg (p.168)	30 ♀ mcg 30 ♂ mcg 30 mcg pregnant 35 mcg lactating	100-200 mcg (p.415)	100 mcg/1000 kcal No toxicity (p.122)
Folic Acid	400 mcg	200 ♀ mcg 180 ♂ mcg (p.153) No toxicity (p. 155)	400 ♀ mcg 400 ♂ mcg 600 mcg pregnant 500 mcg lactating	200 mcg ♂ (p.477) MDR 50 mcg No tox 400 mg/day 5 months or 10 mg/day 5 yrs (p.482)	180-200 mcg (p.141) MDR 50 mcg No Toxicity
Thiamin	1.5 mg	1 mg/day Minimum (p.128)	1.1 ♀ mg 1.2 ♂ mg 1.4 mg pregnant 1.6 mg lactating	.50 mg/1000 kcal (p.272)	.5 mg/1000 kcal (p.116) 1.0-1.2 mg ♀ 1.2-1.5 mg ♂ No toxicity 200 x's RDA
Riboflavin	1.7 mg	1.2 mg minimum intake (p. 134) No toxicity (p.135)	1.3 ♀ mg 1.1 ♂ mg 1.4 mg pregnant 1.6 mg lactating	1.4-1.8 mg (p.303) No toxicity (p.309)	1.4-1.7 mg (p.117) No toxicity
B₁₂	6 mcg	1 mcg can sustain 2 mcg RDA (p162) No toxicity up to 100 mcg (p.163)	2.4 ♀ mcg 2.4 ♂ mcg 2.6 mcg pregnant 2.8 mcg lactating	2 mcg (p.527) no toxicity w/far in excess	2 mcg (p.138) No toxicity
Pyridoxine (B6)	2 mg	1.6 mg ♀ (p. 144) 2 mg ♂ Toxicity 117±92 mg when taken for 6 months to 5 yrs. (p.146)	1.3 - 1.5 ♀ mg 1.3 -1.7 ♂ mg 1.9 mg pregnant 2.0 mg lactating	1.6 mg ♀ (p.368) 2 mg ♂ 2-250 mg/day safe long term (p.377)	1.6 - 2.0 mg (p.130) Chronic use 500 mg or greater can be toxic
Niacin	20 mg 1 mg Niacin= 1 NE 60 mg tryptophan= 1 NE	11.3-13.3 NE (p.139) Toxicity 3-9 g of nicotinic acid per day (p. 140)	14 ♀ mg 16 ♂ mg 18 mg pregnant 17 mg lactating	19 NE ♀ (p.331) 20 NE ♂ Toxicity 3 g/day 3-6 months (p.335)	13-15 NE ♀ 15-20 NE ♂ Toxicity not at 3-6 g/da (p.118)

Nutrient	RDA 1968	RDA 1989 (481)	DRI 1997-98**	Machlin (278)	Linder (275)
Pantothenic Acid	10 mg	4-7 mg/day (p.172) 10-20 mg may cause diarrhea.	5 ♀ mg 5 ♂ mg 6 mg pregnant 7 mg lactating	Estimated intake 5-20 mg 4-7 mg (RDA) 10-15 mg (Krehl's research) (p.442) No toxicity reported (p.446)	4-7 mg/day No toxicity at 10-100 mg (occasional diarrhea) (p.120)
Vitamin E Depending on type of tocopherol 1-1.5 mg=1 IU (Linder, p.168)	30 IU	8 mg ♀ (p.103) 10 mg ♂ can tolerate 100-800 IU (p.104)	Scheduled to be updated in 1999	15 IU (p.127) (In 1974 RDA lowered to 15 IU) No toxicity; 3,200 IU not problem few side effects (p.137)	8-10 mg (approx. 12-15 IU) (p.168) No toxicity 800 IU for 3 years
Vitamin A 1 mg = 3 IU 1 mcg retinol = 1 RE 6 mcg B-carotene = 1 RE 12 mcg mixed carotenoids = 1 RE (Machlin, p.33)	1,000 RE RE = Retinol Equivalent	800 RE ♀ (p.84) 1,000 RE ♂ Toxicity 15,000 mg=50,000 IU	Scheduled to be updated in 1999	800 RE ♀ (p.33) 1,000 RE ♂ Toxicity not clear	800 RE ♀ (p.153) 1,000 RE ♂ Toxicity with prolonged high dose 20-30 x's RDA 200-400 IU (5-10 mcg)
Vitamin D	400 IU	6 mths to 24 yrs-10 mcg (400 IU) (p.96)	5 - 15 ♀ mcg 5 - 15 ♂ mcg 5 mcg pregnant 5 mcg lactating	400 IU (p.85)	
Vitamin K	—	1 mcg/kg/body weight (p.110) Toxicity not observed (p.112)	—	1 mcg/Kg/body weight (p.176) Toxicity not described	60-80 mcg. (p.176) Toxicity little known
Zinc	15 mg	12 mg ♀ (p.209) 15 mg ♂ Toxic chronic ingestion of > 15 mg/day is concern (p.211)	—		15 mg (p.227) Absorb 31-51% Among least toxic (p.229)
Copper	2 mg	1.5-3 mg (p.227) Absorb 36% (p.226) 10 mg/day non-toxic (p.228)	—		1.5 - 3 mg (p.234) Absorb 30-60% Non toxic (p.229)
Chromium	—	50-200 mcg (p.242) Absorb .5% Long term 200 mcg non-toxic	—		10-60 mcg=avg. intake; RDA not mentioned Absorb .5 - 20% (p.216) Least toxic trace mineral (p.250)

Nutrient	RDA 1968	RDA 1989 [481]	DRI 1997-98**	Machlin [278]	Linder [275]
Selenium	—	55 mcg ♀ (p.220) 70 mcg ♂ Toxicity not defined (p.221)	Scheduled to be updated in 1999		50-200 mcg (p.245) Absorb 35 - 85% (p.216) Toxicity 2,400-3,000 mcg likely (p.246)
Iodine	150 mcg	150 mcg (p.215) 2 mg no side effects (p.216)	—		100 mcg (p.254) Average intake 500 mcg Absorb 100% (p.216) 1-2 mg no side effects (p.255)
Molybdenum	—	75-250 mcg (p.245) 10-15 mg=gout-like syndrome	—		150 - 500 mcg (p.240) Absorb 40-100% (p.216)
Manganese	—	2-5 mg (p.232) 8-9 mg safe No toxicity specified (p.233)	—		2.5-5 mg (p.238) Absorb 3-4% (p.216) Non toxic (p.239)
Magnesium	—	280 mg ♀ (p.191) 350 mg ♂ Absorb 40-60% (p.188) No toxicity except for renal disease. (p.192)	**310 - 320 ♀ mg 400 -420 ♂ mg 360 - 400 mg pregnant 310 - 360 mg lactating**		280 mg ♀ (p.194) 350 mg ♂ Absorb 30-40% Toxicity not specified
Calcium	1000 mg	800 mg (p.180) Absorb 30-40% (p.179) 2,500 mg toxic (p.180) Re: Do not exceed RDA	*1,000 - 1,200 ♀ mg 1,000 - 1,200 ♂ mg 1,000 - 1,300 mg pregnant 1,000 - 1,300 mg lactating*		800 mg (p.206) Absorb 30-50%
Iron	18 mg	15 mg ♀ (p.200) 10 mg ♂ Absorb 10-15% (p.200) Toxic 25-75 mg unlikely a problem (p.202)	—		15 mg (p.218) Absorb 5-15% (p.216) Toxicity is situation specific (p.224)
Phosphorus	—	1200 mg 11-24 yrs, pregnancy and lactation 800 mg>24 yrs (p.186)	**700 ♀ mg 700 ♂ mg 1,000 - 1,300 mg pregnant 1,000 - 1,300 mg lactating**		800 mg Absorb 70-80% (p.192-193)

Nutrient	RDA 1968	RDA 1989 [481]	DRI 1997-98**	Machlin [278]	Linder [275]
Potassium	3,500 mg (90 mEq) (p.256) Absorb 90% (p.255)	3500 mg (DRV*) same regardless of kcalories	—		2,500 mg (p.192)
Sodium	500 mg (p.253)	2400 mg (DRV*) same regardless of kcalories	—		2,500 mg (p.192)
Dietary Fiber	—	25 g (DRV*) 11.5g per 1000 kcal	—		—

*Daily Reference Values (DRVs) were established by the Food and Drug Administration in May, 1995. For more information contact the FDA or look on the internet at http://vm.cfsan.fda.gov/label.html.

**NOTE: In this chart when the DRIs are in bold print they represent the Recommended Dietary Allowances (RDAs). When the DRIs are in italic print they represent the Adequate Intakes (AIs). RDAs and AIs may both be used as goals for individual intake. RDAs are set to meet the needs of almost all (97% to 98%) of the individuals in a group. For healthy breast-fed infants, the AI is the mean intake. The AI for other life stage and gender groups is believed to cover needs of all individuals in the group, but lack of data and uncertainty in the data prevent being able to specify with confidence the percentage of individuals covered by this intake. You can get more information on the Dietary Reference Intake (DRIs) on the internet at http://www2.nas.edu/fnb/ or by contacting the Institute of Medicine Food and Nutrition Board:

Food and Nutrition Board
Institute of Medicine
2101 Constitution Avenue, N.W.
Washington, DC 20418

Index